Best wishes

David Morley

Paediatric Priorities
in the
Developing World

POSTGRADUATE PAEDIATRIC
SERIES

under the General Editorship of

JOHN APLEY
C.B.E., M.D., B.S., F.R.C.P., J.P.

Consultant Paediatrician, United Bristol Hospitals and
Bath Clinical Area; Lecturer in Diseases of Children,
University of Bristol

Paediatric
Priorities
in the
Developing World

DAVID MORLEY
M.D., M.R.C.P., D.C.H.

Reader in Tropical Child Health,
Institute of Child Health, University
of London

BUTTERWORTHS

ENGLAND: BUTTERWORTH & CO. (PUBLISHERS) LTD.
              LONDON: 88 Kingsway, WC2B 6AB

AUSTRALIA: BUTTERWORTHS PTY. LTD.
              SYDNEY: 586 Pacific Highway, 2067
              MELBOURNE: 343 Little Collins Street, 3000
              BRISBANE: 240 Queen Street, 4000

CANADA: BUTTERWORTH & CO. (CANADA) LTD.
              ONTARIO: 2265 Midland Avenue, Scarborough, M1P 4S1

NEW ZEALAND: BUTTERWORTHS OF NEW ZEALAND LTD.
              WELLINGTON: 26–28 Waring Taylor Street, 1

SOUTH AFRICA: BUTTERWORTH & CO. (SOUTH AFRICA) (PTY.) LTD.
              DURBAN: 152–154 Gale Street

First Edition . .1973
Reprinted 1974

Suggested UDC Number: 613.95

ISBN: 0 407 35111 6 (Cased Edn)
      0 407 35110 8 (Limp Edn)

Printed and bound
in Great Britain
by

Roydon Printers (Luton) Limited

*Dedicated to the United Nations Children's Fund (UNICEF)
and to all those within and without this organization
striving for the underprivileged children of our World*

Contents

CONTENTS

Foreword

This book covers new ground. It is concerned with priorities in the child health services of the developing world. The exercise of establishing a strict order of priority among a large number of measures, each of which will have an impact on child health, is difficult and painful, particularly when the total sum of money presently available − and likely to become available by the end of this century − for the health services in the developing world is so very small; about $1 per head of population was available in 1970 as compared to $100 per head in the more developed countries. Painful though this exercise may be, it must be undertaken; otherwise childhood mortality and morbidity in the developing world is not likely to decline to levels even approaching those of the developed world. A recent estimate suggests that whereas in the developed countries each year half a million children die during the first 5 years of life, the corresponding figure for the developing world is 20 million; or, expressed as deaths per year per million of under-fives, 625 in the developed countries and 48,000 in the developing countries.

Unfortunately, the principles underlying the provision of health services are not discussed in the undergraduate curricula of most medical schools. They include considerations which fall outside the conventional definition of 'medical'. Social, economic, cultural, ethical and political implications can no longer be ignored.

The first need is for the correct questions to be asked and for the sometimes tragic dilemmas to be presented clearly; this requires imagination, thoughtfulness and even courage, in addition to personal experience gained in the practice of paediatrics in the developing world. The second need is to suggest answers. These cannot be absolute and will have to be reviewed constantly and critically in the light of results achieved and the ever-changing conditions of the community.

FOREWORD

There can be few paediatricians as well qualified as David Morley to undertake the daunting task of writing a single-author book on paediatric priorities which requires some knowledge of several non-paediatric and even non-medical subjects. He has made the health of children in the developing world his prime professional concern. After many years' work in Imesi, in Western Nigeria, which resulted in a remarkable lowering of child morbidity and mortality in that village community and which formed the basis of his many contributions to research into child health services, he became tutor to the Course for Senior Teachers of Child Health from the developing countries, organized by the United Nations Children's Fund and the World Health Organization. More recently he has established a Tropical Child Health Unit at the Institute of Child Health in London.

Whilst working in Nigeria he and Miss Margaret Woodland established a special clinic for the under-fives and designed a weight chart for the prevention of malnutrition. Many countries have now introduced such clinics and are using these charts, with a resulting improvement in child health. In his teachings David Morley stresses that in the developing world most of the children (up to 80 per cent) live in rural areas and that, therefore, priority must be given to provision of services for these areas.

This book will be deeply appreciated by all doctors working with children in the developing world, whether for the whole of their professional lives or for shorter periods. Non-medical health workers, including nurses, will benefit equally and will be pleased to see that full recognition is given to their vital contributions. Politicians, economists, nutritionists, agriculturists and architects will find certain chapters thought-provoking and instructive.

I suspect that paediatricians working in the developed world will also find the book of interest because it is now becoming clear that no country, however wealthy, has the financial resources to satisfy all demands which can reasonably be made on behalf of the health of its community. Hopes that as the health of a community improves, less money needs to be spent on health have proved wrong, and we must face the fact that most advances in medicine will involve additional expense; therefore the need to establish priorities is becoming more and more urgent.

OTTO H. WOLFF
Nuffield Professor of Child Health,
Institute of Child Health, University of London, and
Consultant Physician, Hospital for Sick Children,
Great Ormond Street, London

Preface

In 1956, due to the foresight of John Wright and Andrew Pearson of Wesley Guild Hospital, Ilesha, an approach was made to the West African Council for Medical Research to undertake what at that time was an unusual community-based study. This request was supported in the Council by Dr. John Walters, and in 1956, assisted by their grant, I took up a post as paediatrician to the Wesley Guild Hospital, Ilesha, in the Western State of Nigeria. There I was joined a few months later by Miss Margaret Woodland.

On 1 January 1957 we started to follow up all babies born in the village of Imesi on the edge of the Ekiti hills in the Western State of Nigeria. The study started where possible with the mother early in her pregnancy. Over the next 18 months, 413 children were born into the village, and 404 of these were included in our study and closely followed up at least monthly by Margaret Woodland over 5 years. In this she was ably assisted by Mrs. Bifarin, Mrs. Fasade and a team of loyal and hard working nurses. This longitudinal study was the first of its size to be undertaken in Tropical Africa. I returned to the UK in 1961, but Miss Margaret Woodland stayed on in the village and later at Ilesha until 1970 and during this period I made yearly visits. Since 1961 I have also had the opportunity to travel widely particularly to West and East Africa, India, and also to the Middle East and South America. This book is a direct outcome of this study and the contact with colleagues in these countries, from whom I have learnt so much.

Health planners who have the difficult responsibility to develop health care programmes in developing countries, rightly consider that these plans must be generated from experiences within these countries. Such planners may consider this book as yet another attempt to impose a system from outside. I hope that this work will not be

PREFACE

read in this light, but rather that the book questions many systems that developed in Europe and the U.S.A. and suggests alternatives that have worked in some developing countries. I particularly hope that it will be of help to those planners who are involved in discussions with the 'doctor monopoly' which may be at times conservative in its outlook. In the acknowledgements that follow I realize I will have missed out more names than I have included. To these people, who have helped me so much but I have failed to mention, I apologize.

Dr. S. D. M. Court encouraged me to undertake this book. Dr. W. R. Aykroyd helped me to start writing during my time at the London School of Hygiene and Tropical Medicine, in the late Professor Platt's Department of Human Nutrition. More recently, Professor O. H. Wolff and Dr. G. Newns, the Dean of the Institute of Child Health, have provided me with the facilities to set up a Tropical Child Health Unit that has made this book possible.

Those who are familiar with the writings of Professor Maurice King will find frequent extracts and references to his outstanding work *Medical Care in Developing Countries*. He has assisted with my early draft on this book. Much help has also been obtained from Dr. John Bryant's book *Health and the Developing World*.

In specific chapters, Dr. O. Gish helped with economics; Dr. Mary Thwaites and Dr. V. J. Hartfield with newborn care; Dr. E. Schoemaker, Dr. K. Weston and Dr. J. Breman with whooping cough; Dr. W. P. T. James and Dr. T. Jacob John with diarrhoea; Dr. F. J. W. Miller and Dr. D. R. Nagpaul with tuberculosis; and Dr. Betty Topley with anaemia. Much of the ideas in the birth interval chapter come from Dr. W. A. M. Cutting, and Dr. F. Rosa also helped with that chapter. In nursing, I received much assistance from Miss Shirley Alcoe, Miss Laidlaw, Miss Joan Koppert and Miss Jenny Jeffs. Mr. P. Torrie and Dr. Malcolm Segall gave me many ideas, and I hope I have met some of their criticisms in the chapter on management. Mark Wells gave me help over architectural problems. Dr. Alan Shrank advised me in the chapter on skin diseases.

Others who have helped include Dr. Bankole, Mr. John Rees, Dr. D. Brooks, Dr. Maletnelemea, Dr. Peter Swift, Dr. Paul Snell, Dr. Anne-Marie Gade, Dr. Okeahaliam, and the Fellows of the UNICEF/WHO Course for Senior Teachers of Child Health. Dr. E. T. C. Spooner helped me on a number of points, and Mr. R. A. U. J. Jennings found a number of anomalies in my writing.

Mrs. Priscilla Milton has been the mainstay for typing, although many others, including Mrs. Grace Saldanha, Miss Dianne Hensey and my wife, have helped at times. The tremendous undertaking of duplicating a trial version was carried out by Mrs. Katherine Aresti. My daughter Ruth undertook the binding of these duplicated copies.

PREFACE

In preparation of the art work I am indebted to Mr. Geoffrey Lythe and more recently to Mrs. Gillian Oliver in the Department of Medical Illustration headed by Mr. Ray Lunnon in the Institute of Child Health. My son Robin undertook some of the original art work, and copying this on to the litho plates for the duplicated version. Mr. Brian Kesterton reproduced the illustrations.

I hope there is an occasional touch of humour in this book; perhaps the best examples are found in the two cartoons, *Figures 105* and *140*. Unfortunately, I have mislaid the exact details of their source and so I can only offer my apologies to the originator of these cartoons and their publishers for failing to seek permission to reproduce their excellent and strikingly apt drawings.

I should never have reached the publishers' deadline were it not for Miss Margaret Woodland, who has joined me in London, and who undertook the considerable task of checking references and much of the correcting of the final copy.

Sending duplicated copies of chapters to friends will I hope have avoided some errors, and has certainly led to further useful material being incorporated in the book. Usually a book is a one-way method of communication from author to reader. However, Appendix 1 has been included in order that there may be some possible communication from reader to author. I hope that at least some of my readers will find time to comment on which parts of the book they find useful, and particularly to put me in touch with material that might be useful to others who are involved in the struggle to improve the health care of children in the developing world.

To make this book available to doctors in less prosperous countries, every effort has been made to reduce its cost. The low price of this edition has been achieved by grants towards the cost of printing. For these I am indebted to a splendid old lady who wishes to remain anonymous; to the students of La Sainte Union College of Education, Southampton, who raised a fund; and to the Medical Department of War on Want. In addition I am surrendering any royalties due to me on this edition. Despatch of copies by the organizers of Teaching Aids at Low Cost (TALC) before publication has further reduced the cost. However, my efforts to reduce the cost would have met with little success except for the constant help and advice from the publishers to whom I am most grateful.

I have a special acknowledgement to the United Nations Children's Fund (UNICEF) who in various ways have done so much to help me over the last 10 years for allowing me to dedicate the book to them and their fellow workers.

DAVID MORLEY

CHAPTER 1

Guiding Principles

GENERAL CONSIDERATIONS

The paediatrician in a developing country faces problems that are quite different from those in industrial areas. Firstly, there are many more children — they may comprise 40 per cent of the population. Secondly, a quarter, a third, or, in some rural areas, even one-half of all children born die during the first 5 years of life. Usually one-half of all deaths takes place in the age group below 5 years, in which the major health problems of the country are concentrated. The number of human beings involved is shown in Table 1. More than 97 per cent of all deaths below the age of 5 years took place in the less developed countries.

The world's total population (excluding China) in 1968 was about 3,500 million. These figures come from the Demographic Year Book of the United Nations (63) and can do no more than suggest the order of magnitude of the problem. Deaths under the age of 5 years have been computed at an annual rate of 5 per 1,000 in the more developed countries and 50 per 1,000 for the less, and this latter figure is likely to be an underestimate for most rural areas. Australia, Europe, Japan, North America (excluding Mexico) and Russia have been classified as more developed countries.

In the less developed countries child development and health is dominated by the twin problems of nutritional deficiency and infectious diseases. This blanket of illness that affects so many children is of great importance in human social terms. In the past, medical workers and planners have often assumed that any large reduction of this mortality would need to await an improvement in socio-economic conditions and in environmental hygiene. However, we now realize that doctors with the relevant paediatric training can organize a service which will prevent more than one-half of the deaths in infancy and early childhood without awaiting any great change in environment. Moreover, such prevention must not wait until living standards approach those currently existing in more developed areas of the world.

GUIDING PRINCIPLES

The financial projection given in Table 2 suggests that living standards will change only slowly unless people can be organized to organize themselves and create a behavioural change, as is being witnessed in the

TABLE 1

Total Population and Number of Children under 5 years and the
Number Dying in More Developed and Less Developed Countries

	Population (millions)	Under fives (millions)	Deaths/year under fives
More developed countries	976	85	500,000
Less developed countries	2,510	415	20,000,000

improved environment and sanitation of Ujamaa, a village in Tanzania, and in a few other communities. Once this organization within the rural societies has been achieved, forms of family limitation suggested in later chapters may be acceptable and desired by the parents.

Economic factors

Economic factors, which will be later described in more detail, are so essential that they require mention here. Medical workers who live and work in developing countries are familiar with the stringency of medical budgets, though they frequently do not realize how limited the medical budget would be if it were divided over the whole population; nor do they realize that the discrepancy in this respect between the more developed countries (in whose standards they have normally been trained) and the less developed is likely to increase by the end of the century. Table 2 suggests that the gap between the level of living in the more developed and the less developed regions will widen, and will be reflected in the sums available for expenditure on health.

The figures in Table 2 relate to an 'average' developing country (32). Some developing countries cannot hope even for the limited increase in expenditure on health suggested in Table 2 over the next 30 years. Their GNP may indeed be growing faster than in the more developed countries, but this is likely to be offset by population growth. An increased rate of economic growth depends on more capital being available to provide more jobs, but there seems little hope of this unless there is a move into small scale rural industries.

The bleak economic outlook for developing countries during the next 30 years shown in Table 2 implies that improvement in health

TABLE 2

Gross National Product* (GNP) and Health Expenditure per
Capita ($) in 1970 and 2000

	GNP/capita		Health expenditure/capita	
	1970	2000	1970	2000
More developed countries	2,200	5,800	100	250
Less developed countries	160	325	1	3

*The gross national product is estimated as the total production, either in wages earned, or for the farmer in terms of crops produced, whether these are eaten or sold

services will call for redeployment of resources. At the present time the greater part of the expenditure is divided between central sophisticated hospitals and smaller peripheral hospitals, leaving little for medical care provided at health centres, which combine curative and preventive services. This situation urgently needs to be changed as unless paediatric services can expand along satisfactory lines and provide an assurance to the parents that their children will survive, the worldwide effort to control the growth of population is unlikely to succeed. Alternative systems of delivery of health care have been developed in China, and the available data suggests that many have met with considerable success (231).

The subject and the reader

The present book deals primarily with the common conditions and with the priorities which should be followed in child health programmes. In practice 'tropical' diseases other than malaria account for only a small proportion of child admissions to hospitals in tropical countries and are rarely seen in the wards of European hospitals; the diseases encountered are more related to the material poverty of the people than the climatic conditions in which they live.

Although three-quarters of the population in most countries in the tropics and sub-tropics live in rural areas, three-quarters of the spending on medical care is in urban areas, and also three-quarters of the doctors live there. Three-quarters of the deaths are due to conditions that can be prevented at low cost, but three-quarters of the medical budget is spent on curative services, many of them provided at high cost. Nor have priorities in medical training been properly considered, and many believe that the high mortality is partly due to the inadequacy and irrelevance of much of the training given to doctors and paediatricians who are being taught a form of medical care more relevant to a European country than to their own.

This book is written for the doctor who finds that his training has inadequately prepared him to care for children in developing countries. If as a result a proportion of those who have received such a training start to question what they are doing, and the basis of their training, I shall consider it as having achieved a large part of its objective. For the medical student, this book may provide a complementary account of child care to that which he may receive from other sources. Economists and sociologists who have read draft copies suggest that some in their disciplines will find parts of this book useful. For these reasons relatively more space will be given to a description of prevention and organization, and less to the description of disease, as it is the former that is urgently required in tropical child health. Emphasis will be placed on rural societies, because most of the children live there, and because the type of care that can be developed in rural areas is likely to be substantially different from that suited to urban areas.

Training

A real difficulty arises for the doctor who is responsible for the care of children in a rural community. In the West the training of most doctors and paediatricians is directed towards applying modern medical science to the care of the individual child in a hospital or a well-equipped clinic. They are not familiar with the problems of caring for large numbers of children on a limited budget. The care of the individual child and the care of the many are, of course, both essential, and training in both is needed. Unfortunately, a good training in the former is not necessarily a good training in the latter. The training necessary for each has indeed much in common, yet there are skills, knowledge and attitudes, and even ethical views, relating to the care of all the

4

children in the community, that are not learned in teaching programmes focused on individual children in a hospital setting. In the past
half century the university through its medical school, research units
and teaching hospitals has made much progress in providing the expertise necessary to care for the individual. Only recently have universities
become involved in studying and participating in the total care of a
defined community. As a result of this change in emphasis, the paediatrician in the future should be better equipped to care for children in
rural societies, shanty towns and 'marginados'. To achieve this he will
need to learn skills from disciplines such as 'community development'.

Location of children: urban or rural

Two of the characteristics of child health in developing countries,
namely the large numbers of young children and the small funds available for child health services, have been mentioned. A third characteristic which particularly influences the health picture is locality
(Figure 1). In *Figure 1* the proportion of children living in the rural

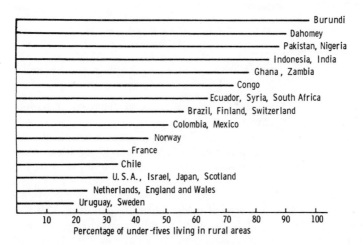

Figure 1. Proportion of under-fives living in rural areas

areas of 15 countries that represent different areas of the world is given;
for this figure a town was considered as containing a population of over
100,000.

In the UK only 22 per cent of children live in the country; in India

88 per cent live there. In the majority of developing countries 60–90 per cent of the population live in these areas. This fact has many implications: the most important is that providing adequate services for rural areas may be more expensive if the services are mobile, due to the cost of transport of material and personnel. This has been emphasized in one of the more effective mobile programmes so far developed (180). Few figures are available on differential mortality in rural and urban areas. Table 3, however, suggests that some differences do exist. The three developing territories given in this table are believed to be fairly representative and suggest that mortality rates may be twice as high in rural as compared with urban areas. Countries with a high level of expenditure on health, such as Norway, can overcome the great problems of difficult travel and the isolation of their rural population, with the result that the rural infant mortality is very similar to that in the

TABLE 3

Infant Mortality Rates in Urban and Rural Areas

Country	Urban	Rural	Country	Urban	Rural
Guinea	189	218	Rumania	41	49
Dahomey	46	115	Norway	16	17
Morocco	100	170	UK	20	17

towns. In the UK infant mortality is slightly higher in urban areas, where pockets of poverty are more frequent, than in rural areas.

Every civilization has eventually led to urbanization; in the future this will be associated with trends in agriculture by which one country-man can feed 10 or more townspeople. Migration into the towns is now increasing in all the developing countries. These countries are experiencing a rapid explosion of city life, and demographers have suggested that Calcutta, for example, may be in the midst of a conurbation of 50–70 million by the year 2000. Emphasis is laid primarily on the services for rural areas but similar services need to be developed in the peri-urban slum or 'favelas'. It cannot be foretold in what manner these 'septic fringes' to the cities will develop but they are likely to be poorly served by existing services. Present services based largely on large city hospitals have in general failed to provide the comprehensive care suggested in this book for rural societies. In some countries, such as Brazil, providing medical care for the population of favelas is a major problem and can only be successfully met by employing workers from these areas in their médical services.

Unfortunately, in most developing countries, the better education, and particularly higher education, is a prerogative of the townspeople and relatively few, if any, of those who receive secondary schooling in rural areas achieve university entry, and particularly entry into the medical faculty. Those few from rural areas who achieve higher education are at present lost to these areas. The more education the less chance there is of them returning. Doctors who have lived most of their lives in urban areas often view the country and country folk with some fear, a little contempt, and usually less understanding; If governments are to be serious in their intentions to supply rural areas with doctors, they must see that more of the equally intelligent but less well-educated young people from rural areas find their way into the medical faculties. The doctor who will be likely to be happy and contented in rural areas is the doctor who has been born, grown up and been educated there. In the future, not only must his primary and secondary education, but also a high proportion of his medical education be undertaken in rural areas. This latter is particularly difficult as the majority of present medical teachers would themselves be at a loss how to provide medical care in a rural setting. This does not mean that the majority of doctors who have grown up in rural areas will want to stay there, but rather that given certain inducements and motivation during their training, they will be more willing to return to serve rural societies than their colleagues who have spent their formative years in a city. In the rural areas they must be joined by representatives of other disciplines who have a university training.

It is fair to say that the majority of the 'elite' or 'upper class' in any country accept as a right their role and their ready access to the best education available in the country. Few are willing to accept that it is through some quirk or accident of birth that they have been chosen as the elite. Unfortunately, while willing to accept the large salary that goes with this position, few are willing to accept the responsibility. Only 6 out of a group of 60 doctors qualifying in the Philippines in 1955 are now working there. The same is true to some extent of many other countries. Ultimately, one might hope that the acceptance of the opportunity of education will involve the responsibility of using that education where it is most needed for the good of the community which has made the education available.

The preceding paragraphs indicate some of the basic facts and problems confronting the doctor concerned with child health in the tropics. But if these are to be realistic, the guiding principles must be clear.

7

MAJOR AXIOMS* OF CHILD CARE

Child care is immensely worthwhile

In every country the most precious possessions of parents are their young children. We now have the technical knowledge and means needed to reduce the mortality among children by one-half. This is the most effective way of winning the co-operation of the local people – a co-operation which can be used to help promote their development in better health and in other disciplines.

In the past it was advantageous to parents and communities to have large numbers of children; today there is some realization that small families of healthy children, with opportunities for education, are to be preferred. In agricultural societies farmers needed many children to provide sufficient hands to work on the land, and in such societies great stress was rightly placed on producing a large family of children as many were likely to die in childhood. At present, in most of the world, increasing attention is being given to the health of mothers and young children and considerably larger funds are being invested in their care. If a country is to make rapid strides in economic and other development, it may well be that this can be brought about only 20–30 years after services have been provided for the medical, nutritional and general care of small children, that is, when these well-cared for children have become effective members of the adult society.

The argument that the best way to improve a nation's health in the long term is through the care of young children and women of child-bearing age is widely held and in this book taken for granted, even if action along these lines is seldom implemented.

An objective and imaginative approach to child health in developing countries is necessary, supported by a knowledge of local customs and practices, without preconceived ideas adopted from industrialized societies

While some specialities of medicine, such as radiology, can be exported with little alteration from Europe or North America, other subdivisions – and here child health is a good example – cannot be so exported. Attempts to do so have the effect of limiting child care to a small fraction of the population. The artificial separation of preventive

---

*King (139) was one of the first to define problems and facilities available for the delivery of health care. Following his example, this book will start by presenting some axioms similar to those that he offers, but suitably adjusted to the special needs of young children

from curative care, which has been a feature of child health in Europe during the last 50 years, is disastrous in the developing countries as has been poignantly indicated by Cicely Williams (282) in the following passage describing a 'well-baby' clinic:

> I have seen a mother trailing dejectedly away from one of these centres. The six-month-old baby on her back, chubby and cheerful, had been weighed, examined and commended. The three-year-old child in her arms was suffering from malnutrition and dysentery. She had been advised to take it to a dispensary five miles away. Is it any wonder that she would not pay much attention to a lecture on washing her hands before eating, or that she did not relish the idea of another ten mile walk, a long wait in an out-patients in order to receive a few pills unaccompanied by any advice on the feeding and care of her sick child who was so desperately in need of it?

•The paediatrician has the great opportunity to pave the way for other disciplines towards a form of medical care dedicated to promote health rather than solely to cure sickness. Unfortunately, although this comprehensive approach has so much to offer, there are still senior paediatricians whose interests and teaching remain solely in the curative field. This out-dated approach, if taught to medical students, acts as a serious brake in developing effective child care services.

The advice given here on this comprehensive child care competes with that from traditional sources, some of which is contrary to the child's interest. If the medical team is to win the confidence of the people, they must show endless patience and avoid displaying irritation or annoyance, however much they feel these are justified. The mother already regards the doctor with awe, an increase of this fear will not be beneficial to the child. The traditional healer, present in all societies, also regards the doctor with suspicion and repeated friendly approaches by the doctor will be needed if he wishes to overcome this fear and win the help and co-operation of the healer in improving child care.

A maximum return in terms of reduced child mortality and healthier and happier children must be obtained from the limited funds available

A child health service that requires funds well beyond the economic means of a rural society will not be beneficial in the long run. And yet this pattern has been repeated in almost every country, as doctors attempt to import services and facilities which they have seen working effectively in another society at different social and economic levels.

Since the young child under 5 years of age is growing rapidly and contracting a number of predictable illnesses, the choice on a basis of cost effectiveness between different measures, all of which will maintain adequate growth and prevent illness, should be relatively easy to make. At the present time such assessment is ineffectively undertaken. For example, the notification of diseases to a central health department does not supply the health worker with any evidence of change of prevalence or indication of the cost effectiveness of preventive measures, such as immunization, undertaken in his area. A simple technique which makes this information available at health centres is described in Chapter 8.

Do not separate mother and child

Up to the age of 5 years the child is heavily dependent on mother and effective health care must do as much as possible to enhance her competence and skill. In rural areas mothers do many things to their children which medical staff cannot understand; as a result the mothers are blamed both by them and by their husbands for contributing to the child's illness. The doctor's function and responsibility are not to pass judgement, criticize or blame the mother. If she does bring the child too late to hospital, the doctor must not blame her but rather try and find out the factors that produced the delay. The medical worker's ignorance of severe measles and how it should be managed can be blamed on inadequacy of his training which did not include a study of local beliefs in depth.

The separation of the mother from the child during a period of hospitalization, which until recently was generally followed in Western hospitals, is now known to be harmful to the child. The mother's presence should not just be tolerated but every effort must be made to look after her comfort and make good use of this as a learning situation. She needs help to improve her knowledge and understanding and above all to give her increased confidence in her own ability to care for her child. The medical personnel caring for the child's health must also be concerned with maintaining and improving the mother's health as an important step in preventing or curing further illness in the child. Where possible, the same doctor should be caring for the health of both.

Care for all children in every section of the community: services need to be near the child's home and differ from those required by the adult

The way of life of the mother in most developing countries is in a stage of rapid transition. She is moving from a rural society with a traditional approach to an understanding of illness and other calamities

10

to a society where science explains the causative agent of the majority of illnesses. During this period, the charms, herbs and incantations she previously placed her trust in are no longer adequate. Her frequent need to be assured that modern medicine is a better alternative may severely tax the medical services. Once an acceptable service satisfying the mother's real and felt needs is available, the demands on it are likely to grow rapidly.

Like the mother, the doctor has his difficulties. In his training he will have absorbed philosophies characteristic of materially advancing nations which in their teaching of child health have focused attention on the individual child. In them the technology of medicine has become so fascinating and so absorbing that it can be easily forgotten that the purpose of medicine is to care for people and to understand disease so as to prevent it. Unfortunately, the developing countries have too often accepted without questioning Western ideas and standards, have been proud of their own ability to match them and reluctant to deviate from them. The result may be a fairly sophisticated service for the children living in urban areas.

The young infant can be carried some distance by his mother but the older child is less easily brought to a clinic. Out-patient or clinic systems designed for adults are not suitable for children. The clinic for the child needs to emphasize preventive care and teaching. Both of these will demand frequent, if brief, contacts between staff and patients. An important step in encouraging brief contacts both in the clinic and in the home has been the introduction of the system of 'home-based' records. This book will describe such a system which includes a record of the growth of every child through the first years of life – a necessary record because monitoring the growth of the child is the most effective way of discerning and averting impending malnutrition, and also because illness in childhood is usually multifactorial and a knowledge of the preceding state of nutrition and illnesses is necessary if the most appropriate measures are to be taken. It has been found that 'home-based' record systems have other practical advantages over the traditional system of keeping records in the clinic.

Child care must be the best that circumstances allow

Doctors and nurses will wish that the child under their care should be treated in the same way as they would hope that their own child, or that of near relatives, would be treated. One of the tragedies of medical care as it has been imposed on developing countries is that many standards exist. Medical care available to the elite 5 per cent of the population which include the doctors is very different from the standard of care available to the rest. Child care imposes considerably greater demands on staff that the care of the older age groups. For example, decisions have to be made without delay because many childhood illnesses develop and kill in hours or a day or two when the same illness takes much longer in adults. If a high standard is to be achieved, the child requires attention from some person, usually a nurse, or a nurse-midwife, who knows him and his mother and has a feeling of personal responsibility for him. This nurse should as far as possible see the child on every clinic attendance and should be responsible for arranging that he is seen by more senior workers when this is necessary. At the same time these more senior workers by this frequent contact will renew and extend the nurse's or medical assistant's knowledge and skill. Caring for children will win the respect of the community. That respect and affection (given to the doctor or nurse in Europe even before they were equipped with modern drugs) must still be a considerable part of the reward of the doctor working in developing countries. Such a reward is more important in rural than in urban societies. It engenders that trust and co-operation through which further services may be developed to benefit the local people. Above all, child health services must be made more just; our great responsibility is the child from the underprivileged family.

Organization of child health services at village level should be a matter in which the senior paediatricians are deeply involved

The pyramid of child health care must be built on a firm base, It should be organized from the bottom up, and not from the top down *(see Figure 155)*. Services provided should not be judged by the presence of chrome and concrete palaces, but by the men and women who provide care, and the extent to which they make effective use of their knowledge and skills and have gained and maintained contact with the mothers and the children in the rural societies.

Unfortunately, the training of many a senior paediatrician has been disease and hospital-oriented and does not prepare them for these function; many do not have any contact with the people at village level or understanding of the organizational problems involved. The challenge to design and evolve services making the best use of the small budget available is worthy of the most intelligent. The paediatric societies and journal of the country may be the most effective channels through which research and participation in work at village level can be encouraged. However, to do this it will be necessary to break the academic tradition which does not encourage senior doctors to examine the methodology of health care, particularly when this care has to be applied at low cost.

Parliamentary democratic societies are under very real difficulties in setting up services at village level. The more vocal section of the community demands from their politicians hospitals and doctors as outward signs of a modern health service. The real need of the community is for health centres and auxiliaries, but these will not bring votes for the politicians even if they consider them a priority. The communist countries are not under such constraints. They have seen the need to invest more funds and effort in maternal and child care. Services have been built up in countries such as China, North Vietnam, Tanzania and Cuba from the village level, which have shown how effectively child mortality can be lowered without having to wait for any great improvement in the economic condition of the people.

The role of the paediatrician

To the young doctor from a developing country the 'blue print' of a successful paediatrician in Europe or North America may suggest that success depends largely on the ability to diagnose the rarities of paediatrics and on undertaking research into obscure and uncommon disease. Unfortunately, the paediatrician in developing countries may attempt to follow a similar pattern of work under more frustrating and difficult conditions. The medical student may rarely, if ever, see him working outside the confines of the hospital.

A paediatrician who is to be effective in improving the health of all the children in the community must be seen by his students to be demonstrating by example how a doctor can work with a team of auxiliaries to whom he is an organizer and a supervisor as well as a consultant. Working with such a team of auxiliaries is difficult at the present time in most large cities where medical schools have developed. These cities and medical schools are frequently crowded with underutilized doctors and interns, and only in the rural areas can the paediatrician demonstrate to his students services run by auxiliaries offering an integrated curative and preventive service which will surpass the largely curative service offered through his colleagues in the city.

The paediatrician, once he has organized and taught his team, can make far better use of his skills. No longer will he be seeing large numbers of children who are brought either because their mother is moving in a transitional society (Chapter 3), and has a pressing need for continuing reassurance, or because they have some minor, common and easily-treated condition of childhood. Such tasks can be undertaken by auxiliaries, who will gain satisfaction in treating relatively simple conditions, and in the realization that the continuing good health of the child is their responsibility. Once the paediatrician has deputed routine tasks to trained auxiliaries, his work becomes more interesting. As mentioned already, he will have a role as manager and teacher. The time

13

that he allots to clinical work is taken up with the diagnosis and management of the less common condition which are beyond the capacity of the auxiliaries and require the skills that the paediatrician has learnt through a long and complex training. In many medical schools the interns are used as auxiliaries to undertake the examination and care of the large number of children who attend the out-patient clinics. The intern is being, and has been, trained to recognize the less common conditions. For him satisfaction will come when he finds a child with some complex and difficult condition, and not in preventive measures and in seeing numerous patients with common diseases.

The large number of children in communities in developing countries, and the need for some source of care within about 5 km (3 miles) from the child's home, demands a network of services. To organize this network and to ensure its efficient functioning, the paediatrician must be both an organizer and a teacher. Such skills are more essential for him than for his colleagues in Europe. The paediatrician who is effective as a manager and a teacher will be more successful in reducing child mortality.

The role of the junior staff

The nurse or auxiliary in developing countries works more in the out-patient or the under-fives clinic than in the ward, but in either her function is different from that of most nurses in Europe or North America. In particular, she should be taught to carry out repetitive therapeutic tasks. Her knowledge needs to be regularly renewed by refresher courses and working contacts with doctors. If she has been well chosen and well trained and is properly supervised, she may soon with practice carry out routine functions such as gallows suspension plasters, scalp vein drips and perhaps even lumbar punctures with as much skill as the doctor. Even though she takes over these duties from the doctor she must retain her concern for the basic nursing skill of providing comfort for her child patients. Especially she must always endeavour to teach the mother, who is never likely to be far from the child.

The paediatrician and his team have an important role as teachers

Greater emphasis is now rightly placed on health education, and it is perhaps to the mother with her young child that this is most usefully directed. In many cultures the male community leaders must encourage their wives and others to examine which practices in traditional child care need to be altered. Better nutrition, the need for cleanliness, the

14

importance of immunization are all subjects that should have a high priority in health education programmes. The paediatrician is likely to be involved in health education programmes, at least as an adviser. He should take every opportunity that may arise to use the mass media of radio and newspapers, and where available also television. If health teaching can be camouflaged as an item of news, it is likely to be more widely absorbed (the locally based community radio station can be particularly effective). We are all teachers persuading people to accept new ideas, develop new attitudes and change their behaviour.

The full-time health educator may have only a limited impact unless he works closely with the paediatric staff. The clinic worker who has just brought a child safely through pneumonia has gained the respect and affection of the mother, and the teaching that she receives from him will be more acceptable than that of the health educator, unless it is clear that the two are working together. Co-operation between the paediatrician and the Institutes of education can be productive. The school teacher, male or female, is much respected in rural areas. If instructed in practical health matters, they have many opportunities to spread them in school hours or at other times, or, in the case of the female teacher, in social gatherings with mothers.

As well as this responsibility for giving help in teaching and in the organization of health teaching for children, the paediatrician has a greater responsibility to train his own staff of doctors, nurses and auxiliaries. Skilled staff must teach the less skilled. Particularly in rural areas, success in reducing child mortality will depend on disseminating the skills of diagnosis and management of the sick child down to the village worker. An excellent example of such training of village workers has been developed in China as the 'barefoot doctor' (231) or the village medical helpers in the Ujamaa villages in Tanzania, in Chile (167) and in Guatemala (313). The community select a suitable mother, whom they are responsible for paying. This woman is given an initial period of training in the local hospital. She is then responsible for organizing the people in preparation for the regular visit of the health team, and holds a small stock of medical supplies to give to the children between visits. The professional levels of nurses and auxiliaries will vary from country to country, but their success will depend more on their receiving a practical training with enthusiasm than their educational background.

CHAPTER 2

Economic Background of Child Care in Developing Countries

The inaugural lecture for the Southampton Medical School (3) drew attention to the theme of this Chapter and Chapter 21.

One starting point from which to consider improvement in medical education is the current shortcomings of the profession. High up on any list, I fancy, would be our ignorance of and contempt for techniques of management and our lack of understanding of the economic constraints within which we must operate.

DEVELOPMENT OF HEALTH SERVICE

The economic constraints for developing countries apparent in Table 2 show that at the present time the developing countries have $1 per head to spend on health per year, compared with $100 in Europe, and it would be unwise to ignore the prediction of economists that in the year 2000 the expenditure per head on health in the developing countries will be only $3 compared with $250 in more fortunate areas. An increase in the proportion of spending on health in less developed countries by the year 2000 is possible if money spent on other items in the budget is cut. Among these, national defence expenditure might well be universally reduced, but this would not materially alter the relationship shown in this table between the developing and materially advanced countries. For this reason in this decade $2 a head can be considered an optimistic figure and throughout this book the reader will be reminded of this by the term 'a two-dollar health budget'.

An example of minimal resources is Bangladesh which in 1972 for a population of 75 million was spending 5 taka, that is 15¢, a head.

The expenditure on health in the more developed countries has increased rapidly in recent years, although the proportion of the national budget spent in this way until the last few years has remained similar. *Figure 2* illustrates how in the UK the amount spent on health has increased rapidly, but only in the last few years has the proportion of the budget spent on health increased.

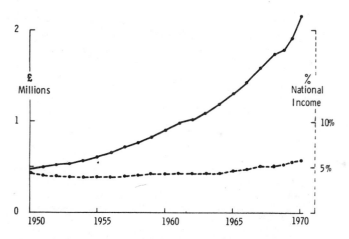

Figure 2. The rising cost of British National Health Service, only recently has this become a greater proportion of the National Income

Hospitals, particularly large hospitals employ many persons with highly specialized skills who are the most expensive section of any health service. Whether this increase in hospital expenditure has been the best outlay of capital and running costs in terms of cost effectiveness in open to doubt (2), even in the UK where an effective system of primary health care exists. Perhaps the hospital has become a satisfactory environment to the doctor, and the rapid growth of hospital rather than domiciliary services is an expression of a 'felt' need of the doctor, and to some extent of society, rather than an expression of a real need. It is perhaps salutary to realize that over the last 50 years, the system of health care in the UK has failed to reduce the discrepancies in mortality between social classes, and recently these differences have even increased (276).

Figures for health expenditure through hospitals and through other means are not readily available for developing countries. However, there are reasons to believe they follow a pattern similar to that in the UK although for many developing countries the proportion spent on hospital services is likely to be much higher. In the National Health Service of the UK, the increased cost of hospital care over a 10-year period and the relative decrease in the services supplied through general practitioners, pharmaceutical, ophthalmic and dental services outside hospital is illustrated in *Figure 3*. The increase in hospital costs in the UK is in

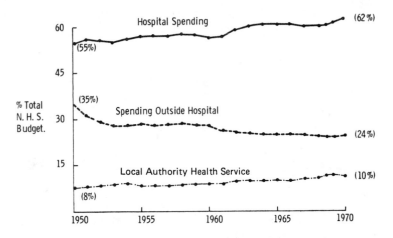

Figure 3. Distribution of the health budget in the UK. The proportion spent on hospital services has increased while the proportion spent through general practitioners has decreased. Administration and other small expenses involving 3–5 per cent of the total are not included

part due to an increase in 'hotel' expenses. Analysis of expenditure within and without hospitals may well demonstrate that reversal of these trends may lead to more effective total health services. One country with a strongly socialistic and egalitarian policy is Tanzania. In her second 5-year development plan it was stated that 'the second plan will increase emphasis on the development of preventive and rural services . . . '. However, the curative institutions are so powerful that in the first year they had overspent their budgets by 20 per cent, while the small preventive budget was underspent by 30 per cent. Similarly, while expenditure in the main teaching hospital had increased in one year by over 100 per cent, all the regional hospital budgets were cut back by amounts varying from 6 to 60 per cent of the previous year. The three large hospitals already established will absorb one-third of the curative budget and one-quarter of the preventive one (243). This failure to execute plans is evidence of the weak medical administration common to most developing countries. This has now been recognized in Tanzania where no further hospitals are to be built until approximately 300 health centres and 900 sub-centres have been constructed. Rapid expansion of auxiliary training has been made possible by freezing the medical school to its present size. The curriculum for, and training of medical students in Tanzania is specifically designed to prepare them to run the health services for a district within 3 years of qualifying. The national expenditure on health does not necessarily reflect what is obtained in return. For example, the USA is currently spending three times as much per head on health as European countries, but there are 18 countries with a lower infant mortality, nor do her citizens survive as long as those of many other countries.

A country setting up a new health system has a number of options open to it, and two of these will be considered. The shortage of economists who have specialized in the economics of medical care both in developing countries and in international organizations limits our knowledge and ability to make effective decisions. Two options will now be considered.

Option 1 – building a large central teaching hospital or many health centres and rural hospitals

A number of countries have opted for the large hospital. This pattern of developing a health service has been likened by one writer to Pharaoh's engineers starting to build the pyramids from the top (151), see *Figure 155*. For example, the choice has recently been taken in Zambia, which is now committed to a £15 million hospital. Experience from several developing countries suggests that the recurring costs of running these large medical institutions each year is equal to around a quarter of their capital cost. Perhaps even more serious than the initial expenditure on their construction is the way these large institutions are likely to have a first call on the national health budget almost indefinitely. Equally serious is their demand for a large number of well-trained staff who are both expensive to train and in short supply (2). Many arguments are put forward in favour of the multimillion teaching hospitals, especially their value in training doctors, as referral centres, and for research into the diseases of the country. These arguments require closer examination *(Figure 4)*.

Training of doctors in large multi-disciplinary units

What is meant by 'doctor'? Should he be trained to sort out difficult genetic and biochemical problems, or work in an open-heart unit dealing with congenital anomalies? Then such a large teaching centre is certainly justified. But the developing country requires a 'doctor' who can not only run a district hospital but can also organize and improve

19

child health in villages through satellite sub-centres and health centres. Doctors trained in large hospitals know how to work in hospitals but will know little about working in health centres where, if he is to be

WHICH OPTION?

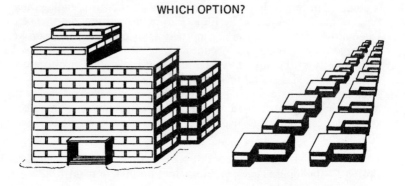

A Vast Teaching Hospital?   OR   Health Centres for the Community?

Figure 4.

happy and effective, the doctor will work closely with other health personnel, usually as leader of the health team. It is likely that doctors trained in countries such as India today may be better equipped, on completion of their training, to work in the British National Health Service hospitals than in primary health centres in rural India. This may be due to the teaching of the present professors having stemmed directly from hospital services which developed in parallel with English hospitals and were not indigenous to India. The medical services in India and most of the developing countries still reflect the origins of their past professors. In the Philippines the medical service resembles that in the USA. Those who are responsible for developing of services perhaps need to look not only at these services, but also at those in China, Cuba, North Vietnam, Kenya and Tanzania. In some of these states, due to ideological differences, medical services have developed along different lines and much greater priority has been given to the mother and her young child. Not only must the regulations be passed and the services provided, but a dialogue between those concerned and the mother is necessary, to discover why apparently excellent services, such as those claimed for Brazil, are not used. Medical schools may also learn from Russian methods by which students can be motivated towards attitudes of service to their community, a subject that has been inadequately studied elsewhere in Europe. Students recounting their time in Soviet Union (4) describe how, early in their course, they undertook full-time nursing duties which brought them in close contact with patients. This experience together with later training, particularly in discussions and outside activities, may lead to a stronger bias towards a concern for the community. Perhaps in the 1970s and 1980s there will be more research into methods by which services at low cost can be provided to 'rural societies' and attract more of the young, highly intelligent and well-motivated doctors of these countries. An indication of a trend away from building further large hospitals is to be found in the University of Ife in the Western State of Nigeria, which is attempting to train doctors in smaller district hospitals and has so far resisted the high cost of constructing and maintaining an enormous hospital and teaching centre. Success in introducing more rational services may be simpler in the more remote unsophisticated areas. At Ilesha, in rural Nigeria, the first Under-Fives' Clinic was established with no difficulty from local authorities. In Lagos, Cunningham required a year, and on Manhattan Island 2 years, before permission from the various authorities concerned could be obtained to establish similar clinics. Developing countries must not ignore the advantages of a 'clean slate'!

The first step in one experienced doctor's opinion (109) when it comes to health planning in developing countries is to be as free as possible from earlier models and inherited systems. Otherwise one may end up with 'snow ploughs for the tropics' as happened in an African country receiving a complete airport as development aid from Europe, including snow ploughs that were part of the standard equipment in the donor country. Or one may have the embarrassing situation of too expensive 'Mercedes-Benz type hospitals' where a 'Volkswagen bug' would be perfectly adequate.

Medical education has similar problems and doctors and nurses trained according to traditional models from affluent countries need a lot of adjustment in order to be fully useful in developing countries. This type of training is like learning to swim and then later being sent to the desert where one is asked to use the newly acquired skills. No wonder then that one either wants to go back to the coast (affluent areas) or tries to build an expensive swimming pool (read: hospital) in 'the desert'. These traditional training models are challenged and changed in different parts of the world, but many people are still not aware of these changes.

The greatest tragedy of all is when a developing country builds a health plan for the needs of tomorrow on the imported solutions of yesterday, and thus fails to use the relative flexibility of its adminstrative and decision-making structures for innovation and pioneering. Many affluent but in their structures more rigid countries are today looking to developing countries for solutions and new methods of delivering health care to all the people.

On a visit to a new medical school recently a doctor from a socialist country made the telling remark 'The doctors look after themselves well here'. Inside this medical school's magnificent exterior there was a large room for each senior doctor with expensive laboratory facilities attached. A senior paediatrician told us that his hospital commitments in service and teaching already precluded him from his responsibilty to supervise and encourage medical assistants in peripheral health centres. How could he find 30 per cent of his time to work in a laboratory? He might reply that he hoped to undertake laboratory work when more staff were available. However, that hospital and medical school already absorbed 160 of the 200 doctors employed by the country's ministry of health. Before this new hospital was built the old hospital complex cost a quarter of the nation's health budget to run. This was achieved by spending approximately $10 on health care per head of population in the capital city and $1 in the rural areas. The offices and laboratories were poorly occupied and used and tended to isolate doctors from one another. Unfortunately, the refectory or canteen where oppportunities arise for doctors to meet informally together with students had not been built.

The national hospital as referral centre

The national hospital cannot satisfy even local demands for child care, and in developing countries they fail in their objective to become referral centres. It is daily besieged by hundreds of mother with children who may account for 60 per cent of all out-patients. The majority are brought with preventable conditions. Hospital rules may allow the paediatrician to spend large sums on treatment, but refuse funds to buy any vaccines. A study in Mulago Hospital, Uganda, in 1964 showed that 93 per cent of all admissions came from nearby districts (105). Even local children will frequently have to be turned away because of overcrowding, and the difficulties for doctors attempting to admit children from more distant areas are considerable. Relatively few parents are willing to bring their children from the village to what to them is a frightening environment in the major city of their country, even if they

22

can afford the cost of transport to, and accommodation in, the strange surroundings.

Research

Large sums have been spent in training doctors from developing countries in research in the affluent countries and on equipping laboratories for them on their return home. However, just as only a fraction of otherwise brilliant doctors in the more developed countries have the inspiration and drive to undertake original research, the same is likely to be true in the developing countries. Research too has tended to be laboratory-based or relates only to patients seen in hospital. Research on community health problems based on a defined population is still uncommon (318).

Most scientific articles on paediatric problems in the developing countries resemble those produced in the early days of paediatric writing in Europe and North America. Undue prominence is given to the rare or unusual case, and genetic conditions get greater prominence than their frequency and importance to the community merit. Articles on the planning of health services or the management of specific common conditions in the community are infrequent, not only in American and European journals but most notably in the journals of developing countries where these problems are particularly urgent. In this reorientation the editors of journals have a heavy responsibility to the children of the country by encouraging articles describing the delivery of child care.

The university, through the medical school and hospital, has developed to a high level the care of individual patients and this is reflected in medical writing. Only in the last few years have universities undertaken studies of how paediatric services can be provided to a defined community within a limited budget. Relevant studies on the organization of such services are still rarely undertaken, and teaching on this subject can only be fragmentary. A description of attempts to develop teaching programmes in communities representing several continents has recently been published (152). In this book a diagram appears which attempts to summarize the relationship and staffing of various levels of medical care in Colombia. This diagram has been simplified and reproduced here as some guide to the form of regional medical services suggested by many developing countries (Table 4). The population given here is only an approximation, and while possible for South America, this regionalization is unrealistic in Africa or India. In India the primary health centre hospital serves a population of 80,000 with only at the most three of four sub-centres.

TABLE 4

Regionalization of Health Services*

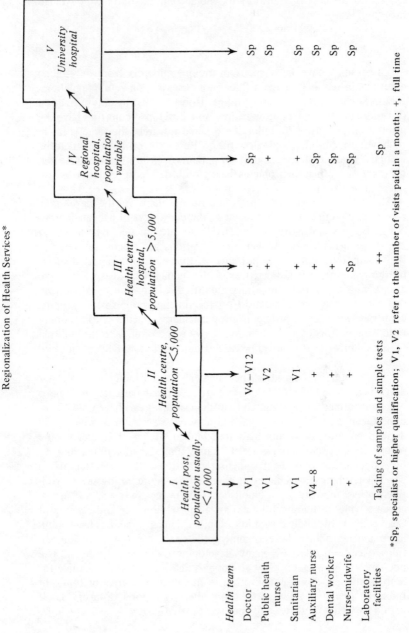

Health team	I Health post, population usually <1,000	II Health centre, population <5,000	III Health centre hospital, population >5,000	IV Regional hospital, population variable	V University hospital
Doctor	V1	V4–V12	+	Sp	Sp
Public health nurse	V1	V2	+	+	Sp
Sanitarian	V1	V1	+	+	Sp
Auxiliary nurse	V4–8	+	+	Sp	Sp
Dental worker	–	+	+	Sp	Sp
Nurse-midwife	+	+	Sp	Sp	Sp
Laboratory facilities	Taking of samples and simple tests		++	Sp	Sp

*Sp, specialist or higher qualification; V1, V2 refer to the number of visits paid in a month; +, full time

Economics of capital spending on health in urban and rural areas

The possible economic effects of building in the city or in rural areas must be considered. The experience of the last 20 years has led some economists to believe that money spent in the rural areas of developing countries is likely to be more effective in promoting the economic growth of the whole nation that the same amount spent in urban areas. Most developing countries still rely heavily on their agricultural products for their overseas purchasing power. The subsistence farmers who have small cash crops are the essential primary producers of these exports, except for those connected with large plantations. These farmers are not encouraged to increase the amount they produce unless there are either rural shops in which they can spend their money, or other ways in which they can see that increased effort on their part will raise their own and their families' standard of living. *Figure 5a* is a simplified diagram of the movement of goods. Economists have claimed

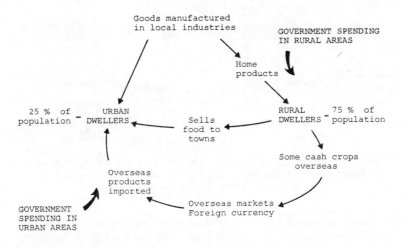

Figure 5a. If emphasis in government spending is shifted to the rural areas, the purchasing power of rural societies will encourage urban industry. This will help the whole economy of the country

that money spent in rural areas by the government should lead to an increase in the farmers' purchasing power and increase the demand for goods produced by local industries in the towns, including such articles as cloth, soap, cement and cycles. Money spent in the urban areas is more likely to lead to a demand for imports. The smaller urban population will quickly become saturated with the articles produced by local industry.

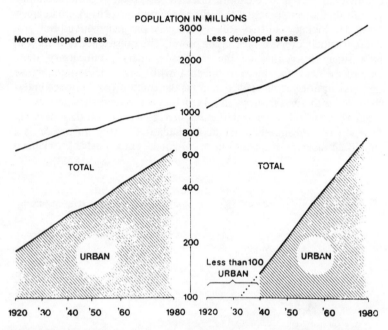

Figure 5b. Trends and crude projections of total and urban populations (reproduced from Kleevens, 1971, by courtesy of the Editor, Transactions of the Royal Society of Tropical Medicine and Hygiene)

These arguments hold equally strongly for health care in general and even more for child care. Money spent in rural areas will go largely on salaries, and health services can play their part in absorbing the unemployed. In the UK the National Health Service employs more people than any single industry. Money spent in urban areas on the highly specialized services will employ fewer people and is likely to lead to greater import demands both of equipment and skills with concomitant higher salaries. The basic requirements of health services can be supplied by personnel with limited training using equipment and medicines some of which may be produced locally or obtained by bulk purchase imported at a low cost. If the health services in the towns continue to outstrip those in rural areas, the drift from rural to urban areas will grow even faster.

The urban drift

One worker (303) has emphasized the magnitude of the drift from rural to urban areas. In a period of 50 years the urban population of developing countries will have grown from under 100 to over 600 millions and by 1980 may exceed the urban population of economically advanced countries *(Figure 5b)*. Maintaining this flood within reasonable limits is an enormous social problem. There are many means of making rural life more attractive, profitable and of equal status to urban life. Among these, maternal and child health services and better schools for children are of great importance. In those areas in which satisfactory rural child health services exist, mothers and their families are more likely to stay.

The building of health centres, particularly if local methods of building are used, is one way of increasing income in rural areas. Capital costs are likely to be low and will not include much imported material. Local methods of building may require more upkeep and care, but this is preferable to a high initial capital cost. Upkeep will provide some continuing employment in the rural areas and the total allocation of resources will still be less.

PAEDIATRIC PRIORITIES

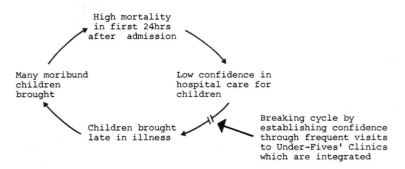

Figure 6. Paediatric priorities: a vicious circle in the medical care for children

In some countries the hospitals have absorbed most of the health budget with only limited expenditure on local clinics. Probably as a direct result of this policy over 50 per cent of the deaths in the children's ward occur within 24 hours of admission. Local medical workers refer to them as being 'brought too late' and their death indicates a need to improve the confidence of the community in the ability of scientific medical care to help their children. A vicious circle exists in which a high mortality leads to the belief that children may die in hospital *(Figure 6)*.

Frequent contact between the mother and the health service in a clinic providing comprehensive care, such as the Under-Fives' Clinic (Chapter 19), will do much to build up the necessary confidence and to identify severe illness in an early and more treatable stage. As a result the morale of those working in children's wards will be raised by reducing the number of children brought in at a terminal and irreversible stage of illness.

Cost of hospitals

The large teaching hospital will have a high capital cost of probably £5,000 per bed and perhaps as much as £8,000. A considerable proportion of this may be spent on imported structural materials, sophisticated equipment, expatriate architects and contractors' fees.

One economist has suggested that the teaching requirement should not, however, be allowed to determine the facilities construction programme, even when large groups of students have to obtain part or all of their clinical experience at a distance from the medical school (2). Unlike the teaching hospital in district centres, hospitals may be built by local contractors. The cost for each bed or child's cot in the district hospital may be £1,000, while in the health centre the cost may be only a half of this.

Equipping and running a hospital

Figure 7 shows how little of the capital cost is usually spent on equipment (139). The major expenditure is on building the hospital and accommodation for staff. Building methods which make use of units manufactured on the site to produce a functional structure can, however, greatly reduce the cost. A hospital built in Benin, Nigeria, cost less than a quarter of a hospital of a similar size constructed in Ibadan 10 years previously. In the developing countries, where the International Labour Organization estimates that 20–30 per cent of adult males are unemployed, a low-cost building which requires a larger maintenance staff is clearly preferable to a more costly building that requires minimum maintenance. The low-cost building can easily be adapted as the

28

demand for medical service grows and the service is modified to meet an ever-changing situation.

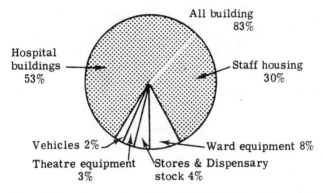

Figure 7. The economy of a rural hospital. Distribution of the capital cost of £53,000 (reproduced from King, 1966, by courtesy of Oxford University Press)

It is necessary to ensure that reduction in the capital cost of the building will allow more to be spent on equipment, so that more effective care can be provided. Much of the hospital equipment can now be produced at low cost within the country by local personnel trained in welding and other skills (72). The above figures give perhaps a fairly average distribution of capital costs under present methods of planning and construction. A more realistic approach would be to use suitably adjusted low-cost local building methods and spend approximately as much on equipment as on the building.

Staff salaries are the major proportion of the running costs in all countries *(Figure 8)*. The efficiency and spirit with which the staff work will depend heavily on the doctor's training and ability as a health team leader and manager (described in Chapter 21) and the help and support he receives in this side of his work from his seniors in local and central health administration.

The economist rightly requires that interest on the capital expenditure must be included as a recurring cost. The high proportion of the total cost spent on salaries suggests that increased productivity can be most effectively produced by regular staff training, delegation and motivation at all levels (Chapter 21). In the developing countries a breakdown of the salary structure of the hospital shows that usually a large proportion goes to the senior medical staff *(Figure 9)*, suggesting the need to employ less skilled health workers wherever possible.

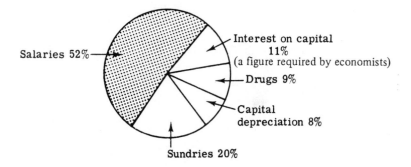

Figure 8. The economy of a rural hospital. Distribution of the annual budget of £25,000 (reproduced from King, 1966, by courtesy of Oxford University Press)

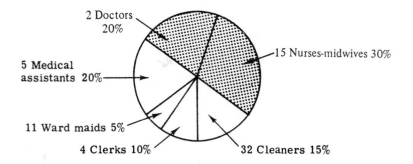

Figure 9. The economy of a rural hospital. Distribution of the staff budget of £12,000 (reproduced from King, 1966, by courtesy of Oxford University Press)

This dependence on less skilled workers should be particularly high in paediatrics, as so much of the management of the common illnesses and preventive measures such as immunization or improving nutrition can be carried out by staff with only limited formal education who have lived all their lives in the society they are serving. Professional pride will be difficult to overcome if a rational reappraisal of function suggests greater use of less qualified staff. With his present tradition and cultural role, the doctor is unfortunately poorly equipped for the leadership of the health team. Few doctors will easily accept this new role, and yet on their ability to adapt in this way will depend the chance of rapidly spreading health services to rural societies.

Further evidence of how money may be differently spent comes from Tanzania. In their national programme of planning for health care, research has been undertaken to compare investment in hospital and health centres. A comparison of an option of investing in one regional hospital or 15 health centres (322) is set out below.

	Capital cost	Running cost	Admissions	Out-patients	Population covered
	(Millions of shillings)				
Regional hospital	6	2.0	9,000	400,000	10–30,000
Fifteen health centres	6	2.0	15,000	1,000,000	300–500,000

There is clearly a great need for the health centres which are likely to care for the rural population. At the present time in Tanzania only 6% of the population live in the cities but they make up 30% of the inpatient and half the out-patients using present facilities. Although a hospital can offer care not available at a health centre the latter is more likely to offer a balanced curative and preventive package for children.

Option 2 – more doctors or many auxiliaries?

The youth in developing countries when deciding what career to take up before entering university have usually been more in contact with teaching and medicine than any other professions. Of these two, medicine attracts many of the best students. They consider medicine, and perhaps law, as the professions with the highest prestige which are also associated with material prosperity. Entry to the medical school is much sought after, and the top section of the Science Sixth will sometimes seek it 'en bloc'. The majority of those entering medical school will never question their right to spend their working years in towns, even though the funds used in their training have been generated by export of agricultural products from rural areas, and it is in these areas that their skills will be required.

On what basis should doctors be paid?

The tendency for doctors to be trained around the world with an overall similar curriculum has led to an economic problem which is depicted in *Figure 10*.

31

Two men develop an identical abdominal emergency. The tractor driver in the developed countries earns a large salary and will be operated on by a team led by a surgeon earning $20,000 a year – four times his own salary.

The man working with a hoe in a developing country earns no more than $50–100 a year. How much should his surgeon earn? Just four

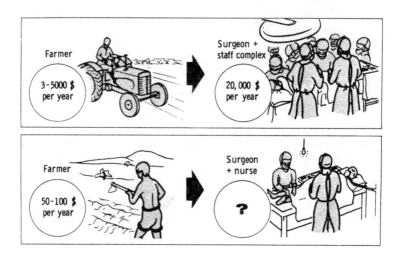

Figure 10. Same abdominal operation in a developed country and in a rural developing area

times his salary, as in the case of the tractor driver? The surgeon operating on him needs more, and more diverse, skills than his colleague in the developed country. He has no team to help him, probably not even an anaesthetist. He alone may be responsible for organizing the delivery of health care to a population of 10,000–50,000. In many countries he earns an income by spending some of his time caring for the private sector patients, but in the long run it is the public sector that will suffer. In China (294) the differential in levels of salary is established at only three times the minimum level for the best paid. Even there the senior doctors have contrived to establish a 'special case' and earn six times the minimum salary. Both in China and in Cuba some senior doctors have voluntarily reduced their salaries. Some limitation of migration of doctors from the developing to the industrialized countries is clearly necessary. Eventually this may be achieved by creating a curriculum in the developing countries designed to produce a doctor with the diverse skills required for the effective delivery of health care in that country. A broader training and a 'better' training than that offered to medical students in the medical schools of industrialized countries — a training that will amongst other things teach the student to create his own team of workers to whom he is always handing on his skills. So far few universities and their medical schools accept such an objective for their doctors.

After an existence of only a few years it is a matter of prestige for most universities to establish a medical school. In South-east Asia and South America universities have existed for 50, or in some instances more than 100 years. Over the last two decades with government support these universities have been turning out doctors in ever-increasing numbers. The argument was put forward that if doctors were sufficiently plentiful, more of them would move into rural areas. So far this expectation has not been fulfilled, and the number of doctors in rural areas has remained low. Most tend to settle in the towns *(Figure 11)* and where there is excess relative to demand in the towns, emigration to other countries increases. In 1969 about three-quarters of the doctors qualifying in one university in Thailand were leaving for the USA, and even if they returned to Thailand they might well be less suited to serve in the under-doctored rural areas than when they left. There is, on average, a doctor/patient ratio of 1/2,500 in the world (316). In the industrial countries their ratio is better than 1/1,000. In Asia it is 1/6,000 and in Africa 1/8,000, and three-quarters are concentrated in the towns.

Drift from rural areas

During a recent visit to a developing country, a doctor expressed the view that all their 'best' doctors left for industrialized countries. Such a view measures 'doctor value' by their clinical ability in diagnosing and managing unusual conditions and is evidence of a failure to appreciate that universities and medical schools have a responsibility for moulding attitudes. Surely the 'best' doctors will appreciate that their skills are part of the capital investment and assets of their country achieved by a general and medical education supported directly or indirectly by their nation. When they leave on the 'brain-drain' these assets are being squandered, for selfish reasons.

Figure 11 emphasizes that the drift from rural areas is the important stage in the dissatisfaction of doctors with work in their own country. The diagram is intended to suggest that effective steps to prevent the medical 'brain-drain' from developing countries can only come after investigating why doctors trained in the conventional manner find work in the rural areas so unsatisfactory. This has been undertaken in India

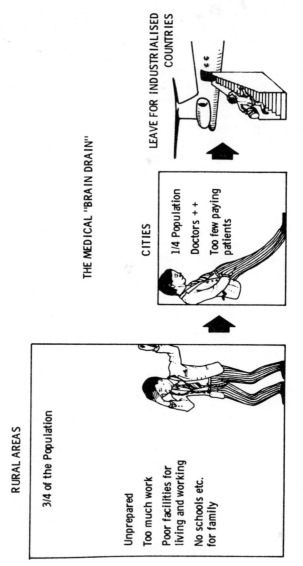

Figure 11. Distribution of doctors in developing countries. In the 'Brain Drain' our concern should be with the drift of doctors from rural areas to the cities rather than on doctors leaving the country

where a team investigated the problems of staffing the health centres (262).

Large numbers of doctors in urban areas may lower standards of medical care. The majority will be looking for an income from private practice and as the number increases, the overall standard of medical care may for a number of reasons decline rather than improve. A large number of doctors seeking fees leads to an erosion of the public sector. There is evidence in some countries that there are pressures from members of the medical profession to weaken the public sector, that is, the hospital-based services, so that more patients will make use of the private fee-paying services available from the doctors' own consulting rooms. A good argument exists to make all hospital doctors limit their practice to hospital patients. One Indian state government introduced such a law, but the doctors and their elite patients stirred up so much resistance that the order was reversed within 3 months. Because of a fear that a patient may be taken to another doctor polypharmacy occurs, and treatment by injections is preferred Over-treatment will increase iatrogenic disease and is also a waste of powerful and expensive drugs which have to be imported or manufactured at considerable cost to the country. Other abuses that may arise are 'split fees' and unnecessary surgery, for example the referring doctor and the surgeon may share the fee for an unnecessary tonsillectomy. For those with specialist degrees life is more secure, and so in some countries almost every doctor is seeking to master some speciality, spending valuable years in another country chasing a higher degree. This may gain promotion and greater security for the doctor, but the additional skill and knowledge he has obtained may not be sufficiently required by his home country. Lastly, if there is an excess of under-utilized medical manpower in the cities, there will be a strong but subtle pressure against the introduction of medical assistants. Such cadres of workers offer the only solution to bringing services to the slums and remote areas, but doctors will see their creation as a threat to themselves and their income.

The few doctors who go to the rural areas are encouraged to move to the cities, and perhaps overseas, by a number of factors, and the importance of each will vary from country to country. The majority of doctors have grown up in towns and even if their early years have been spent in rural areas, they are likely to have spent most of their school years in the urban areas. As the competition for places in the medical schools is enormous, scholars from rural areas are unlikely to obtain them. The doctor who takes a post in a rural area finds that he faces a situation for which he could hardly be less prepared. Few of his teachers have ever experienced it and the majority would be unable to cope with the problems that present. Nor will they encourage a career

35

in rural work, nor do governments. In a national medical research council in one Asian country additional payments are given to those who undertake research based in the capital city, but none are given to thos prepared to undertake research in a village environment. Not only will the doctor working in rural societies feel the lack of skill, but also the lack of preparedness for the situation and the decisions he must take. The situation which then arises has already been described. Attempts to enforce periods or a lifetime in rural areas after the present system of training are not likely to be successful. A hidden aspect of this so-called 'brain-drain' was recently reported (293). The tragic loneliness and failure of preparation for service in rural areas were highlighted by the suicide of two young Indian doctors placed in remote villages. One had just returned from taking his Fellowship in surgery in the UK.

The problems that are met with in medicine are not perhaps all that different from those met in other fields. A study has been made of the development of small-scale industries for developing countries, and an analysis of some of the problems that affect the industrialization of these areas of the world (158). The major points that are mentioned have been set down in Table 5. Against these have been set some of the similar difficulties that exist in the field of health care. This may help to illustrate the similarity of the problems facing the different ministries in a developing country.

> The technologies of the advanced countries which are usually capital-intensive and labour-saving are not fit for the resource endowment of the developing countries whose main characteristics are shortage of capital and abundance of labour. These two features require an opposite kind of technology. With unemployment and underemployment of human resources looming ahead as perhaps the biggest economic and social problem of the developing countries in the '70s and '80s, the indiscriminate use of labour-saving technologies and methods of production can only lead to further aggravation of the employment situation.

This was written in reference to the need for intermediate technologies in developing countries (251). There is the same need for a labour-intensive health service run largely by auxiliaries with limited training (231).

Selection and training of doctors for work in rural areas

A part of the solution to the problem of doctors leaving rural areas and drifting to the cities and overseas is likely to be found in their selection and training. Those who are accepted for medical training should be made fully aware of the requirements of the mass of their

TABLE 5
Comparison between Industrial and Health Problems in a Developing Country

Man–machine confrontation	Man–medical care confrontation
Small-scale industrialization involving men with simple machines leads to an appreciation of how machines work.	The effectively run health centre, involving the treatment and prevention of simple and common conditions, allows a good basis for the understanding of health.
Colonial policy looked to developing countries as sources of raw materials and a market for exports.	Colonial policy made available medical care for those in government. This developed into providing hospital services in the cities.
Developing countries as a solution have sent large numbers of young men to technical universities abroad, or opened such universities. Here they learn advanced engineering skills irrelevant to a developing country. On return they cannot set up their own industrial activity, but have to wait for the government to do so, or become over-educated over-seers in the Ministry of Works. They find little option but to stay away and join the brain-drain.	Lack of medical services has led developing countries at first to send doctors to train overseas and then adopt a similar curriculum in their own medical schools. Both these trainings are largely irrelevant to working in and running of health centres where doctors are needed, and so once the places in the teaching hospital and private practice are full, there is increasing pressure to join the brain-drain.
Foreign large-scale factories are built. They may have some effect in raising the Gross Domestic Product. Their impact on the development process is negligible. The highly sophisticated enclosed machinery does not lead to man–machine confrontation, and highly trained manpower is needed which most developing countries can hardly supply. Even if the manpower can be supplied, only a few will be needed and this will not help the massive urban unemployment.	Foreign-type large hospitals are built. They raise standards of medical care available to the fortunate few, but have little impact on the level of delivery of health care. The patients in these large medical institutions cannot distinguish between investigation and treatment, and a 'man–medical care' confrontation is not achieved. Worse, the hospital may be 'dehumanizing' by treating the individual as a thing rather than a person. Routine procedures may be undertaken without explanation, and no concern is felt for the effects of separating a patient from his family and home. Money is spent on employing a few highly skilled personnel, rather than the many less skilled ones who could be productive.

37

Man—machine confrontation	Man—medical care confrontation
To employ one person in this type of industry will require an investment of about £10,000, and in a small industry £1,000.	To treat 100 children with malnutrition in a large hospital may cost £9,000, and £2,000 in a nutrition rehabilitation centre (49).
These industries are concentrated in the large cities and attract away from the smaller cities and towns, capital and human resources.	Large hospitals are concentrated in large cities and attract away from smaller cities and towns the nursing and auxillary staff trained and needed there.
The alternative is small-scale industry employing 1–50 persons and having a simple managerial system, with a total investiment of £2,000–£10,000. These distribute a knowledge of machines and industrial skills and create an infrastructure on which large-scale industry may be built.	The alternatives to large prestigious hospitals are locally constructed health centres, supported by efficient district hospitals. These distribute an understanding of health care delivery on which the health of the nation can be built.
There is a lack of information in the technical know-how of small industries. This is a type of information not easily taught from books, but by a 'master' and handed on.	There is a lack of knowledge as to how health care can be best delivered, as this has not yet become a subject for study in depth by universities and their medical schools. Nor may they be capable of it in their present institutionalized form.

fellow countrymen who live in rural areas. In their training programmes more emphasis will need to be placed on attitudes which will encourage work away from the cities. At least 2 years' obligatory work in rural health centres should be a universal practice. As the distribution of intelligence in towns and rural areas is not dissimilar, a large proportion of students should have received their education in rural schools. Because of deficiency in their early training such students may not excel at least in the present conventional curriculum, although if chosen on grounds of high intelligence they are likely to catch up with those from the schools of the cities. If the desire to work in rural areas can be maintained in them, they are likely to be of great value to the rural society that has largely paid for their education. The type of education must reflect these needs; it is far too late to change the pattern of a doctor's life after he has qualified. Living, schooling and medical training in the country's capital city are preparation for work in that city or emigration to a city in another country. If all his teachers and in fact all the leaders in medicine live and work in the cities, that is where he will plan to live. If larger numbers of doctors are to be recruited from rural areas, then more attention will have to be paid to the effect of catapulting a student from a relatively unorganized rural society, rich in oral traditions and culture, into a Western-oriented scientific milieu.

Society needs to recognize that the doctor who designs and executes an effective system of medical care in a rural area is more worthy of recognition than for example the doctor who designs a system of renal dialysis centres. Probably two-thirds of the doctor's time should be taken up with organizing, training and supervising health centres, or running a small hospital. For this he needs the managerial skills described in Chapter 21. Once he has set up the health team he will no longer spend time diagnosing and arranging treatment for the common conditions, except when training new members of the team. His time will be given in part to diagnosing and managing the difficult cases for which his specialized training has prepared him, and in part to training and supervising the team who will be responsible for managing common conditions and for carrying out most of the preventive work. A doctor who works in this way will need to receive much of his training away from a large hospital.

Health is basically inseparable from justice and consequently from political participation. It is also inseparable from concurrent development in rural societies in other fields such as education, communication, water supply, sanitation and total economic development. Once governments are determined to retain doctors and other professionals in rural areas, then there are means in their power which enable them to do so. Examples are tax relief, good housing, and help or preference in schooling for children. Alternatively, those working in rural areas might well be paid more than the specialists who remain in the cities. This would do something to reduce the pull of the town. But more important that the above-mentioned factors is a satisfying and useful professional life, one in which the lowering of mortality rates is regarded as being of equal importance to the highest clinical expertise, China is facing the same problem by encouraging a third of all doctors who live and are based in the cities to be working in the rural areas at one time.

An expert suggests that what is most required is the doctor trained and equipped to lead a team of medical auxiliaries (95). These teams should be part of a health centre service (under a director of health services) acting as the main carrier of health measures in the country. The health centre service would be the basis upon which all other health activities in the country would rest. The focus of medical attention must be shifted from the big teaching hospital on the capital city hilltop to the unobtrusive health centre in the middle of the village, constructed by the villagers themselves and managed by a comittee on which they are well represented. This would be an ideal community relations approach. With a more even distribution and some increase in finance, working through such teams it is possible to provide a comprehensive service across the country. How these services should be financed is still an open question. Central financing through governments has proved unsatisfactory and the 'free' services available are not respected by the people. At the other extreme, fee-for-service systems prevent the group most in need from utilizing available services. Other methods of collecting funds need to be found if equitable services are to be provided; small community-based insurance schemes have many advantages. Investigations in Thailand showed that in a rural area the Government were spending $0.20 per head on health, but the people themselves $1.20. One project in Central Java was run on a contribution of less than $0.03 a month (314). The investigator believed that basic health care could be provided for $1.40 per head per year.

Friends whom the author respects suggest that the case for services in the rural areas has been overstated here. He would justify this presentation both because rural areas have previously been neglected, and because services in the peri-urban slums need to be similar in character.

Economics and child care

The points raised so far in this chapter relate to medical care at all ages. The sums available for different age groups have not yet been calculated in developing countries. Table 6 presents a breakdown of

TABLE 6

Expenditure by Age Group (53), UK National Health Service

	0–14 years	15–44 years	45–64 years	65+ years
Expenditure (£/caput/year)	16	22	29	67

expenditure by age groups in the UK (53). Those who have less life in front of them receive more help. Perhaps as communities become more concerned to receive greater benefit from health expenditure, there will be a shift to greater expenditure on the preventive side of medical care in the earlier years of life.

Corruption

The problems of underdevelopment have been well documented in contrast to the little that has been written on corruption (198). Corruption has been defined as the use of power for profit, preferment or prestige, or for the benefit of a group or class in a way that constitutes a breach of law or standards of high moral conduct.

This is a subject on which little is written and little research has been done, and yet corruption is one of the causes of administrations being so cumbersome. Corruption in the developing countries can be usefully compared with corruption in the past in the UK and the forces that led to its decline (295). Difficulties arise over deciding what should be included as corruption, and what excluded. In a medical service, it is the example given by the doctors which will set the standard for honesty in dealing with patients. If it is known that the doctor makes a large income by giving injections to all those who come to his home for treatment, is it surprising that the male nurse or orderly will also be quietly doing the same on the side? The doctor claims that because of his qualification, giving injections is legal, even if by general standards of medical treatment injections for that condition are unnecessary.

Myrdal makes a plea for research into the general nature and extent of corruption in a country, its incursion upon various levels and branches of economic life, and any trends that are discernible. The same is true in medical fields. The effects of corruption are far-reaching in that they do much to limit the delivery of health care to the populace at large. Because some private doctors charge high fees, the general population assumes that the delivery of health care from state hospitals not associated with such high fees must be of an inferior quality. Similarly, the fear of being charged these high fees is at least in part to blame for the unwillingness of many from the less well-off sections of the community to come forward for medical care. By charging high fees in the large cities some senior doctors gain for themselves and their families a standard of living totally different from that possible to doctors dependent on government salaries. Unwittingly such action corrupts the ideals of many other doctors who come in contact with them, particularly during their student days.

Some nationals have given a vivid description of corruption in their own country, both in the medical services and elsewhere (23). However, such information, while important in building up the 'folklore' of popular beliefs about corruption, is less valuable than scientific examination of this subject, which is so necessary.

One writer examines corruption in Thailand (274), and suggests a number of ways in which this can be investigated. Unlike others he thinks that most approaches to corruption are ethnocentric and arise from the presumption that the world is governed by a single moral code. In describing the situation in Thailand, he describes how the whole Thai society is enmeshed with a system of 'patron and client'. Each person seeks out a patron and also takes unto himself a number of clients. From the patron he expects to receive economic, social and political favours, and in return he expects to contribute finacially or in any other way that he is able to do so. Each patron will himself be a client of another, more senior, patron, and each client may well be a patron to others lower in the rank system of Thai culture.

It is suggested that these relationships are maintained by gratitude and respect, and corruption is conversely linked with ingratitude or disrespect. The latter in our terms would be failure to 'know one's place'. From a study of the thesis on this subject comes an understanding that the concept of corruption, like most other concepts, may vary enormously from culture to culture. It was suggested that in the Thai society corruption as we know it may be a force which maintains the integrity of the culture, and removal of corruption would lead to a disintegration of the society which is based on this patron—client system. However, as Thailand has opened her doors to world economic arrangements so a different view of corruption has had to be accepted, at least in some quarters.

Corruption is a force in all societies, which certainly in the medical field does not lead to the optimum use of resources for the benefit of the whole of the community. Some would claim that the present pattern of health care is largely determined by the 'class' nature of the society. In this present position various levels of care exist, and parents wishing to obtain the best for their children are liable to be involved in furthering corrupt practices.

CHAPTER 3

Beliefs and Attitudes to
Child-rearing and Disease

GENERAL BACKGROUND

As children, we are born into a culture which is all around us,
and we absorb it unawares as we grow up. If, say, an Indian child and
an English child were exchanged at birth and brought up in Bristol and
Bombay, as adults they would resemble citizens of their adopted rather
than their native country. The Indian child who had grown up in
Bristol, except for slight differences of pigmentation, would be English
in his attitudes and beliefs, while the English child who had grown up in
Bombay would have absorbed the culture of India. Such culture is so
much a part of us that it is only the educated, and particularly those
who have travelled and have had the opportunity of living in other
lands, who begin to understand some of the differences.

Culture is the sum total of customs, beliefs, attitudes, values, goals,
laws, traditions and moral codes of a people. It will, of course, include
their language and art, as well as how they express themselves in what
they make, from the shape of the canoe to the shape of the jet aircraft,
with all the noise and fumes the latter emits.

Many of these differences are quite obvious from only a short visit
to a country. Unfortunately, even after a longer stay in a country other
than one's own, one may limit observations to the obvious and visible
differences between that country and one's homeland. As an Indian
sociologist remarked, 'They see only what is not there'.

'The almost inevitable human tendency is to accept the visible parts
of a strange culture and unconsciously graft on to them invisible
elements from the observer's own culture, howbeit in a very incomplete
and haphazard way' (139). To progress farther along the road to a real
understanding of a strange culture requires a determined effort and
some knowledge of how to approach the subject. These are needed
both by the doctor from Europe and by the doctor indigenous to the
country. The doctor who has had a Western training may assume that

43

the parents of the children he cares for accept that measles is spread by 'droplet infection', as he understands it. Even if he realizes that they do not appreciate the method of spread of the disease, he will seldom realize the full significance of the beliefs about this disease which they hold. He may know that his patients seek other sources of medical advice and care, but is frequently unwilling to find out more about these because subconsciously he may feel that their popularity threaten his position as a doctor. He may resent the freedom of the individual to seek help from a herbalist or other traditional healer. He seldom asks himself why the patient went elsewhere and what was done for him. The educated but sociologically untrained person living in a strange culture will develop a view based on the visible elements of that culture, plus some of the invisible elements of his own culture.

The urgency to acquire a cross-cultural knowledge

Doctors only rarely practise among people with a homogenous culture identical to their own. In the tropical world this is particularly true. Even the few doctors who have been born in rural societies will have undergone a prolonged schooling and medical training in the city, so that they have become to some extent alienated from the culture they have been born into. Many doctors have practised, and still practise, with a limited knowledge of the culture and the beliefs of the people among whom they work. The author has recently had an experience that illustrates this point. In one part of Asia the belief is held that a child grows not because it eats food, but as a result of the sun's rays. If a child wastes, then a shadow has fallen on him. One of the first signs of this is a recurrent diarrhoea and sunken fontanelle. As a result, the people believe that it is right to take a child with mild diarrhoea to hospital for 'Western medicine', but not the child who has green stools and a sunken fontanelle. He is better treated with a special bark in the home, or by being taken to the priest. The author discussed this belief in one major teaching centre, and the paediatricians were amused that communities in another distant part of their country should hold such a view. Later in the day, during a visit to some slums close to the teaching centre, two out of the three households visited were found to have this belief, which clearly was widely held in the community but unknown to the doctors. A rather similar belief is held in one part of Africa where undernourished babies with sunken fontanelles are considered to have 'arram'. They believe such infants should not be treated in hospital but by indigenous medicine.

An understanding of the patient's view of himself and the reasons why diseases afflict him is needed by medical workers everywhere, but its importance is emphasized in only a minority of medical, nursing and auxiliary training schools. The present tendency for the medical profession to be drawn almost entirely from the 'elite' or upper social class will be mentioned on a number of occasions in this book. One result of this is an almost complete ignorance among many doctors of the culture and customs of the people in the working classes. One experienced professor of paediatrics in Asia regularly asked her paediatricians to answer a questionnaire on local culture and customs. Most were unwilling to complete it, and those who did had few significant replies to make.

Antibiotics work similarly in any human society, and a surgical operation has the same structural effect on the body whether it is undertaken in Newcastle or Dar es Salaam. But medicine should be more than just the application of techniques, and the patient's culture must be understood as it relates to his health. Particularly is this necessary if the doctor is to move out among the people and accept responsibility for the health of the whole community, rather than for only those who come and seek his help. It may, for example, enable him to understand why a child is taken from hospital when he develops measles, or why the mother is so anxious when she sees a blood specimen being taken from her child. With knowledge of her beliefs, he and the medical team can hope to reduce her anxiety over the blood specimen, and sometimes persuade her that the child with measles will be better cared for in hospital. He may have to encourage her actively to observe traditional rites or function in the ward, just as a Jew is permitted to carry out a traditional circumcision in a ward in England. The doctor who encourages this or any other rite to be performed does not believe in the need for it for the patient's direct physical benefit, but rather that the maintenance of family and traditional beliefs undoubtedly speeds recovery.

Doctors who have received their medical training in Europe or the USA, and who are going to work for a time in tropical areas, usually think that the great difference they will find will be the nature of diseases in tropical areas. Although this difference clearly exists, there are greater differences in the culture of the people with whom they will be working, and in their approach to life and, more important to the doctor, to health and disease. The beliefs are not only held by those living in rural societies. An eminent surgeon from one country who held a higher degree from the UK went back to his village herbalist for treatment of his jaundice. A senior health teacher, who regularly lectured to school children on ventilation, when back in his own village carefully shut up and barred his house against 'evil spirits'. The doctor from another culture will need to study these beliefs and attitudes if he is to be effective in providing health care, particularly if he is to gain any contact with that large secion of the community who still do not usually reach hospitals. Even the doctor indigenous to the area needs to study these differences, because he will have grown up in a sub-culture of the main cultural stream of his country, and because most of his training will have been undertaken among the comparatively small population of urban areas. For many doctors, indeed, their closest contacts are with fee-paying private patients who are unrepresentative of the inhabitants of the country as a whole.

UNDERSTANDING ANOTHER CULTURE

To gain a real understanding of another culture one requires the tools and knowledge of the sociologist and the anthropologist. As a start, there are in all parts of the world, including England (206), written descriptions available of traditional customs and beliefs. Examples are records from Burma (80), Malaya (42), the Pacific (35), East Africa (91), New Guinea (174), Thailand (106) and from Mali (122). To date, the majority of these studies have been undertaken by expatriates and many of the more recently established medical schools in the developing countries have not as yet accepted the collection of such material as an important requirement of the societies they serve. A classical collection of studies, *Health, Culture and Community* (220), has shown how a lack of knowledge of traditional health beliefs can be disastrous for an embryonic medical programme.

Frequently, local novelists have given a vivid description of a culture. Examples of these are *Blossoms in the Dust* in India, and the books by Chinua Acheb and Wole Soyinka in Nigeria. Although such works, and the more detailed studies of the anthropologist, provide a useful background, the student is likely to obtain worthwhile basic knowledge only if he undertakes a definite study of the culture of his own town or village. For this, the methods used by an educationalist (17) in Ghana were simple and direct, and could be applied by teachers in other disciplines. During their periods of vacation, the student teachers were sent out with specific questions, relating for example to the attitude of the community to punishing a child, to enuresis, to how a child should be fed, when the father sees the child, and what place he has in its early upbringing. The student who goes to gather this information is expected to talk to his old relatives and others in the village, to obtain answers to his questions, and to discover how these vary between different old people, and their attitudes, emotional and otherwise, towards them. At the end of their holiday studies, the students, whether they are teachers, nurses, medical auxiliaries or medical students, sit round a table and as a group discuss their findings. They will usually discover how generally similar are the beliefs in different parts of their country, although these will always differ in detail. This wealth of knowledge about the child needs to be integrated with knowledge of the family and its composition, the age of marriage and how frequently divorce occurs, what are the emotional ties with and obligations to distant relatives, and particularly what is the status of women within the family. Such data about the family must in turn be set in a picture of the community as a whole. King (139) gives a list of further areas on which information needs to be sought. The medical student will then be in a position to start the difficult synthesis of traditional beliefs and attitudes with those that they are being taught during their training in medical care.

'Conspiracy theory' or witchcraft

A common cause for all disasters is inferred in the following quotation.

> For if any adversity, grief, sickness, loss of children, corn, cattle, or liberty happen unto them; by and by they exclaim upon witches. As if there were no God that ordereth all things according to His Will . . . but that certain old women here on earth, called witches, must needs be the contrivers of all men's calamities . . . in so much as a clap of thunder, or a gale of wind is no sooner heard, but either they run to bells, or cry out to burn the witches.

Reginald Scott (240), who wrote this in 1584, was an unusual man, particularly in those days, both because he had the insight to distinguish superstition and reason, and also because he had the courage to speak his mind. This was a period when anyone expressing disbelief in witchcraft or criticism of the practice of witch-hunting might himself be burned at the stake along with the so-called witches.

Anyone who works among people who are still involved in the process of evolving from the primitive stage, as was the case in medieval Europe, will realize that what Scott said in 1584 still very much describes the attitude towards disease and calamity in most tropical societies today (207). The emphasis may be on witches, ancestral spirits or malevolent gods. These beliefs of course persist to a small extent in European and American societies, and may even be on the increase in these. In tropical societies, life is not governed by predetermined laws of nature, but by the relative influence of good and bad fortune, and both can be modified by the people's behaviour. It is difficult for people of any country to believe that 'we' are so unimportant that 'nature' can take its course. Most of us live in our own little world which is the centre of the universe and everything revolves around it. The idea that many events are completely outside our control, and that 'nature' works on us in the same way as gravity works on a falling stone, is difficult for those from any society to accept, and is offensive to us and our *amour propre**. This difference in beliefs regarding the causation of disease was well exemplified in a statement by a health inspector who remarked: 'You know, Doctor, with us it is not a question of what caused me to get sick but who caused it'.

Witches

Belief in witches is still occasionally found in rural areas of most industrialized countries and is common in tropical areas. It is necessary, however, to distinguish between the 'witch' who does not exist except in man's imagination and the 'witch doctor' or 'traditional practitioner' who may have an important part to play in society even today. The witch is believed to be a normal person by day, but by night she gathers with others of her kind and plots pestilential calamities in the community, or in some parts of it. The tragedy arises when the person who is imagined to be a witch is persecuted. In some areas of the world it is a criminal offence to call someone a witch; it is the duty of the more educated members of a society to prevent any person being named as a witch or the equivalent. If a doctor tells a Zulu patient that he is coughing up millions of tubercle bacilli and thereby infecting others, in terms of modern medical concepts this is in fact true, but in terms of the traditional ideas of disease the doctor has made the worst possible accusation in African society – that the patient is a witch (48). Western medicine is well equipped to answer the question 'How did a disease arise?' but not 'Why?' It is this question that is usually asked, and witchcraft can often give a more satisfying answer than modern medicine. There may be many reasons 'why' the same disease occurs. Conversely, an 'evil spirit' may cause any of a wide variety of diseases, and under these conditions classification of disease as we know it is unimportant.

People in the developing countries may be most unwilling to offend any other person because of the fear that they may be offending someone who, unknown to them, is a witch and may have the ability to place some sort of curse upon them. Even bumping into someone or upsetting a tray in a market place may in retrospect be regarded as a

---

Amour propre (Fr.), Self-love, exaggerated self-esteem

cause of illness. This accounts in part for the 'anxious-to-please' attitude that is frequently met. Those who undertake studies in remote
areas should realize that fear of what the outsider may do to them is
one reason why 'good co-operation' is achieved.

Origin of beliefs and attitudes in the individual

Because these beliefs and attitudes are so strongly held by adults, it
must be suspected that they were learned at a very early age. The child
in the first 5 years of life in the developing countries suffers from a
great many illnesses; in many of the rural areas of these countries
between a quarter and one-third of the children born die before their
fifth birthday. For every convulsion or attack of diarrhoea that a child
in Western society is likely to get, the child in the developing community is likely to get five or ten. Every time the child is sick (a time
when he is particularly close to his mother), his mother is likely to seek
help from 'traditional practitioners' or wise women, who will almost
certainly instil in her, and through her in her child, the idea that the
disease arises from giving offence to some spirit or god, and this idea
sticks. Often no amount of later education will completely change these
deep-seated beliefs in the causation of disease. One method through
which this attitude to disease and calamity can be prevented is the
provision of simple, understandable but scientific medical advice and
care offered in a concerned and friendly atmosphere. This will counter-
act the spoken and unspoken messages the child receives about spirits
and other influences in the home, at a time when he is beginning to
understand himself but is still close to his mother and learns so much
from her. In the Under-Fives' Clinic or similar service the worker can
prevent a large number of the common illnesses and has simple treatment available for many more. In this way, the child, through the clinic
worker and his mother, may learn to have a more rational approach to
disease and other calamities, and as a result may be more stable and
reliable in his decisions as he grows up. It is even suggested that in
developing countries a magicomythical world view is an obstacle to the
emergence of creative scientists, although it does not interfere with the
training of competent practitioners of scientific techniques (210).

Comprehensive child care through the Under-Fives' Clinic, if
examined in this light, plays a part in promoting the general well-being
and education of the population, as well as in reducing morbidity and
mortality in young children. To be effective in moulding the beliefs of
this age group, frequent although brief attendance at the clinic is required. These visits allow the mother to gain the reassurance she needs
from someone she trusts.

Western medicine as an alternative form of medical care

'Go in search of your people.
Love them.
Learn from them.
Plan with them.
Serve them.
Begin with what they know
Build on what they have.'

As medical workers in the study village of Imesi, Nigeria, Margaret Woodland and the author of this book believed that they were introducing medical care as something new. As their knowledge grew, they came to understand that they were not so much introducing something new as introducing an alternative system from that to which the people had been accustomed. Medical care is a social activity, present in some form in every community that has been studied. The mother appreciates the many dangers which arise for her small child in the early years of his life; she seeks to overcome and perhaps obviate these. For example, the mothers regularly used a medicinal herb tea for their children. With the advent of the Western medical care the preparation of these teas in Imesi has declined and they are now little used. The mothers also purchased bottles of medicine — few of which contained any active substances — from various itinerant salesmen. Frequently, neither the vendor nor the mother could read the label. If the child was ill, the mother would take him to the local 'traditional practitioner', who would listen briefly to what she said was wrong with him and then, by some means such as throwing bones on the floor and studying the pattern they produced, decide on the most suitable herb treatment.

The medical worker must realize that he is offering an alternative to these other methods, and whether his alternative is acceptable or not will depend both on how successful these measures are and also on his approach to and particularly his sympathy for the child and the mother. In the first of these, that is in successful treatment, the medical worker should have a considerable advantage. In the second, that is the approach to the patient, the 'traditional practitioner' is likely to be more experienced, to have more time, and be more successful in gaining the confidence of the mother. The medical worker needs to know and understand and appreciate the people's beliefs, and particularly the beliefs of the mothers and how they believe disease is caused. The 'traditional practitioner' believes that diseases are due to evil spirits, spells, shadows, or the evil eye. These may afflict the child through an evil person, a 'witch', or an inanimate object which is believed to contain a spirit. Such beliefs are handed down from generation to generation, continually reinforced by the 'traditional practitioner'. He may make a valuable contribution to the community, particularly in the field of adult psychosomatic medicine. The belief that in child health he had little to offer received support from the apparent readiness with which he referred sick children to the clinic. The overcoming of these beliefs and the introduction of the idea that disease is due to physical factors and infection by germs is an important function of the Under-Fives' Clinic. In these clinics an alternative explanation of disease is offered to the mother. Too little interest has been taken in the whole question of approach in traditional health education. The objective has been to change beliefs and attitudes with maximum rapidity, paying little consideration to such things as the patient's view of himself, his environment, his beliefs concerning disease and how slow the process of attitude change will be. A description of the natural history of disease needs to be included in health education. There may be less difficulty in teaching the mother that fluid loss from diarrhoea leads to a sunken fontanelle, than there is in explaining the need to wash hands. The first of these lessons may be more important in preventing death from diarrhoea. Perhaps in health education one can more readily teach the management than the prevention of diarrhoea.

If a child has been convinced in the first 5 years of his life that fever, for example, is due to evil spirits, it is most difficult to teach him in school the importance of malaria. Among African (219) and Indian (165) university students research has shown that university education has little effect on practices and taboos learnt in their family circle. Even students undertaking a scientific training retain their magico-mythical beliefs. Conversely, if a child has received sympathetic treatment for his fever by someone in an Under-Fives' Clinic who knows its cause, then the basis of a future scientific explanation of malaria has been laid. As well as the general beliefs about the causation of disease, communities have beliefs about the management of life in general. These are particularly important at certain periods, such as pregnancy, parturition and in the early years of life. The beliefs arise because experience has taught the people that at these times calamities are most likely to occur and they believe that these may possibly be warded off by some of the rituals which custom demands that the mother should carry out (126).

PRACTICES AND BELIEFS CONNECTED WITH CHILD-REARING

Every community has ideas and practices relating to child-rearing that are passed down from mother to daughter. Educational, social and medical workers with a westernized education unfortunately tend to deplore and discourage many of these when they come across them in developing countries. A detailed knowledge of local beliefs and practices and the extent to which the population hold and follow them is, however, needed, and students should study them during periods of vacation as already suggested.

Differentiation of practices and beliefs

Many beliefs and practices have intrinsic value. An attempt should be made to separate customs into the following groups.

(1) Beneficial practices: for example, carrying the infant on the back, true 'demand breast-feeding', the continual physical contact between the infant and adults, giving simple tasks to children so that they feel needed.

(2) Innocuous practices: for example, wearing beads and bangles, rubbing the infant with oil, failing to name a child when it is first born, most food fads in European countries.

(3) Practices believed to be harmful: for example, in some areas children's feet are subjected to heat when they have a convulsion, or concoctions which cause coma may be used. In measles, herbs may be applied to the eyes which damage the conjunctiva. The newborn may be swaddled, as by the Lapps, American Indians and Malays, resulting in an increased incidence of congenital dislocation of the hip. Use of pigment containing lead sulphide as an embellishment on the eyes in parts of Africa may possibly be a cause of lead poisoning. Such pigment as kajal, widely used in Asia, is satisfactory if prepared in the home, but many of the commercial preparations have a high lead content. Harmful practices are by no means limited to developing countries. In Europe, particularly the isolation, loneliness and boredom of an infant left by himself in the early months of life should be mentioned.

(4) Practices about which too little is known: for example, force-feeding or hand-feeding, circumcision, use of local medicines, swinging children in hammocks, as in India, bouncing them in hammocks on springs as in some Chinese areas.

Such differentiation is important. The nurses and health workers should appreciate the value of many local practices and make efforts to retain them. Numerically, there are many beneficial or harmless beliefs and only relatively few that are harmful. Otherwise they tend to adopt a 'superior' and discouraging attitude which reduces the mother's trust in the services provided for her child. The doctor should set an example; he should try to discover how the beliefs arose, and when they are harmful offer an alternative practice such as the application of cool water to a child with convulsions to replace the heating of the child's feet. At all times he must avoid letting his staff undermine the mother's faith in her own ability. By offering her an alternative and better practice one can avoid implying that what she did before was bad or wrong.

Epidemiological approach to cultural beliefs

In any field study in medicine, one learns the need to obtain a satisfactory sample before the results of the study are inferred to the whole community. In obtaining views on cultural beliefs, this is equally necessary. For example, in the context of attitude towards medical care, there are usually four classes in the population which are dealt with (48).

(1)   The hospital- and clinic-orientated population.

(2)   The private physician-orientated population.

(3)   The 'traditional doctor'-orientated population. These are staunch believers in the 'conspiracy theory' or witchcraft.

(4)   Certain religious populations which believe in divine or faith healing, and are very different in their orientation from 1, 2 or 3.

It is the first two of these groups that the majority of doctors are in contact with, and most closely with those who seek medical help as private patients, because culturally the doctor can communicate more easily and effectively with this group. Frequently, the last two groups who never even visit the health services are the largest in the population, and observations made from the first two groups will give very little insight indeed into the beliefs and attitudes of these groups.

The failure of confidence in present health
delivery service

In many rural societies of developing countries the existing clinics and hospitals have done little to take over health care from the traditional practitioner. The individuals in the community tend to be more flexible about the acceptance of treatment than in their beliefs about causation. The individual considers that his illness has a spiritual cause and the proper person for treating this is the traditional doctor, but this does not prevent him from attending the modern clinic or hospital for medical treatment. But if he is cured, in his mind it will the the traditional practitioner who will have done this. The treatment given by hospital or clinic is considered similar to that offered by a herbalist and is supportive, the real curative agent being the counter-charms, amulets and incantations of the traditional practitioner. The mother with a sick child frequently does not get what she is looking for as she attends the Western-type hospital. She has a double requirement; she needs not only treatment for the organic illness of her child, but also some answer to the question why her child is sick. It is understandable that medical workers often fail to give the understanding and reassurance hoped for. The dispensing of medical care by overworked personnel with varying levels of training in a crowded but ill-staffed clinic does not allow for the creation of personal rapport between the medical worker and the patient. The traditional practitioner has the advantage of a more leisurely procedure which allows him to devote a great deal of time to each patient, hear them out and give the psychological satisfaction wanted. This engenders trust and knowledge of the role of each in the process of treatment. Above all, patients want to know why the sickness has happened, and the traditional healer, with the same cultural concepts of disease, can give the answer. The doctor in the expensive hospital has much to offer in therapy, but because he fails to delegate, has little time for each patient. The workers in the Under-Fives' Clinic (Chapter 19) will work in simple surroundings more familiar to the mother, offering only simple therapy. A 'talisman' is supplied in the form of the road-to-health chart. The medical workers in this situation should be adequate in number, so that they have time to listen, talk and to sympathize with the mothers.

The traditional practitioner works in simple familiar surroundings, has little therapy to offer, but can give of his time and succeeds in maintaining the trust and love of the patient. The modern medical worker has much to learn from him.

CHAPTER 4

Priorities: The Doctor's Dilemma

THE DOCTOR'S ROLE

Priorities in the care of mothers and children need to be considered in the context of the whole health programme. Only recently doctors in developing countries have accepted their role and responsibility to the whole community. Such an acceptance demands a critical appraisal of their role in the maternal and child health programme. The following quotations (30) illustrate many of the issues involved.

The general picture

We can move closer to these problems by joining a young government physician as he arrives at his first assignment. He has just finished his internship and has been assigned to serve in a rural district. His district is 20 miles wide and 30 miles long and contains about 70,000 people. He is the only doctor. The hospital has 70 beds, and there are 110 patients. The nurse — there is only one — shows him around.

A large crowd is in the out-patient clinic, and he learns that 200 to 400 patients come each day. Two medical assistants are looking after them. The doctor will be asked to see the difficult problems. As he walks by, malnutrition, anaemia, skin problems and eye diseases are obvious. The hospital is clean and well kept. A midwife is taking care of two women in labour; no complications. There is an x-ray machine that will probably work when the tube is replaced. There is no x-ray technician; someone will have to be taught. The pharmacy is neat but poorly stocked; of the last drug order they received no penicillin and only half the chloroquin. This is an area where infection is common and malaria is endemic.

The refrigerator is not working. A little lab has a small microscope, a hand-driven centrifuge and some unlabelled stains. There is no technician, but one of the medical assistants has expressed an interest in brushing up on his microscopy and working in the lab. The operating theatre is simple and adequate. The medical assistant who had been giving anaesthesia was transferred, but one of the

55

others would be happy to learn. The nurse could give rag-and-bottle ether anaesthesia if needed.

The staff of the hospital consists of the doctor, the nurse, two midwives, two auxiliary nurses, four medical assistants, and various ancillary personnel including two drivers. The office of the District Health Inspector adjoins the hospital. In this district are four health centres, each staffed with auxiliaries, and each has a Land Rover, though these are occasionally grounded for lack of petrol.

As they look around, the nursing sister tells him of a new patient, a women who has been in obstructed labour for two days and now has the signs of a ruptured uterus. The operating theatre is ready if he needs it. The regional hospital with a surgeon is 140 dirt-road miles away.

The medical assistants are having difficulty setting a shattered fracture of the leg. A boy is comatose with what they believe to be cerebral malaria; his father is a local chief of considerable importance. The traditional healer from the village is with the boy now. A message was received last week from a medical assistant at one of the health centres about two cases with fever, headache and mental confusion — it could be sleeping sickness .

For whom is the doctor responsible?

The young doctor whom Bryant (30) describes above has to make certain immediate decisions about his responsibilities. In the first place, is he responsible only for the patients who come to hospital, for those who come to the health centres, and for those who come to neither?

The difficulty and importance of these decisions are increased by the fact that the people in the greatest need of health care may not realize their need, and will frequently not seek it, either in the health centre or hospital. No longer can we expect to go on giving the answer 'I have no choice in what I do'. Perhaps the various sections of the population, in relation to their take-up of health care, can be thought of as belonging to three groups, as shown in *Figure 12*.

Group A in *Figure 12* is the smallest. The members of this group have a good understanding of the need for curative care, and some understanding of the part that preventive care should play, particularly with respect to their children. It includes many of the leaders and the more wealthy members of the population. These will be literate, and many may read fairly widely. They will usually possess transistor radios, and will listen to the health talks.

Group B includes between 30 and 60 per cent of the population. They will make relatively good use of the curative services, although they will not understand them so well as group A. However, they will make little or no use of the preventive services. They will be economically less well off than the members of group A, and in many countries their literacy rate will not be high, and even when literate this group will read little.

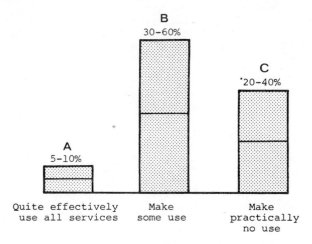

Figure 12. Users of the Health Services in the average developing country

Group C may vary in size, and receives little or no Western type of medical care for a number of reasons. Among these will be the distance that its members live from the hospitals and health centres, which are usually concentrated in urban areas; also their poverty and, most important of all, their lack of understanding of the need for health services and what they can do for their families. A recent study in a village close to New Delhi showed that only 7 per cent of illness came to the attention of the medical services (92). Domiciliary and home visit services, when available, should concentrate on this group and encourage them to understand that they will be welcomed at the clinic. How these children can be discovered is described in Chapter 8. Achieving success in reaching this group will involve community concern and action. The better-endowed mother will need to become more concerned with her underprivileged 'sister'.

Studies of the use of all services offered in a community have been made, and one from the rural Punjab (132) is given as an example (Table 7). The table emphasizes the relatively small proportion of all contacts for health care made to the primary health centre, and that more services are supplied by the indigenous medical practitioner who

TABLE 7

Medical Care Given by Different Types of Practitioner in Rural Punjab (132)*

Type of practitioner	Factors influencing continuity of practice	Number available and use made of services
Folk practitioners (spiritual healers, bone setters, spirit-mediums)	Significant role in treating children's diseases which are considered super-natural. Not important in adult disease. No cash paid. Highly trusted. They adhere strictly to cultural guide-lines. Their practice will last as long as traditional beliefs continue	150/90,000† popula-tion.

Utilization is quite low because use limited to certain diseases |
Registered indigenous medicine practitioners; some have institutional Ayurvedic or Unani training	May specialize in certain adult diseases or treat all ages. Paid in cash or credit. Fairly well trusted. Adhere to cultural guide-lines. Qualified doctors when available will compete with them	60/90,000 population, achieving 221 contacts per 100 population. The majority of these visits are to those without institutional training, practising 'popular' medicine with a wide range of treatment. These are accessible and highly used
Qualified doctors; private sector	Treat all age groups. Immediate cash payment. Adhere to cultural guide-lines except when they conflict with the modern concepts of disease. Highly trusted. Role is likely to increase as long as private sector is encouraged	5/90,000 population, achieving 14 contacts per 100 population. Low utilization due to small number
Qualified doctors. Primary health centre and staff with sub-centres; Public sector	Treat all age groups. Negligible payments. Cultural guide-lines. frequently neglected. Often poorly trusted (depending on individual practitioner). Significant only close (2–3 miles) to centre. Only services capable of team approach	2/90,000 doctors (5–15 other health workers), achieving 89 contacts per 100 population per year. Medium utilization due to poor facilities and poor quality services. High potential if team given leadership. Still limited to immediate locality

*The facts given here have been rearranged and condensed from the original article
†This was the size of the block being investigated

has not undergone institutional training to become Unani or Ayurvedic. These indigenous medical practitioners are flexible and offer a popular form of care involving the use of antibiotics and other substances purchased locally. The presence of these indigenous practitioners is an expression of a felt need by the people (316).

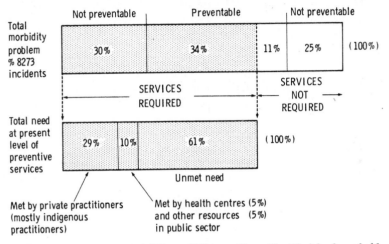

Figure 13. Distribution of 8,273 morbidity problems identified by household visits in Punjab villages

In another study (216) the health needs in terms of over 8,000 episodes of illness were related to the facilities available and the unmet need measured *(Figure 13)*. From this, the proportion for which services are required is further broken down and the large unmet need is apparent. The relatively large volume of care given by the indigenous medical practitioners is again emphasized. In a further breakdown the authors suggest that if all episodes of disease that are preventable are excluded, the present service could cope with 84 per cent of what remains. These figures come from an economically well off area of a state in which peripheral services are better planned than in most other developing countries. Studies in other areas are likely to demonstrate an even higher proportion of unmet need. Even in the industrialized countries, a significant proportion of need remains unmet.

In Egypt which has a more widely distributed health service than India, one study showed that only 20–25 per cent of families made use of National Child Health centres and up to 80 per cent of mothers were dependent on traditional midwives for delivery (315).

Only by such studies of the differential uptake of medical services in a defined population will we come to know the size and importance of these groups, the economic, geographical and cultural factors underlying them, and how we as doctors and leaders of teams of health workers can overcome the barriers which prevent more effective use being made of health services. The division of limited resources is unequal. Those with some knowledge of disease processes (group A in *Figure 12)* whose need is least, receive the largest share, while the ignorant and deprived (group C) receive little. If, however, medical resources are to be re-allocated on a more equitable basis, one cannot avoid making a choice; this is the heart of the matter. In doing this, the doctor is deciding who shall be served and who shall be deprived, which means deciding who shall live and who shall die, or live in a state of disablement. The difficulty comes in considering what criteria the doctor should use, what system of values should guide him in choosing, for example, whether to improve the health of the mothers and the children, and then which children, or to what extent should the fathers receive help, as they can contribute most of the nation's wealth. Can a doctor attempt to answer all these questions? One of the first steps is to examine his method of decision-making and how he defines his priorities.

PRIORITIES AMONG HEALTH PROBLEMS

The subject of priorities in health problems will be considered in greater detail in the chapter on management. It is suggested that the following sequence (31) should be followed *(Figure 14)*. In this cycle the two most essential steps are the setting of priorities among the many health problems, and assigning priorities among the population groups.

System of criteria

A useful technique for setting priorities among health problems is illustrated in Table 8. Four criteria are used: community concern, which includes knowledge, attitudes, feelings and the degree of urgency; prevalence, which refers to the frequency with which the problem occurs; seriousness, that is its destructive effects on individuals and society; and susceptibility to management, which takes into account the availability of methods for management as well as the cost and difficulty of applying them. In considering this susceptibility to management, special preference will be given to management within the community, partly for economic reasons, but mainly because the community will be involved.

In the absence of numerical data, these criteria can be weighted intuitively, using a scale of + to ++++. A score for each health problem

60

is reached by multiplying the individual weightings. This simple method for setting priorities is used by groups of medical and nursing students working in rural Thailand. Increasing experience will stimulate thought

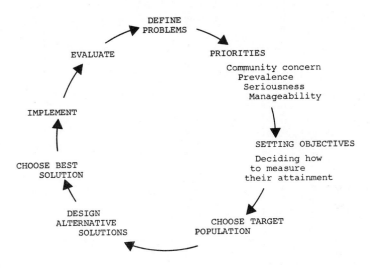

Figure 14. Bryant's problem-solving cycle (31)

on the criteria chosen. Those given in Table 8 are the author's for a West African rural community. Other workers, from this and other societies, will no doubt lay different emphasis on these criteria. Notice that community concern is placed first, even if this concern is for non-medical help, or their requirement has to be assessed as a low priority. The very fact that their concern has been shared and considered will help to get the problem solved. Community concern will change and develop as the community awakens to its problems.

The method is directed toward health problems rather than population groups. Particular groups are implicitly involved in some instances — for example, malnutrition is found largely in small children, and pregnancy involves only women — but otherwise the method does not take into account special groups in the population. It does not, for example, lend itself to criteria that might be suggested by an economist whose major objective is the country's development. For him, health care priority might be given to males between the age of 15 and 50 years because of the contribution of their labour to the gross national product. However, over the last decade economists have been dissatisfied with this index and many consider that expenditure on health

61

TABLE 8

Criteria for Building Priorites in a Rural Society

Health problems	Community concern	Point prevalence	Seriousness	Susceptibility to management	Total
Malnutrition	++	+++	++++	+++	72
Inadequate antenatal and obstetrical care	+++	++	++++	++	48
Large and poorly spaced family	++	+++	++++	++	48
Specific diseases					
Pneumonia	+++	++	++++	+++	72
Whooping cough or measles	++	++	+++	++++	48
Tuberculosis	++	+	+++	+++	24
Leprosy	+++	+	++	++	12
Dental problems	++	++++	+	+	8
Common cold	+	+	+	+	1

62

should not be regarded as a 'capital investment' giving small returns, but that 'health needs no justification'.

The points assigned to different criteria will depend on the area and on the training of the worker. Trying to reach decisions will require each discipline to see their objectives in relation to those of others. However, by such methods one is beginning to widen the criteria by which such decisions are made, and moving a step beyond the stage of working on 'hunches'. Such a method is different from initiating a health service by building many hospitals of different sizes. By so doing decisions have already been taken – and not necessarily the right ones – even if the hospitals are soon overcrowded with patients.

In Asia the problem of the large family is more serious for each nation than in Africa, where there is still space, and where concern for the adequate spacing of children is more accepted. Malnutrition heads the list in Table 8; it is always present. It may be an immediate cause of mortality, but more important is its effect on physical and intellectual development of children (54). Associated with infectious disease, poor nutrition can be responsible for a high mortality. How readily malnutrition can be prevented varies widely, and will depend on other sciences such as agriculture, education and transport. Many of the causes have been pin-pointed in the 'Food Pathway' (141).

Choosing 'target' populations

Setting priorities among health problems has two limitations in helping to decide whom to serve when all cannot be served. Firstly, as noted above, it does not take into account special population groups; secondly, even when it seems right to attack a specific disease, resources may be inadequate to care for all who have that disease, for geographical and other reasons. Thus, malnutrition may be given high priority but if two-thirds of pre-school children are malnourished, resources may be adequate to care only for those who are most malnourished, or perhaps efforts should be concentrated on children with malnutrition in their first year, whose intellectual potential may be permanently reduced.

Death and disability due to complications of pregnancy and childbirth is a serious problem throughout the developing world. If resources will allow only 25 per cent of pregnant women to receive care, which 25 per cent should it be? In practice it is usually those who seek medical assistance, whereas it can be argued that it should be the 25 per cent whose health is most threatened by pregnancy and childbirth, and that we must find means to select these and get them to 'maternity villages' attached to hospitals.

The concept emerges of a system for searching through the population for those most in need, that is those already afflicted or those most threatened (the 'high-risk' group described in Chapter 9), and bringing limited resources to prevent or overcome their special problems.

Dividing-up health resources in a population of 2,000

The village that will be considered consists of 2,000 people, and by the standards of a developing country is exceptionally well served by a medical assistant and an auxiliary nurse—midwife*. A community development approach will aid in the identification of the rural society's need. An assessment of the identified need, the means of satisfying it, and the consequences of this satisfaction will be an appreciation of the whole issue. In the light of this approach their health problem will be closely looked at.

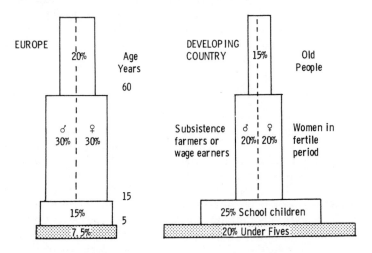

Figure 15. Simplified population pyramids

Age distribution is very different from that found in Europe. Most services and training programmes in developing countries are designed to serve a 'European-structured' population — a point illustrated in

*Unfortunately no satisfactory and generally accepted terminology exists. These workers will have had around 2 years of training in both curative and preventive care. The word 'nurse' may be considered a synonymn for 'medical assistant' in such circumstances.

Figure 15. In this figure the population pyramid has been simplified to aid in memorizing the figures. For comparative purposes, a European type of breakdown of age distribution has been used. However, this is unsuitable to other areas. For example, in many developing countries the majority of so-called school-age children will be not at school but working on the farms. A rought estimation of the size of the various groups in each population is a necessary step in planning, even if this has to be achieved by a sample survey. There are likely to be 2–2½ times as many children in the under-five group in developing countries. This very high proportion is due partly to the large number of births, but also to the number of deaths, so that one-third of these children do not pass on into the school-age group. It is also large because the population is expanding rapidly. In the study village there are likely to be 350–400 out of the 2,000 who will be children under 5 years of age. There will be 400–500 children of school age. Women in the fertile period will number 300-400, and there will be a similar number of men, the majority of whom will be subsistence farmers as it is an agricultural area. Lastly, there will be approximately 200–250 old people.

Health needs of various population groups

To the sick villager life is miserable but he believes and trusts that his health may improve. Death, on the other hand, is final. A dramatic change in the number of deaths in a village, particularly through the removal of well-known killing diseases such as measles or whooping cough, is more significant to him, and more noticeable, than a general improvement in health. Since illnesses which are likely to cause ill-health are also likely to cause death, the general health of the people will be improved by preventing deaths. Prevention of death answers a fundamentally felt need in that it maintains and safeguards the family unit.

The prevention of deaths should therefore remain the primary aim of the health service. In a village of 2,000 the following are likely to die each year: 8 old people, 6 people in their working years or in the school-age group, 1 mother, and perhaps 25–30 children under 5 years of age. These various groups will now be considered.

The 8 old people. — Neither the old people nor their relatives are likely to seek or expect medical care in an attempt to delay death.

The 6 people in their working years. — These people belong to the group of greatest economic importance in the village. Their health is the concern of the medical assistant or his equivalent, rather than the

65

PRIORITIES: THE DOCTOR'S DILEMMA

TABLE 9

Measures Taken by a Nurse–midwife to Overcome Maternal and Perinatal Mortality

Cause of death	Prevention of death
Disproportion or malpresentation (hours ++)*	*Referral* to a hospital, or better a 'maternity village' will be necessary as the facilities and experience of the nurse–midwife exclude local delivery. The midwife may sometimes diagnose these in the antenatal period. However, in practice this is rarely achieved at present. Greater attention to objective measurements such as the woman's height and the careful taking of obstetric histories are usually needed. Those mothers who are likely to have a normal delivery may be cared for by the traditional attendant if she has received minimal training and is supervised. In some societies these traditional attendants also live with the mother to help and support her in the days after delivery, in a way that would be impossible for the few trained midwives
Infections (hours +)	*Local.* – The prevention of malaria and the immediate treatment of such acute infections as pneumonia in the mother. In the newborn, the prevention or early treatment of umbilical sepsis and other acute neonatal infections, and the prevention of neonatal tetanus by giving the mother toxoid during her pregnancy

Referral is needed for most of the antenatal and puerperal infections |
Anaemia (hours +++)	*Referral* is required. The WHO Technical Report on nutrition in pregnancy and lactation (289) deprecates the administration of iron as a routine. If the midwife can diagnose anaemia before symptoms develop, she will need to use a routine therapy designed for the common conditions of that area
Toxaemia and eclampsia (hours +++)	*Referral* is necessary. Prolonged albuminuria as a sign of toxaemia and pre-eclampsia is not commonly found in West Africa. The onset of eclampsia may be diagnosed only by relative hypertension and albuminuria shortly before or at delivery. Routine urine testing is, therefore, of limited value, and if undertaken can be very time-consuming
Haemorrhage (hours +)	*Referral* is needed after 'first-aid' treatment

*The (hours +) or (hours ++) refers to the relative time taken by the nurse–midwife if she is to prevent one death from this cause

66

nurse—midwife, and they will not be considered further here, although this group and its health are of great importance.

The one mother. — With this mother can be grouped 4 of the 30 children likely to die — these 4 representing the proportion of infant deaths in the perinatal period Prevention of maternal and perinatal deaths is the task of the nurse—midwife. She can achieve this either by measures she undertakes herself, or by persuading the mother to attend hospital, that is by 'referral'. The survival and good health of the mother is of course important also for her older children. However, in communities where there is a long birth interval, it is unlikely that there will be more than one other child under 5 years *(Figure 102)*. Only under the age of 5 years will the death of the mother have a serious effect on the health of the child. The principal causes of maternal and perinatal deaths in this village are listed in Table 9.

Deaths from disproportion and malpresentation call especially for prevention. This will take up a fairly large part of the nurse—midwife's time in obtaining a history which may, however, be relatively quick if her records are good and the mother has been seen for previous deliveries. With the standard of training that she will have received, one must question and evaluate whether the amount of time that she may spend on antenatal palpation will reveal sufficient information about disproportion and malpresentation to make it worthwhile.

With respect to infections, this is a malarious area, and therefore by giving monthly antimalarials the nurse can do much to improve maternal health and reduce maternal and perinatal mortality at a low cost in terms of resources. Certainly the antimalarials that she will give will be a most effective use of her resources. In the management of anaemia her resources can be expended less well. It is doubtful whether the routine use of iron is to be recommended unless evaluation of local anaemia in mothers has confirmed that this is due to iron deficiency. In some areas routine iron administration with or without folic acid may be desirable.

The early diagnosis of toxaemia may be difficult. Several hundred samples of urine would have to be tested before an abnormality in one would be discovered, and diagnosis through taking large numbers of blood pressures will again be uneconomic of the nurse—midwife's resources. Maintaining maternal weight records may also be difficult.

Lastly, in the management of antenatal and postnatal haemorrhage, the nurse can clearly play little part, and in this and other fields her success will depend on the referral system and whether there are facilities to move the mother to a hospital. Only too frequently the hospital will be so far away and transport so difficult that transfer will be unlikely.

PRIORITIES: THE DOCTOR'S DILEMMA

TABLE 10

Measures Taken by a Nurse–midwife to Prevent Infant and Child Deaths

Cause of deaths	Proportion	Prevention
Protein–calorie deficiency (hours ++)*	12%	*Local.* By the use of a weight chart supplied to every child, the nurse–midwife can detect a failure of growth which will precede the syndromes of kwashiorkor and marasmus by many months. By encouraging the mother to give the children better and more frequent food, and where necessary by the use of food supplements, she may bring about a satisfactory weight gain. Referral will be necessary only where there is persistent failure to gain weight adequately and the nurse is unable to identify the cause of failure to grow.

Protein–calorie deficiency may sometimes be acute in onset, often following acute infections such as measles and whooping cough. The nurse–midwife will help prevent these infections by arranging immunizations, and will treat them in their early stages at the Under-Fives' Clinic |
| Pneumonia (hours +) | 12% | *Local.* The nurse–midwife will be supplied with sulphadimidine and antibiotics for administration in the early stages of lower respiratory infections of childhood. She will need to receive continuing education so that she can better distinguish early pneumonia from a mild respiratory infection |
| Diarrhoea (hours +) | 12% | *Local.* The nurse–midwife can play some part in prevention, particularly by improving the nutrition of children, which will be shown by their weight curves. In general, however, prevention must await the availability of improved sanitary facilities, particularly piped water supplies to each house.

Diarrhoea and dehydration. There are good reasons for treating dehydrated children locally in a simple way in the home or Under-Fives' |

68

PRIORITIES AMONG HEALTH PROBLEMS

TABLE 10 *(cont.)*

Causes of deaths	Proportion	Prevention
		Clinic. The medical and sociological reasons for this in West Africa are likely to be as important elsewhere, and will be given in Chapter 10
Measles (hours +)	8%	*Local.* By preventive inoculation. The nurse—midwife's responsibility may be to immunize or to see that the mother and child attend on the day the mobile immunizing unit visits her centre. This and other immunizations may be administered by mechanical injector rather than by syringe. She will know that a specific percentage of those at risk in her community need to be protected if epidemics are to be avoided
Whooping cough (hours +)	8%	*Local.* By preventive inoculation in the first 3 months of life
Malaria (hours +)	8%	*Local.* By giving pyrimethamine monthly and making chloroquin available whenever the child attends with fever. In many areas of the world conditions other than malaria are responsible for anaemia, and this contributes to mortality. Control of this will also depend on local preventive methods
Tuberculosis (hours +)	5%	*Local.* By preventive inoculation early in infancy with BCG vaccine by the immunization staff.
Smallpox (hours +)	5%	*Local.* By preventive inoculation
Remaining conditions	30%	Through her continuing in-service training the nurse—midwife will come to understand the management of many of these conditions. Even in those that have to be referred she can supervise the treatment of many locally. Others, if common, she may be able to prevent as, for example, neonatal tetanus by immunizing the mother

*As in Table 9 the (hours +) represents the time taken to prevent one death. Because death is so common in all these conditions, only one + has been given. The nurse—midwife will have to spend more time in promoting better nutrition, but this is immensely worthwhile, as better nutrition reduces the chance of death from so many of these conditions

An excellent method of overcoming some of these difficulties is through the development of a 'maternity village' close to a hospital, where the mother can not only be under observation during the last few weeks of her pregnancy, but can also be involved in health education and preventive care.

The spectrum of disease associated with maternal and perinatal mortality described here is that found in West Africa (39). Some differences are likely to exist elsewhere. In most regions, however, the training of the midwife has been based largely on the Western spectrum of maternal disease in which toxaemia and iron-deficiency anaemia predominate. As a result, much of her effort has been directed to such questionable activities as the testing or urine samples and the distribution of iron tablets. It is doubtful whether the resources of her time and those of the medical services spent on these activities are justified.

Suppose 80 women in the village community under consideration give birth to an infant each year. The majority of these will experience a pregnancy relatively free from disease followed by a normal delivery. The services which the nurse-midwife can offer will have little effect on their health or the outcome of pregnancy. Her main responsibility lies in detecting the small number of mothers — perhaps 10 per cent — in whom the complications of pregnancy are likely to occur and who will usually need referral to obtain adequate care. Her second responsibility will be in the field of family planning in most countries. Her approach to this problem may be through adequate child spacing, using the 'road-to-health card' as described in Chapter 18, the objective being to improve the health of the children rather than to limit the family size.

The 25–30 children who die under the age of 5 years. — The spectrum of disease described here is that of the early 1960s in West Africa. Since then it has changed; in particular smallpox is no longer a problem. The argument is not, however, effectively altered. Seldom does a child die of a single condition; more usually two or more are combined. Table 10 gives an approximate idea of some of the common causes of death.

Comparison of Tables 9 and 10 demonstrates a considerable difference between the prevention of most maternal and child deaths. Most maternal deaths require hospital resources if they are to be prevented. Most child deaths can be prevented in the village by a nurse—midwife with vaccine, simple therapy and equipment, with the skills to use them.

THE NURSE—MIDWIFE

Traditionally, the female worker has been trained largely in the field of midwifery, and within the limitations of her training has striven to help rural mothers, The emphasis on midwifery has been in response to a felt need in the local community for care in the antenatal period, and to a lesser extent during delivery, and also for the care of the mother in obstructed labour. The community know that a woman with severe haemorrhage or obstructed labour will almost certainly die, and such women are brought to hospital even by the population in group C in *Figure 12* who usually do not make use of hospital services. Just as long as the doctors stay within their hospitals, they will see and help these mothers but fail to respond to the many other needs of the community.

Her function and training

The functions of the nurse—midwife need to be reconsidered. Her training can only be limited in scope, and her resources at village level will remain small. These resources could, however, be more scientifically deployed, and her training redesigned to give her skills which are more applicable to the needs of a rural society. Much more of her time could be spent with the under-fives, and also in helping the mother to maintain adequate birth-spacing through family planning. In these activities she will remain largely self-sufficient if given adequate supervision and repeated teaching. She can probably prevent the majority of deaths in children under five within the confines of the village. Because of the advances of science she can be more effective than the best trained doctor of 30 years ago. She will retain her function as a midwife, but greater emphasis will need to be placed on the criteria by which the 'at risk' pregnancy can be recognized by her and the mother removed to the maternity village or hospital.

This retraining and redeploying of resources linked with the health centre and sub-centre make good sense, both economically and also in building up the strength of the family and community. The process of health education and the mother's and child's understanding of disease will come about through the nurse—midwife in the village more readily than through the sophisticated hospital. Just as national leaders in many developing countries are laying fresh emphasis on the wholesomeness of village life, so in the medical sphere, maintaining and improving the health of the rural society must be emphasized as a function of members of that society. Unfortunately, only a few documented examples of this approach exist (6), (252), (134), (314), and yet these are the most promising pointers to how the health and well-being of rural societies may be rapidly improved. The doctor holds a key position. Only as and when the doctor recognizes and respects the nurse—midwife working in the rural area as an essential colleague through whom the greater part of medical care can be provided

71

(Chapter 20), will the rural society come to respect and trust these workers.

TRAINING PROGRAMMES

If this simplified comment on the health of a community of 2,000 even approaches a true statement of what is happening, and it is accepted that the teaching of medicine must be with reference to the needs of the community, then the balance of training needs to be shifted heavily towards solving the problems of community child health. Some countries now recognize child health, along with surgery and medicine, as one of the three major specialities required by their medical undergraduates. In others, a year or more of the training of a large proportion of their doctors is spent in study of child health. These longer periods of training should prepare the doctor to be more effective in the frequent situation in which around 50 per cent of all his work is among children. However, this emphasis on child health in the medical curriculum is still limited to a few countries which have appreciated healthy children as their most valuable asset. A planning cycle for educational programmes has been suggested that needs to be followed in an ever-changing situation (31) *(Figure 16)*. This approach is different from

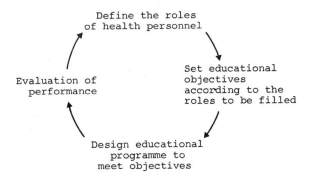

Figure 16. Planning cycle for educational programmes

that currently in use. The role (and function) of health personnel needs to be scientifically studied. From this, well-defined educational objectives can be set and suitable programmes designed. The success of these programmes will be re-examined as the roles of the health personnel are redefined in a rapidly changing society.

If medical services through auxiliaries are to be available for whole populations, statements such as the following, written by a doctor in the Congo, will become more commonplace: ' . . . assistant nurses often with two years or less of secondary training, plus two years' nursing training. With experience and informal instruction over the years, they become competent for example at cross-matching blood and giving a transfusion without supervision, coping with most minor surgery, and if pressed major surgery. During my recent leave, these assistant nurses successfully performed nine lower segment Caesarean sections and relieved four strangulated hernias. This may not be ideal, but lives are saved, and there is a shortage of doctors in all rural areas' (168). If the doctor is to become involved so closely in a team with auxiliaries, this must be recognized from the early days of his training. A Ghanaian (4) describes how, during his training in Russia, he was involved early in the course in a period of nursing patients. The subjects given in this course included 'basic nursing care, removal of bed pans, cleaning and sterilization of instruments, nursing of very ill patients . .,. '. This and similar experience in the training he believes were of considerable value to him in preparing him to be involved in the further training and supervision of a health team largely composed of auxiliaries. In Denmark, medical students may undergo a rather similar experience, as in their vacation periods, during their period of pre-clinical studies, they are strongly encouraged to undertake nursing duties.

New approach

A new approach to the training of doctors which is being attempted now in a number of countries runs into many difficulties. Just as the airport and parliament buildings must be prestigious, so must be the teaching hospital. The new medical school will recruit largely expatriate staff, chosen for their skills as anatomists, neurologists, surgeons, and so on, coming from a variety of developing countries. They all consider their own education to be the best and try to pass this on to their student. Under such circumstances, one professor found considerable resistance to community medicine (142) (Table 11). The 'blue' opinions of many expatriates are strongly reinforced by the immediate consumers, the urban-educated elite civil servants and others, many of whom have experienced 'fee for service' hospital-based medical care during time spent overseas.

PRIORITIES: THE DOCTOR'S DILEMMA

TABLE 11

Medicine, Red and Blue*

? ? ?	Right (blue)	Left (red)
How important is community medicine in the curriculum?	What is it?	Vital
What can medicine give the rural poor?	Their needs are economic	Much
Should student's training be different?	We must maintain standards and comparability	Radically
How important is rural field-work?	Complete waste of time	Essential
Should there be bonding?	Infringement of liberty	Why not. the cost of their eaucation is borne by the poor
Doctor's car?	Mercedes	VW
Responsibility for whom?	Patients who request our services	For those who ask and those who don't
Medical School to train whom?	Doctors	Whole health team
Is teaching hospital essential	Yes	Modify district hospitals
Conditions costly to treat?	Let's be a centre of excellence	Compassionate palliation
Should writing basic English texts be an important academic activity?	Gram described his stain in about 1880. No need to do it again	Yes

*Freely adapted from King (142)

Private practice

Any remarks on the subject of private practice are likely to be resented by the vast number of doctors in many developing countries who earn most of their salary through private practice. A great many doctors maintain their families by a few hours' private practice while giving their services free or almost free during the morning hours.

Private practice unfortunately concentrates doctors in the cities and is open to many abuses. The doctor in private practice usually acts as an individual and is seldom part of a well-constructed health team. If a doctor is to divide his time between service in a clinic, administration, teaching, research and private practice, then at least one of these will be inadequately undertaken. If there is to be greater equality of opportunity for what services are available, then that absorbed into the

74

'private sector' must be limited. However, both the doctors and those politically vocal are at the present time the main beneficiaries of a system of private practice and resistance to any change can be expected.

Probably each country will find its own solution and abolition of private practice by decree is unlikely to succeed. Interesting developments are taking place. In Rajasthan, (North India) junior hospital doctors have been on strike in 1972 against their consultants being involved in private practice. In both Cuba and China, junior doctors have pressed those senior to them to limit their salaries.

CHAPTER 5

Care of the Newborn

Many children sicken and die during the perinatal and neonatal periods in the developing countries. These are periods of great emotional significance. The delivery of the mother and the birth of the child are subject to more beliefs and superstitions than any other period of life.

GENERAL OBSERVATIONS

Morbidity may be particularly sinister during this period because of its long-term effect in later life. A good example is the newborn infant who develops an acute infection of the head of the femur, with involvement of the hip joint. In the rural society of a developing country, such an infant may show insufficient evidence of serious illness to prompt the parents to seek help from a medical assistant or a busy doctor. Equally, the severity of the condition may be overlooked by medical workers until the process has reached the stage at which the head of the femur is irrevocably damaged so that even if the infection is halted, the child will grow up with a destroyed hip joint in a society where walking is essential, problems with his toilet will be embarrassing and a limp will make farming difficult. Until a satisfactory level of confidence in the health service is achieved many children with treatable congenital abnormalities will be hidden away due to the feelings of 'guilt' that such children commonly inspire in their parents. Even more serious is the possibility that failure of adequate physical growth in the early months of life may be associated with impairment of the potential intellectual development. The brain grows rapidly at birth, at the rate of 1 mg per minute, and any limitation of growth of the individual is likely to influence the growth of the brain, and presumably also of the intellect.

In Chapter 3 a division of health care was suggested and the need to consider the total child population as the denominator was emphasized, with the possibility that children at special risk should receive a larger proportion than the general population of any services that are available. In considering the care of the newborn, such a division is even more necessary. The facilities for care of the newborn in developing countries have often been divided up as follows:

facilities for newborn care
_____
babies born in the maternity hospitals

Relatively efficient care may be provided for infants during their stay in hospital. However, if the facilities available can be divided up to reach as many of the children in the community as possible, they will have a far greater impact in reducing morbidity. A more appropriate division of services in developing countries should perhaps be:

facilities for newborn care
_____
all the babies born in the community that can be reached

In the rural society, close contact between the mother and the young infant is crucial; the mother is a source of warmth, humidity and nourishment and emotional support. In the Western society, this role is often overlooked, and during the last 50 years the infant has been removed from his mother and placed in another cot or even in a separate nursery where warmth and humidity are perhaps less well controlled, and where breast-feeding is expected to depend on the clock. More recently the tide has turned and the newborns have been moved back beside their mothers where they belong. The importance of close contact in developing that relationship which is so vital for the first years of life has been rediscovered. This close relationship is even more important if the baby is to survive the hazards of infancy and childhood common to all developing countries. We are now beginning to appreciate the depth of the emotion of 'longing to belong', and that if this sense of 'belonging' can be established early in the first hours and days, the effect will be long-lasting and of importance throughout life.

The perinatal and neonatal periods can be influenced more readily by simple yet expert care than at other periods. In the village of Imesi in Nigeria, West Africa, Miss Woodland, a nurse with training in midwifery and community work, leading a team of five local nurses and supported when necessary by the Wesley Guild Hospital, 25 miles away, reduced the neonatal death rate by 1966 to less than a third of the figures prior to 1957 (Table 12).

Study of these figures shows that the neonatal and infant mortality fell dramatically. No doubt circumstances other than the presence of this team played a part; for example, a road was built to the village,

TABLE 12

Child Mortality Rates, Imesi Ile, Western Nigeria

	Prior to 1957	1962–1965 (3 years)	1966 (1 year)	1966 (UK)
Still births/1,000 total births	41	36.4	21.7	15.3
Neonatal deaths/1,000 live births	78	21.9	22.2	12.9
Infant mortality/1,000 live births	295	72.0	48.1	19.0
1–4 years mortality/1,000 alive at that age	69	28.1	18.9	0.84

secondary schools were established, and there was an increase of prosperity in the area. But the continuing high mortality in surrounding areas suggests that Miss Woodland and her team, using simple and well-established methods of child care, played a major part in the reduction in mortality at Imesi.

If perinatal and neonatal care is to be planned on a community basis, special attention must be given to the following:

(1) Maternal health and antenatal paediatrics.
(2) Infection after birth.
(3) Delivery and the environment of the child in the first weeks of his life.
(4) Nutrition in the early months (considered in the chapter on breast-feeding).

MATERNAL HEALTH AND ANTENATAL PAEDIATRICS

Causes of low birth weight in infants

The diet of the mother during pregnancy is vital for her own health and that of her child. However, the idea held in many communities and by many doctors that the size of the infant at birth depends on the amount of food eaten by the mother cannot yet be substantiated. Only in conditions of extreme starvation, when amenorrhoea is common and pregnancy unusual, such as may exist during sieges, does under-nutrition lead to a smaller infant. In general, the size of the infant correlates well with the height and size of the mother, and perhaps most closely with her heart size (118). The size of the mother depends not only on genetic factors, but also on her own diet in infancy and childhood, and also surprisingly on her age, as in malnourished communities growth is not completed until the age of 18 or 19 years and mothers are commonly pregnant at 17 years. This a major reason for the small babies of primiparous mothers, and also for the infrequency of caesarean or instrumental deliveries (11). The size of the infant at birth therefore depends on the early diet of the mother, rather than the diet during pregnancy. The smaller size of babies in less developed countries is due to many factors causing dysmaturity rather than premature birth. It is suggested that up to the age of 32 weeks the Indian foetus is similar in its growth to the American foetus, and only then grows more slowly (93).

Malaria

Malaria is a major cause of low birth weight in Africa, and one of the easiest to prevent. During pregnancy, an alteration in the normal immunological mechanisms of the mother diminishes her previously well-established immunity to malaria. A proportion of mothers develop a heavy infection of the placenta which results in macroscopic changes, the malarial pigment present making it darker in colour. The malarial infection of the placenta is more common in the first and early pregnancies and less frequent in mothers of high parity, presumably due to increased maternal immunity. There is clear evidence that babies born of mothers with infected placentae are lighter in weight than those born of mothers whose placentae are normal. Malarial attacks during pregnancy may also induce abortion and premature delivery.

Falciparum malaria is an established cause of low birth weight in areas where it is endemic, and the giving of monthly or weekly tablets of antimalarials is an important step in antenatal care. In a study involving 400 mothers (185) the weight of babies born to mothers who had had regular monthly doses of pyrimethamine was compared with that of babies whose mothers had not had regular antimalarials, but only chloroquine when they attended with fever. The birth weight of children born to those mothers who received regular pyrimethamine was 157 g (5½ oz) greater than those born to mothers who had not received regular pyrimethamine. This result suggests the need for giving regular antimalarials to all mothers in areas where malaria is still endemic. For economic reasons, if these drugs are to be used widely, monthly administration (50 mg of pyrimethamine) is to be preferred, although as in other fields further cost−benefit studies will be required before a final decision can be made on the merits of weekly over monthly therapy.

Anaemia

Anaemia in pregnancy is common in the tropics and is a frequent cause of premature labour. In holo-endemic areas malaria, together with a secondary folate deficiency, and frequently an iron deficiency, is the likely cause. In non-malarious areas iron deficiency can be the principal cause; this is probably due both to poor iron intake and to hookworm infestation, although the high iron content of many tropical soils and of the foods grown in them suggests that protein–calorie malnutrition may limit iron absorption. Satisfactory programmes to overcome anaemia, both in mothers and in their young children, are hampered by the lack of satisfactory equipment for measuring levels of anaemia. Electric colorimeters currently available have proved unsuitable because of high expense and difficulties in standardization and maintenance. Probably the methods most likely to prove satisfactory at health centres, for use with both mothers and children, are low-cost micro-haematocrit methods which are currently being developed. A standardized treatment is needed for each region. In the individual child the success of this would be checked by the microhaematocrit, and only those who failed to improve would undergo further investigation.

Other causes of low birth weight

The serious effect of smoking during pregnancy in reducing the birth weight is now well established and will increase in importance with urbanization. Other chronic infections, such as urinary infections and parasitic infestations, may also prove to be important. The effects of maternal smoking during pregnancy are still discernible when the child is aged 7 years. He is likely to be 1.3 cm shorter and be 4 months behind in reading (61).

As in other societies, premature delivery, frequently for unexplained reasons, is an important cause of low birth weight also in developing countries.

Co-operation between paediatricians and obstetricians in the antenatal period

One field for co-operation between the paediatrician and the obstetrician is the routine giving of tetanus toxoid to all mothers in areas where neonatal tetanus is common. This is proving to be the most practical method of preventing neonatal tetanus. Three injections are required at monthly intervals; the last must be given at least 5 days before the birth of the child. Only a booster will be required in future pregnancies. Two tetanus toxoid injections will prevent 80 per cent of cases, and complete protection can be expected from three injections (239). At first, to achieve a high level of cover, a campaign may be undertaken, but eventually most of these inoculations should be given as a routine measure in the antenatal service.

The health of the baby in the first few months of life will depend to a large extent on effective co-operation between the obstetrician and the paediatrician. The paediatrician will be concerned that all mothers with chronic diseases, such as, tuberculosis, leprosy and renal disease are identified as early in their pregnancy as possible, so that they may receive treatment and that when the child is born the paediatrician is forewarned of the mother's condition. Where this co-operation exists, the paediatrician will hope that all mothers delivered by midwives and doctors will automatically receive the 'road-to-health' chart with teaching on the importance of this record and how it will last their children through the first 5 years of life. On this any problems that have arisen in pregnancy will be recorded, so that the paediatric services are forewarned. Co-operation will also lead to the mother in rural areas being attended by the same nurse-midwife during her pregnancy and in later years, with the effect of interlinking the health services given to the mother and her child. The paediatrician will be concerned to ensure that when the mother is again pregnant, she brings her previous child to the clinic, so that it receives adequate attention during the dangerous period associated with the birth of a sibling. For this reason, the Under-Fives' Clinic needs to be run in close contact with the antenatal clinic, to enable both the mother and her previous child to receive attention on the same visit, given where possible by the same nurse—midwife. Similarly, both the paediatric and obstetric staff, knowing the common birth interval in the community, will wish to maintain and extend this, and encourage the mother to space her births well. Facilities need to be available for family planning. Details of the way in which the health and weight chart may be used as a record system for family planning are described in Chapter 18.

BIRTH AND THE FIRST DAYS OF LIFE

Paediatrician—obstetrician co-operation

The paediatrician's responsibility during this period will vary. In some areas he will take over entire charge of the newborn, as in Europe and

North America, where the obstetrician desires the paediatrician's assistance from the moment of birth. He will be responsible for resuscitation following a caesarean section or mechanically assisted delivery. Such close involvement in the care of the infant has many advantages in those areas in which the level of staffing is sufficient to make it feasible. However, such involvement of the paediatrician carries one serious disadvantage. The obstetrical officers, during their training, may gain insufficient experience and training from a paediatrician in the care of the newborn, and this should be guarded against in all such units. When they leave the large hospital to staff small hospitals in the country, they are unlikely to have the same close co-operation with the paediatrician as in city hospitals. The need for effective co-operation through a team approach is repeatedly stressed in this book, but this is seldom more important than in the perinatal period. Here the team must include doctors responsible for maternal and child care, medical assistants and particularly their nursing colleagues. Weekly meetings to discuss the perinatal deaths and disorders can be particularly helpful in training and creating understanding within the team.

Measures taken immediately after birth

The staff concerned with the infant immediately after birth will pay particular attention to the following procedures.

Timing of birth

Should resuscitation be necessary, it will be important to know the exact time of birth, so that resuscitation can be undertaken if natural breathing fails to be established. Incidentally, in some Asian communities accurate timing of birth will be a valuable record for horoscopic purposes.

Treatment of eyes

The eyes should be swabbed immediately on birth of the head. In areas where gonococcal ophthalmitis is a problem, 1 per cent silver nitrate drops should be instilled into the eyes (Crede's method). Silver nitrate should be used only if it can be freshly prepared each week and the old material discarded. Unfortunately, these drops may themselves produce a chemical conjunctivitis. Pencillin has also been used, but this is difficult in most smaller hospitals as the penicillin drops must be freshly made up and stored between use in a refrigerator.

Sucking the baby out

For this a soft Nylon* or polystyrene catheter is needed, which may be attached to a glass chamber. An alternative is the use of old pencillin bottles. Soft nylon tubing is introduced after a hole has been drilled with a cork borer.

In most developing countries this apparatus may be made in a local technical school, or in the hospital, and large numbers are necessary, so that they may be used only when sterile. They may be suitably sterilized in a polythene envelope (*Figure 17*). These simple techniques are

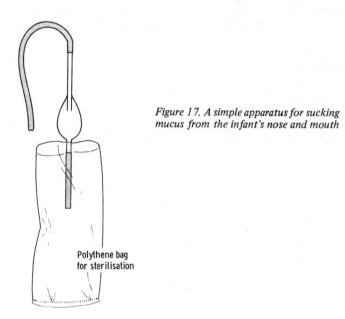

Figure 17. A simple apparatus for sucking mucus from the infant's nose and mouth

Polythene bag
for sterilisation

better than mechanical suction which may be too violent for the tender mucous membrane of the infant's nose and mouth. In addition to sucking out the pharynx, the nostrils must also be cleared, as it is only through the nostrils that the newborn baby can breathe during the first month or so of life.

*Available from Portland Plastics Ltd., Basset House, Hythe, Kent, Great Britain

Delayed clamping of the cord

Immediately after birth the baby may be momentarily suspended upside down to drain liquor from the stomach, but thereafter he should be placed on the same level as the uterus, or slightly below, so that he may receive blood from the placenta. Up to 100 ml of blood can be received by the baby in this way. This is particularly important in countries where anaemia is frequent since the blood is a further source of iron for the infant. It is not enough to wait until pulsation of the cord finishes, as the pulsation of the cord is only an indication of the baby's own heart action, and of blood being pumped from the baby. Clearly drainage from the placenta will last longer than this. If possible, clamping of the cord should be left until the baby has taken several good breaths and until at least 2 minutes after delivery. In many societies, tying of the cord in any way is discouraged until after delivery of the placenta itself and medical workers too need to be patient.

Tying the cord

The traditional methods of tying the cord, using tape or thread, are unsatisfactory in some infants. Either the cord is poorly tied, or because of the contraction of an oedematous cord, serious haemorrhage may result. For this reason, methods have been developed involving the use of either metal or plastic clamps, or some form of rubber band or ring. A low-cost system is shown here in which a small section of rubber transfusion tubing is used. If the right size cannot be obtained, special tubing* can be bought.

The tubing is first slipped on to the clamp *(Figure 18a)*. The clamp is then put on the cord, and the portion of rubber ring is slipped from the clamp on to the cord *(Figure 18b)* and the loop of string cut and removed (*Figure 18c* and *d*). The tubing must be of good quality rubber as if it is perished, it may not be effective. Note that 1½–2 inches of cord should be left free, in case there is any herniation of abdominal contents into the cord (especially important in African children). The tubing will not slip off the cord, and this eliminates the danger of haemorrhage. Bleeding from a young infant is particularly dangerous. One ounce (30 ml) of blood will appear as a stain only a few centimetres across, and although this may represent 10–20 per cent of the child's

*Medication tubing (Amber), 1/8" bore, 1/16" wall, from Al Medicals, 1649 Pershore Road, Birmingham 30. One metre costs 25p, and 200 can be made from one metre

blood, the nurse may well not appreciate the danger of this level of blood loss from an infant.

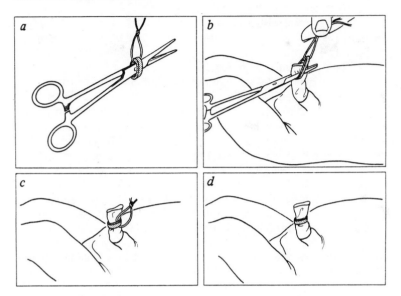

Figure 18. A simple reliable but economic method of 'tying' the umbilical cord

Resuscitation methods

Wherever babies are regularly being delivered, simple apparatus for resuscitation is essential. The need to 'plan ahead' is never more necessary than in preparation for the first few minutes of life. If relatively simple equipment, facilities and skills are available during this dangerous period, mortality can be considerably reduced. All labour wards should be equipped with the following simple apparatus for resuscitation for the newborn (16).

1   Mucous catheter (rubber, open-ended, 15 French gauge – FG)
1   Funnel
1   Nasal catheter (rubber, open-ended, 8 FG)
3   Endotracheal tubes (sterile, disposable, 12 FG)
1   Curved stilette (for stiffening endotracheal tube in difficult intubations)
3   Suction catheters (sterile, disposable, 6 FG)
1   Magill infant's laryngoscope with spare bulb and batteries

Nalorphine, vitamin K or Vandid to be used sublingually when infant is shocked

1   Ventilatory bag (Penlon*)
2   1 ml syringes with needles
Adhesive tape
Scissors
1   Oxygen cylinder with flow meter
1   Water manometer or a simple form of resuscitator with safety valve and rubber bag

It is essential to have somewhere to put the baby, where it can be kept warm, and where the person responsible for resuscitation can be seated. The best place for this is a shelf fixed to the wall, with a cupboard beside it which contains all the essential apparatus, and can be locked. This should be on the operator's right, and the flap of the cupboard should let down to form a table on which the necessary instruments can be placed (*Figure 19*). Above the table, on the wall behind it, there should be simple instructions about the routine of resuscitation. If electricity is available, a movable light, with a 100 watt bulb which will supply both light and warmth, should be placed immediately over the table. Fixed to the wall there should be a simple plastic water manometer (16), through which oxygen can be bubbled. Oxygen is connected by plastic tubing of a suitable bore through a 'T' to the laryngeal tube. From the T-piece a plastic tube descends to a depth of 40 cm in the water manometer *(Figure 20)*. Hence if there is any obstruction to the flow of oxygen down the laryngeal tube, oxygen will then bubble through the water as soon as the pressure in the laryngeal tube rises above 40 cm. A small hole is cut in the side of the plastic tubing just proximal to where it connects to the laryngeal tube. By placing a finger over this hole, the oxygen is connected directly to the laryngeal tube. The finger is placed momentarily over the hole and then released, so that the baby receives intermittent respiration under controlled pressure.

Even the most junior member of the obstetric staff and the midwives should be familiar with the technique of this procedure, and all the apparatus required for it. To make this possible, they should all have ample opportunity for training in the intubation of stillborn infants, so that everyone present at the birth will be capable of intubating and supplying oxygen to a baby with evidence of asphyxia. As well as checking the equipment, the staff should turn on the light, so that the cotton blanket in which the baby will be placed is thoroughly warm.

*Penlon equipment available from Longworth Scientific Instrument Co. Ltd., Abingdon, Berks. The Cardiff Box No. 50312 is a complete box including laryngoscope

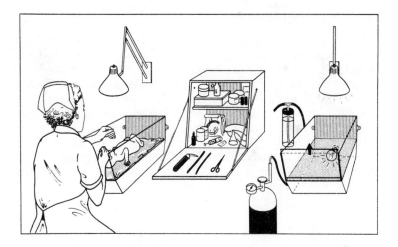

Figure 19. A shelf attached to the wall on which the baby is placed after delivery, this is warmed by an electric bulb underneath or an overhead lamp. The operator sits on a high stool or stands. All the resuscitation apparatus is within easy reach

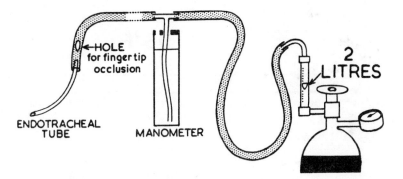

Figure 20. Diagram showing a simple plastic water manometer through which oxygen is bubbled. When the baby is respired with this method, the pressure in the system cannot exceed the depth of the tube in the column of water. For inflation of the unexpanded lung, the tube is pushed to the bottom of the column (40 cm of water pressure). For ventilation of the expanded lung 10 cm of water pressure is used (reproduced from Barrie, 1963, by courtesy of the Editor, Lancet)

All children who are limp or filled with meconium should be laryngo-scoped and sucked out or, if the cords are open and flacid, intubated. Reliance may also be placed on the Apgar score.

Protection against hypothermia

The frequency of hypothermia in tropical areas has only recently been recognized. It occurs not only in the newborn, where it is well recognized in temperate climates, but also in children suffering from malnutrition. The most likely cause is that less care is taken to wrap up small babies at night. Staff and the mothers often do not appreciate that hypothermia is a hazard, even in a tropical environment. Low-reading clinical thermometers* (*Figure 21*) should be available in every maternity unit. Only by using these thermometers will the frequency and importance of this condition be recognized. Unfortunately, they are difficult to obtain in many developing countries, although they should be standard medical equipment.

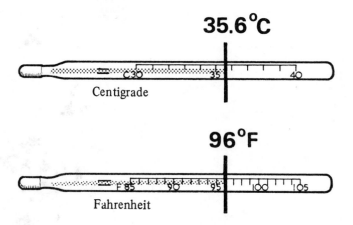

Figure 21. Low-reading clinical thermometers, essential equipment in all tropical hospitals for children

In some regions hyperpyrexia of newborns may arise in very hot weather. A modified 'desert cooler' consisting of an electric fan behind a wet screen may be a simple but satisfactory method of cooling.

The risk of hypothermia will arise in any institution where babies are separated from their mothers, and particularly if there is a drop of temperature at night, or during a cool season, or when bathing in cold

*Available from E.C. Smith & Sons Ltd., 13 Oldfields Road Trading Estate, Sutton, Surrey. All thermometers for rectal use should have a blue tip

water is allowed Infants kept close to their mothers are unlikely to suffer from hypothermia.

If the temperature is taken shortly after birth as a routine, the possibility of imperforate anus will be excluded.

Infection in the newborn

Most infants are born healthy and uninfected in rural areas of developing countries, and yet during the first few months of life they will be in danger of developing a number of infections. Much of the neonatal mortality prior to 1957 in the village of Imesi was due to this (see Table 12). A better understanding of how infection occurs in this age group has made it possible to prevent these infections, particularly those due to the staphylococcus. These methods of preventing infection cost less than those currently in use, many of which can be abandoned.

Prevention of umbilical stump infection

The umbilical stump normally becomes infected with the organisms in the child's environment within hours of birth, and will pick up any virulent staphylococci or *Escherichia coli* that are on the hands of the child's attendants. Among ways by which the umbilicus and the rest of the skin can be colonized, infected dust droplets, droplets from the nose and mouth of the carrier, and direct contamination of the skin are all likely. However, the hands of attendant staff provide the main route of staphylococcal infections from the environment to the infant. Armed with this knowledge, it is possible to set priorities in measures to control infection in the newborn infant.

Agents applied to the stump.—First priority may be on the routine for the umbilical stump. A variety of agents may be used. The most effective are the aerosol sprays, but these are relatively expensive, and may be so efficient that the umbilical cord does not separate quickly. An umbilical cord that remains attached for more than a week will worry mothers in a developing country, making the method unacceptable, because the neonatal service will become unpopular. A cheap but adequate method is the use of 0.33 per cent hexachlorophene* dusting powder on the umbilical stump, particularly if this can be supplied in small individual containers or envelopes separately sterilized so that several infants do not use the powder from the same container. A

*Hexachlorophene, like many other useful substances, is toxic in high concentrations: in a 0.33 per cent powdered use around the umbilical stump it is perfectly safe (323)

further method, which is quite satisfactory, is the use of a 1 per cent aqueous solution of gentian violet to paint the umbilical cord. Alternatively, brilliant green and crystal violet paint (BNF) in 50 per cent alcohol dries more easily. These dyes, however, are likely to stain linen and clothing and everything else. No dressing is needed. Binders are costly, may conceal umbilical sepsis, and if put on soon after birth may inhibit respiration, as the child starts to swallow and air enters the large intestine. Mothers are often fearful to touch the binder put on by a nurse or doctor.

Washing facilities for the attendants. – Since it is the hands of attendants that are responsible for carrying organisms, washing facilities must be widely available – not easy to arrange in countries where a bar of soap is precious and water scarce. Drying the hands also presents problems. A communal towel is a dangerous source of cross infection. Paper towels are expensive, but offcuts from newspaper may be used. An attitude of mind on the part of the staff needs to be developed which ensures that no baby is ever touched without the hands first being washed. Further protection is provided by the use of a suitable antiseptic; the only one that is fully acceptable is hexachlorophene as a 3 per cent solution. There are many reports on the effectiveness of this preparation in cutting down the spread of infection (24). This strength is safe on adult skin, but nothing stronger than 0.33 per cent may be used on infants.

Reduction in the number of staff handling the infant. – As far as possible the number of staff who handle the child should be reduced to a minimum. Newborn infants will soon share the organisms carried by the mother. If they are kept in a nursery, they may be handled during a week by 10–20 staff members who will be handling also many other babies. As mentioned later, the baby should be beside the mother, preferably in bed with her. The mother can do all the necessary feeding and care, and once delivered nurses should rarely handle healthy newborns. Unlike European girls, young mothers in developing countries are experienced with babies. Even when primiparae, they are highly competent in their breast-feeding and general care if only encouraged. Society should be educated to limit the number of relatives who handle small babies, both in hospital and after discharge. Such advice is particularly needed in areas of India where grandmothers believe they gain merit by bathing the infant, and will happily do this twice a day. The old practice of frequent or even daily baths has been shown to be a potent source of infection and is unnecessary. Meconium and blood are removed with sterile wool at birth. The vernix acts as a protection and should if possible be left to be absorbed. If the mother stays in hospital for 4 or 5 days, she should give the baby the first bath under the supervision of the nurse just before they go home.

If these steps are taken, then relaxation of other widely employed anti-infective measures is possible, and expense involved in the use of hexachlorophene can largely be made up by the reduction in expense in these other fields. In particular, the use of caps and masks, hair-nets for nurses, scrubbing brushes for the hands (but still needed for the nails), gowning techniques and exclusion of students and parents from the nursery have all been shown to have no effect on the rate of nasal colonization and infection rates amongst the newborn (24).

The one disadvantage of relying heavily on hexachlorophene in the prevention of infection is that infections with Gram-negative organisms may become more frequent.

The environment of the child

Sudden death has occurred in early infancy from the beginning of time. When it takes place at night, the mother thinks that death was due to her lying on the baby. This explanation was readily accepted in the last century by medical workers, and appeared to be confirmed by the absence of gross post-mortem findings. These deaths were called 'overlaying' and, in an attempt to prevent them, it was commonly taught that children should always be put in separate cots and not allowed to sleep in the same bed as the mother. The separation of mother and child did not, however, prevent these deaths, and during the last 20 years 'cot deaths' have received quite intensive study. Pathological and epidemiological investigations suggest that one common cause is an acute fulminating respiratory infection. Pathologists believe that the proportion due to suffocation by overlaying is less than 5 per cent.

Separating the baby from the mother, moreover has serious disadvantages which probably far outweigh any advantage. There are three major advantages in keeping the infant and his mother together.

Warmth and moisture

Sleeping next to the mother, the baby is kept naturally warm, and it is known that without such warmth babies are in danger of developing hypothermia.

Suckling

The baby who sleeps apart from the mother is less likely to suckle through the night, and because the mother's breasts are not frequently emptied, she is likely to wake up early in the morning with congested and slightly painful breasts. Every time this happens there may be a decline in her output of breast milk. Before long, the supply may be too small for her infant. In most villages in developing countries the infant sleeps with his mother and suckles through the night without waking either. Substantial quantities of breast milk may be obtained while the infant and mother are sleeping. The separation of the baby from the mother may be an important reason for the decline in breast-feeding in the more developed countries, a reason that has received little attention.

Close physical contact with the mother

For many years it has been known that low birth weight babies in later years will do less well in school and have more problems than heavier infants. Until recently, this has been largely blamed on the direct effects of prematurity, but the suggestion is now being made that many of the later difficulties of these babies may arise from the lack of stimulus that the mother received immediately after birth from the close proximity of her baby. Without this stimulus a close and satisfactory mother–child relationship may not develop adequately. This has recently been studied by a number of workers (13), and they make a point of ensuring that even the most premature baby is regularly handled by its mother, even if she must handle it within the incubator. Studies in animals show that the first few hours after birth are crucial and separation in that period may lead to complete rejection or poor maternal care. Studies in mothers suggest that those separated from their babies immediately after birth handle them less well and show less affection. The mother in America, when she is first presented with her newborn infant goes through an unconscious regular pattern of behaviour, in which she touches the baby first with her fingertips and then with the palms of her hands. She wishes to see the baby's eyes open, and to look directly at his eyes (144). Another study (237) illustrates a further possible advantage of close physical contact with the mother. Groups of newborn babies were exposed to a number of sounds — those of recorded heart sounds, a metronome ticking at 60 per minute, and songs. Babies who could hear the recorded heart sounds went to sleep more quickly, and gained weight more satisfactorily, than babies either hearing no sounds or hearing either of the other two — the metronome or songs. If the baby is against the mother's body, he is nearer to the situation in which he was before birth, and is more likely to be contented and satisfied, and perhaps more able to accept the vast increase in stimuli which assails him after birth.

For many people, the need of the infant for the mother in developing countries is only too clear, but the idea of the mother needing the infant is perhaps less obvious. The extreme examples may be cited where in one hospital in Asia and one in North Africa the premature infants were kept separate from the mothers. After 3 or 4 weeks' intensive care, the staff were a little surprised that the mothers were no longer willing to accept their babies and take them home. These mothers had experienced no physical contact with their children, and had hardly seen them during their stay in the special care unit. As a

TABLE 13

Comparison of Survivals by Birth Weight between Birmingham (20)
and Imesi, Nigeria

Birth weight (g)	Stillbirths/1,000 total births		Neonatal deaths/ 1,000 total births		Mortality 1–12 months/ 1,000 total births	
	Birmingham	Imesi	Birmingham	Imesi	Birmingham	Imesi
−1,000	448	429	931	750	118	1,000
1,000−	436	—	612	200	64	444
1,500−	192	95	224	211	37	286
2,000−	87	47	77	49	18	103
2,250−	46	14	36	13.7	19	111
2,500+	10.6	22.9	6.8	15.2	8	38
All weights	22.1	27.2	15.8	24.9	9	54

result, their instincts of love and mother care had not been developed, and even if they had taken their babies home the chances that they would have survived are perhaps remote. Due to the difficulty of follow-up, few attempts have been made in developing countries to discover whether children nursed in 'special care' or 'premature' units have managed to survive. In one institution where such a study was undertaken, where there is an excellent programme for the hospital care of premature infants, with survival rates comparable to those in North America, a follow-up showed that 70 per cent of the infants discharged from the premature nursery were dead within 3 months (298). Miss

Woodland (Table 13) showed how simple sympathetic care in a village mud-block dispensary, from which the mother can maintain close ties with her community, can give excellent chances of survival for low-weight infants. Sophisticated and expensive services can be justified only when many more low birth weight infants survive beyond the first year than were shown in this study.

Table 13 records the survival by weight of children in Imesi. The figures are compared with those published for 91,656 births in Birmingham in 1951-55 (20). The infants in Imesi were mature 'light for dates' which in part explains the lower neonatal mortality rates between 2,000—2,500 g in the neonatal period. Much of the credit for this must go to the team of Nigerian locally trained nurses.

Nursing position of the infant

The position in which the infant is placed is important. If he is nursed in a position with the knees drawn up and the face to one side, preferably on a cellular cotton blanket, he will go to sleep more quickly and cry less. This position is satisfactory for the infant to breathe, safe

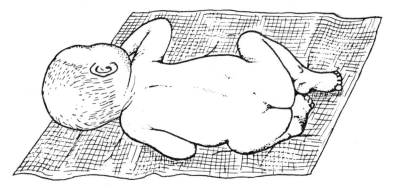

Figure 22. Preferred position for nursing of the newborn, lying on a cellular cotton blanket

from the possibility of inhaling vomit, and approximates more closely to the position *in utero* (*Figure 22*).

Special care units in developing countries

Special care units, or as they were then called, units for premature babies, developed in Europe and North America at a time when the neonatal mortality had already been reduced. By then low birth weight babies had become the largest cause of mortality in this age period. In temperate climates, one of the first needs was to supply these small infants with a warm atmosphere, as the temperature in the homes from which they came was usually low, and cold injury was likely to arise. Earlier generations in Europe had maintained the warmth of the infant by close bodily contact with the mother. This danger of cold injury was particularly great in the badly heated homes of the poor, where the majority of low-weight infants were born. As well as warmth, these infants required extra humidity, since raising the temperature of the room led to a decrease in the moisture content of the air. A minority also require tube-feeding for a period of days or weeks, and for a very few oxygen might be life-saving. In these societies the child who is artificially fed usually fares as well as the one who is breast-fed. Maintaining the mother's breast-milk supply is not essential to the survival of the infant, and the objective of the special care unit in Europe or North America is the production of a healthy, sturdy infant weighing 2–2.5 kg (4½–5½ lb), obtaining milk either from the mother or more usually from a bottle.

A different problem presents in developing countries. Infant mortality is still high, particularly in rural areas. The baby is almost entirely dependent on his mother for everything, and this dependence lasts for well over a year. The likelihood of survival through the first 3 years depends on a close emotional and physical relationship being established between the mother and her child. The visible and most vital part of this relationship is successful breast-feeding. Outside observers may believe that breast-feeding is easily established and maintained, but if the mother is disinterested, as when she has had puerperal depression, this will not happen. Artificial feeding on the other hand is dangerous or impossible in most developing countries, except for the small minority of the population who live in large cities and have all the requirements for artificial feeding described in Chapter 6. In developing countries, to take the child off the mother's breast is equivalent to signing his death sentence. In other words, the low birth weight infant, in common with all infants in developing countries, must be breast-fed if he is to have a chance of survival. Of 20 infants artificially fed in the Punjab, only one was surviving at the age of 2 years. This means that special care units cannot and must not be patterned on those in the Western world where artificial feeding produces no major difficulties. If special care units are to be anything other than show places prolonging the survival time of small infants, then arrangements must be made to breast-feed all the infants they house.

Objectives of special care units

The objectives of special care units for low-weight infants in developing countries may thus be defined as:

(1) establishing close ties between the mother and her infant and achieving complete suckling at the earliest opportunity; and

(2) training the mother in the care of her low-weight baby. In particular she should be taught what steps can be taken to minimize the chances of infection, and what symptoms can be expected should infections arise, so that she may seek help at the earliest opportunity.

The criterion of success in a special care unit in Europe or North America is measured partly by the proportion of babies from differing weight groups who survive their time in hospital. A similar figure in a developing country, as already stated, is meaningless, and a special care unit in these tropical areas must aim at a follow-up for at least 6 months.

'At risk' infants in developing countries

Apart from newborn infants at risk for conditions recognized in Europe and America, some additional hazards should be noted.

Orphans

The orphan with no mother to breast-feed him has little chance of surviving unless there is another woman able and willing to suckle him, or there are nursing and medical staff prepared to teach and supervise the family caring for him, week by week. A full-cream milk powder may be beyond the purchasing power of the family. If no source of an infant milk is available, the orphan can be reared on a skimmed milk (10 volumes), oil (2 volumes) and sugar (1 volume) mixture, as long as a preparation containing vitamins A and D is given. The ingredients are mixed in the 'dry' state without water and can be stored for 2–3 weeks in a tight-fitting container. Some doctors employing this mixture have used up to twice as much of either sucrose or oil to increase the calorie content of the mixture when the child is over 3 months old, depending on the local availability of these ingredients.

Whatever milk is used, feeding should be done with a cup and spoon, or alternatively with a traditional feeding cup in countries such as India, where these exist. Maintaining a feeding bottle in a hygienic condition is not feasible in rural societies or the less prosperous city areas of the developing countries. Due to difficulties in artificial feeding and the deprivation infants may receive from too little handling, orphanages are a low priority. Where possible, a relative should be taught how to care for the child at a nutrition rehabilitation centre, and then carefully supervised by the local Under-Fives' Clinic as she attempts to rear the child on artificial foods.

Visible congenital abnormalities in the child

An infant with any major congenital abnormality, such as a meningomyelocoele, is unlikely to survive, and the mother will not wish it to live. However, mothers may be very anxious about infants born with naevi. Infants born with cosmetically serious skin conditions that could be effectively treated later may not survive because of the attitude of the society towards them. For this reason, surgical treatment needs to be undertaken early whenever feasible.

Mother's illness

As described in Chapter 6, acute (breast abscess, phenumonia, typhoid) or chronic (tuberculosis, leprosy) maternal infections are no bar to successful breast-feeding and are not an indication for taking the infant off the breast. The successful care of infants born to mothers with chronic illness will involve measures to encourage breast-feeding, such as maternal food supplements. The problems of attempting to teach the mother to bottle-feed her infant will almost certainly be greater than the 'drain' on her body of suckling her infant.

Twins

In some areas of the world, twinning may be two to three times as common as in Europe. Among the Yorubas in Nigeria (146), for example, it reaches a level of 10 per cent of pregnancies in mothers over parity 7. Twins, because they start life small and may have to share their mother's breast-milk supply, are at a considerable disadvantage, particularly when they are born to an elderly mother. A careful watch needs to be kept on their weight charts from an early age, so that supplementary foods can be given when necessary. Twins are a source of special beliefs and superstitions. In some areas twins are so feared that they were destroyed even less than 50 years ago. The literature on twins is now extensive, and health workers caring for them need to know the local child-rearing beliefs.

97

Jaundice in the newborn

In tropical countries, too little is known about jaundice in the neo-natal period. Among the reasons for this are early discharge from hospital, the lack of follow-up, and the difficulty of identifying jaundice in a dark-skinned child.

Jaundice in the first 24 hours is particularly significant if Rh or ABO incompatibility is a problem, but where infection or glucose-6-phosphate dehydrogenase (G6PD) deficiency is the main cause, jaundice may be serious when it develops later.

Neonatal infection is the first cause that must be suspected in any ill and jaundiced neonate. Rhesus incompatibility is uncommon in Africa, and is also seldom found amongst American blacks (241). Other factors that may be important include haemoglobinopathies, and particularly deficiency of glucose-6-phosphate dehydrogenase (221).

In rural areas where bilirubin estimations are difficult or impossible, the icterometer* (*Figure 23*) has proved to be useful. It is now used as a check on clinical assessment in Great Britain. Due to pigmentation, this instrument may not be satisfactory on the skin. However, firm pressure on the mucous membrane of the gum will force out the blood. This simple instrument can then be used on this blanched mucous membrane, and serves to identify children whose jaundice is reaching dangerous limits. Once identified, they may then be referred to centres where bilirubin estimations and exchange transfusions are feasible.

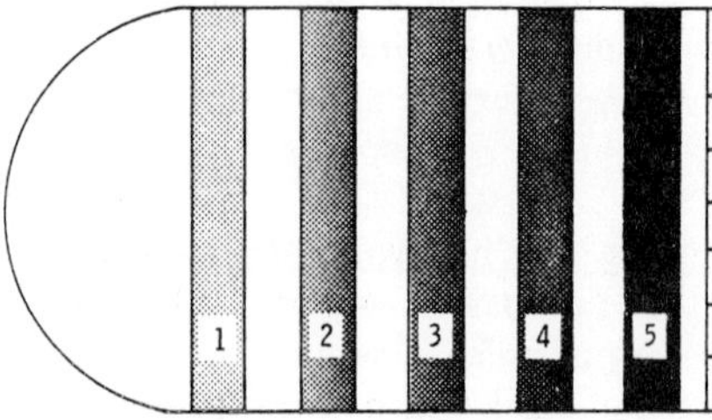

Icterometer Grade	Serum Bilirubin Mean	Mg% Indirect + 2 S.D.
2	5.55	8.7
2½	7.57	12.11
3	10.03	14.58
3½	12.31	17.31
4	15.73	21.8
4½	19.06	26.8

Figure 23. The icterometer

Immunization during the newborn period

Bacillus Calmette-Guerin (BCG) vaccination is essential in the newborn period. In countries where smallpox still exists, this should also be

*Available from Thos. A. Ingram, Santon Works, Prescott Street, Birmingham 18

given in the newborn period, and it is possible that in the future the first dose of triple antigen may also be given in this period. As the newborn period is the first contact that the medical services have with the baby, and sometimes with the mother also, good use of it must be made both in giving immunizations and in teaching the mother and the relatives the need for regular attendance at the Under-Fives' Clinic. The mother will receive the 'road-to-health' card, and health education may well centre round this card.

Unattended births

Births away from all medical facilities will be those most in need of help. In what way the medical services can help these infants and their mothers will depend on the environment and other circumstances. Certainly facilities should be available designed to encourage mothers giving birth at home to bring or send their infants to be seen by a medical worker as soon after birth as possible.

CHAPTER 6

Breast-feeding and the Difficulties of Artificial Feeding

BREAST-FEEDING

Breast-feeding has great emotional associations. This may be the reason that in spite of its enormous importance in infant nutrition, it has been the subject of so little scientific research and observation. In 10 years the *Journal of Tropical Pediatrics* published 303 articles: among these 69 were on the subject of nutrition, but in only 13 did the title suggest that the content of the article in any way referred to breast-feeding. Hitherto, most medical writing has been undertaken by men. As more articles are written by women, perhaps this subject will receive increased attention as in one excellent review of the subject (108). Breast-feeding has some marginal advantages in an affluent and educated home. One is the slightly lower incidence of infective disease. A possible more important long-term advantage is the prevention of arterosclerotic disease later in life which may be influenced by the early ingestion of cow's milk protein (62). Breast-feeding is essential in the rural homes of developing countries. In the past in the UK and now in Asia and Africa doctors appreciate that if a child is not breast-fed, it will die.

Breast-feeding and the national economy

The need for a new approach to halt the decline in breast-feeding has renewed emphasis (128). Three main reasons are stressed.

(1) The developing countries in which breast-feeding is on the decline see a change in the type of malnutrition towards the 'marasmic-diarrhoea' syndrome. This occurs in the first 18 months of life, at a time when the brain is actively growing, and carries with it the inherent dangers to the intellectual development of the individual.

(2)   On a national scale, nutrition planners now question the wisdom of politicians permitting the entry of salesmen of imported infant foods. Even when these foods can be produced within the country, their economic priority may be low. In most developing countries there is a protein 'gap'. Artificial feeding will widen this gap even more, and encouraging breast-feeding needs to be a priority for the economist as much as for the nutritionist in their efforts to close this gap. Developing a milk industry should not be placed high in a nation's list of priorities. It will do little to close the protein gap as cow's milk is displacing human milk. In some countries, excessive bottle-feeding is leading to future obesity, while in others there may be an insidious malnutrition of the child which is being bottle-fed. Among the poor too much of the already stretched family food budget may be spent on the purchase of an expensive artificial milk. All artificial milks are similar in their suitability for infant feeding; however, the most expensive milk frequently outsells the others, the producers spending more on subtle advertising.

(3)   As described later in this chapter, and in Chapter 19, a reduction in the period of breast-feeding is associated with a shorter birth interval. Those countries in the developing world in which breast-feeding is fully maintained have a lower rate of population growth than those in which artificial feeding has become the rule.

Duration of breast-feeding

This chapter will deal with those aspects of breast-feeding which are of particular concern to a doctor working in a rural society in the tropics. As most doctors come from families and cultures where breast-feeding is maintained for no more than 6, or at most 9, months, the word 'prolonged' has crept in to describe the 2 years of breast-feeding which is probably the 'normal' period for *Homo sapiens* as a mammal. A distribution curve for the duration of breast-feeding in a rural society (163) is given in *Figure 24*. The duration of breast-feeding in this group of village women is representative of societies in which cow's milk plays a limited part in infant feeding. Among the 291 mothers, the mean period of breast-feeding was just under 24 months, and the majority discontinued breast-feeding when their infants were between the ages of 21 and 27 months. Only a few stopped before the infant had reached 15 months, while a further few continued almost to the child's third birthday. In this society, no domestic animal suitable for milking can be kept, partly because of trypanosomiasis and also because of the lack of suitable animal foodstuffs.

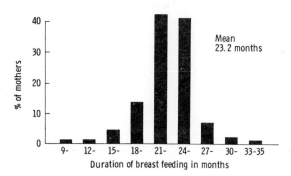

Figure 24. Study on duration of breast feeding in 291 mothers in a West African village

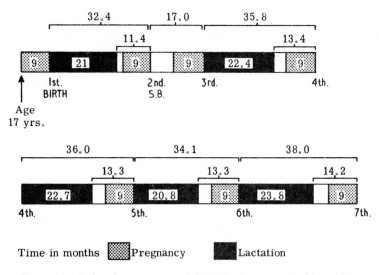

Figure 25. Cycle of pregnancy and lactation in women in West Africa

A more detailed study of the records of these mothers, their pregnancy and subsequent breast-feeding was made, and from this a profile of breast-feeding in this community (192) was constructed by taking the average for the various periods *(Figure 25)*.

Figure 25 shows how pregnancy follows on lactation with an interval of at first 2½ months and with later pregnancies 5 months. Mothers breast-feed if they have successive pregnancies for approximately two-thirds of their fertile period, that is, they are breast-feeding for perhaps 14 years compared with a total of 1–2 years in the few European mothers who breast-feed their babies.

Breast-feeding and birth interval

Among the studied group, the median interval between births was 34 months. This is reduced to approximately 17 months if the baby is stillborn, or dies soon after birth. In the diagram there are gaps representing periods between the end of breast-feeding and the time when the mother became pregnant again. This finding was a surprise to those involved in the study, as the majority of mothers when they finished suckling stated that this was because of their pregnancy. Yet the next baby was not born until more than 9 months after that date. Clearly these mothers who menstruated irregularly, and frequently had prolonged amenorrhoea, would not know they were pregnant until the third or fourth month after conception; when they said they were pregnant they meant that they had finished breast-feeding, were again cohabiting with their husbands, and hoped they were pregnant. In this and some other traditional societies there is a taboo that inhibits coitus during breast-feeding. As a result these societies achieve a satisfactory birth interval of 3 years, producing moderate-sized and well-spaced families (317).

Milk production

The mother's reflexes

In the mother, two reflexes are responsible for successful lactation.

Prolactin reflex. – The prolactin reflex is the main hormonal influence in milk production. In this, sucking by the newborn leads to impulses passing from the nipple areola up to the vagus nerve to the anterior pituitary, which leads to secretion into the circulation of prolactin, responsible for the secretion of milk (130) *(Figure 26a)*.

Let-down reflex. – The second reflex is known variously as the let-down reflex, the draft reflex, or the milk-ejection reflex *(Figure 26b)*. For all those concerned with mothers in the early stages of establishing lactation, it is essential to appreciate that this reflex is psychosomatic, with a physical component which can be powerfully influenced by the mother's emotions. The physical component of the let-down reflex is again through the infant sucking the areola. The impulse passes up the vagus nerve, but on this occasion it is passed to the posterior pituitary which releases oxytocin into the blood stream. The action of the oxytocin is on the muscle cells or myo-epithelial cells of the alveola, squeezing milk out of them and propelling it down to the terminal lacteals where it is easily accessible to the infant. It is this reflex that can be so easily disturbed in the farm yard by a 'strange' milker, or in the mother by a sudden emotional shock, which has been well known to dry up a woman's milk. Conversely, a girl who has grown up amongst women satisfactorily suckling their infants, will have the

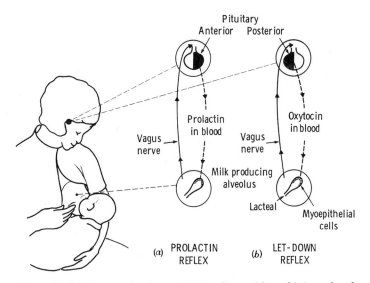

Figure 26. (a) Diagram showing prolactin reflex and how this is produced; (b) the let-down reflex, highly sensitive to the mother's emotions (reproduced from Jelliffe, 1967, by courtesy of the Editor, Journal of Tropical Pediatrics)

confidence that leads to an unimpaired or even an enhanced let-down reflex. The mother feels this draft or let-down reflex as a prickly sensation in the breast and its presence is a reassurance to her of the success of breast-feeding. She will notice that when she is about to breast-feed the baby, the milk may start to drip from her breasts, and soon after she has started breast-feeding from one breast, milk may be discharged quite powerfully from the other breast. Soon after delivery, she may also experience uterine cramps at the time of breast-feeding, because the oxytocin which has stimulated lactation also acts on the smooth muscle of the uterus.

Suckling: the infant's reflexes

The sucking of the infant is only a small part of the total suckling process which includes the following stages. The mother's breast on the infant's cheek is a stimulus that leads to the 'rooting reflex' by which the infant's head turns to the side on which the nipple is felt, the mouth opens and the nipple is drawn into it. The process is illustrated (200) in *Figure 27*. In *Figure 27a* it will be seen that the nipple is being sucked into the mouth. The sucking is assisted by the tongue *(b)*, which draws the nipple deep into the oropharynx. Once the nipple is deep in the oropharynx *(c)* the infant starts a rhythmic movement of the mandible *(d)* which applies pressure to the lacteal sinuses under the areola. This leads to the expression of the milk. Similarly, when a cow is milked by hand *(Figure 28)*, the milker's thumb presses on the lacteal sinuses.

The process of suckling needs to be understood if medical workers are to help the mother prevent cracked nipples and a breast abscess. In a mother whose nipple does not protract well, there is a likelihood that the baby may press with his gums not on the lacteal sinuses behind the nipple, but on the nipple itself; this is particularly common in a primiparous mother. The resulting trauma to the delicate nipple may result in a painful crack frequently only visible with a magnifying glass. This crack is liable to infection which may spread back into the breast. As a result of the failure of suckling, the breast is already partly congested, and the distended ducts are an ideal site for the multiplication of bacteria, leading to an inflamed and tender breast, and the first stages towards a breast abscess. Fortunately, if well managed at this stage with antibiotics and stilboestrol (5 mg once only by mouth, or for short but speedy action by intramuscular injection) to relieve congestion, breast-feeding may be successfully re-established.

The ability of the average baby to suckle is high immediately after birth, and then wanes for a period of hours. The baby should therefore be put to the breast as soon after birth as possible, both for the reassurance of the mother and because the act of suckling promotes the resolution of the uterus. The mother needs to be taught that as her baby sucks, she is likely to experience some abdominal pain due to contraction of the uterus. The suckling of both breasts early in the puerperium is critical in establishing successful breast-feeding. African mothers have a natural ease and ability to express milk directly into the mouths of infants initially too weak to suck. Sucking stimulation, however, has been shown to be the best galactagogue, and the only effective method of increasing the milk supply. Artificial sucking stimulation either by manual emptying of the breast or with the use of a machine, has been

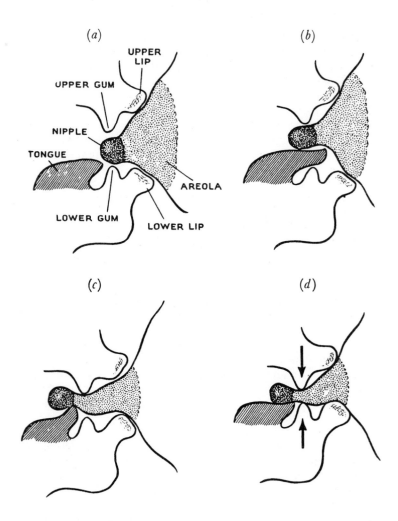

Figure 27. Infant's milking action, wrongly called 'sucking'. (A) The nipple is drawn into the mouth by the buccinators and the sealing action of the lips. (b) The tongue thrusts forward over the lower gum. (c) The tongue is rapidly drawn inwards, bringing the nipple behind the gum edges. (d) The jaws bite and cause the gums to nip the breast on the areola, behind the nipple, and over the collecting sinuses (reproduced from Naish, 1956, by courtesy of Lloyd-Luke Ltd)

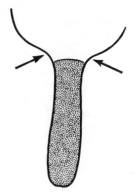

Figure 28. The arrows indicate the point at which farmer's first finger and thumb apply the first pressure in milking (reproduced from Naish, 1956, by courtesy of Lloyd-Luke Ltd)

recommended as a method of increasing milk yield where the infant cannot suck. In a study of over a thousand neonates (236), the observation was made that infants on true self-demand feeding showed the most rapid weight gain and were nearest their birth weight at one week. In the African baby who is allowed unlimited suckling, little or no weight is lost (268). Unlike infants in Aberdeen, and elsewhere in Europe and North America, African infants show a steady gain of weight from the first day *(Figure 29)*. The same was seen in the majority of infants in the village of Imesi, and frequent feeds from as soon after birth and for as long as the baby wishes is physiologically sound advice. Initial suckling usually occurs more easily if the suckling reflex has not been inhibited by medication given to the mother in labour. Those infants permitted to suckle soon after birth took significantly less time to establish feeding, and lost significantly less weight than those who did not suckle for the first 24 hours (74).

Suckling has been shown to be the most effective method of decreasing the amount of soreness felt by mothers feeding their infants. The almost unlimited suckling allowed to the baby in rural societies of most developing countries is beneficial both for the mother and her infant. Except in extremely hot climatic conditions, unrestricted breast-feeding is an adequate source of fluid, and sweetened water from a bottle is a real deterrent to successful breast-feeding. The absence of the need for thumb-sucking is another of the benefits for the infant. The method of frequent suckling and the upright position of the baby when carried probably explain the great infrequency of any regurgitation by these infants.

Thumb-sucking which is common amongst European children is rarely seen in the African village, except in orphaned children. No doubt the uninhibited suckling available to most African children over

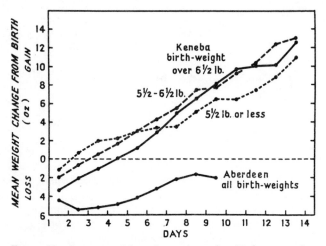

Figure 29. Average weight gain or loss after birth, comparison between Gambian and Scottish babies (reproduced from Thompson, 1966, by courtesy of the Editor, Lancet)

the age of 2 years provides adequate oral satisfaction. One study (145) of adult smokers found that those who could successfully give up smoking were weaned later than those who were unable to give it up, suggesting that the experience of longer periods of suckling may have advantages to the adult.

Composition of human milk

There is variation in the composition of milk from species to species, from mother to mother in the same species, between one part of the day and another, and early or late in a period of suckling. Among nursing mothers, the largest variation occurs in the fat and calcium content. Other nutrients show much less variation, unless the mother is on a deficient diet. A study of the milk of mothers of different ages at the seventh day (11) showed *(Figure 30)* that milk from many older mothers was less in volume and contained rather less fat than milk from younger mothers.

Figure 30a shows that the majority of mothers aged 15–19 years were secreting more than 400 ml of milk by the seventh day of lactation, while among mothers over the age of 30 years relatively few could produce this amount.

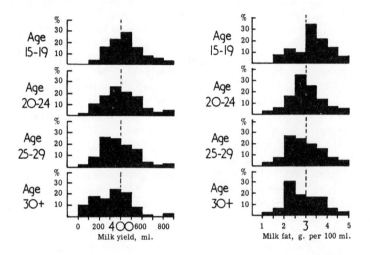

Figure 30. (a) Effect of maternal age on the volume of milk produced on the seventh day after delivery in 509 Aberdeen primiparae. (b) Effect of maternal age on the fat content of milk produced on the seventh day after delivery in 509 Aberdeen primiparae (reproduced from Hytten and Leitch, 1963, by courtesy of Blackwell Scientific Publications, Ltd)

Figure 30b shows that a higher proportion of the older mothers secreted milk with less than 4 per cent of fat, and the total secretion was less than 300 ml. The infant born to the mother aged over 30 years is likely to receive too little milk of low fat content, and therefore obtain too few calories and later develop marasmus. These studies were confined to primiparous mothers, and it is likely that the multiparous mother may perform better when she reaches the age of 30 years, although from the author's experience the old mother of high parity is not so effective at breast-feeding as her younger sister, and the infant of the older mother who has had 7 pregnancies is more likely to show an unsatisfactory weight gain (192). One study showed a high proportion of marasmus in infants born of elderly high-parity mothers (79).

109

Colostrum and transitional milk

In the first 3–6 days the milk secreted by the breast consists of colostrum. It is yellowish in colour, transparent and contains more protein but less sugar and fat than milk. The globulin content is high, and in some species of animals, such as the cow, much of the protective antibodies is passed in the colostrum to the young at this stage. This is not so in human species. The infant is itself born with a high store of protective immunoglobulins received through the placenta and smaller amounts of antibodies are absorbed from either the colostrum or milk.

Although immunoglobulins are poorly absorbed by the human infant, they still have an important local protective function and may be recovered from the faeces. For example, antiviral antibodies may inhibit the effectiveness of poliomyelitis vaccine, and therefore presumably polio virus, by preventing the virus from multiplying. There is evidence (124) that it is the poliomyelitis-neutralizing antibody in human milk that is responsible for the low (40 per cent) success in immunizing with oral poliomyelitis vaccine in tropical areas. Antibodies to *E. coli* traverse the infant's intestinal tract without appreciable change, affording probably some protection against coliform infections to breast-fed infants (137).

Mature milk

The speed at which the young animal grows is reflected in the type of milk that is produced. Mouse milk is high in protein and minerals, and the suckling mouse doubles its birth weight within a matter of days. Cow's milk contains more protein and ash than human milk and the calf grows more quickly than the human baby. There is also some difference in the type of protein present in human milk; the casein content is only a sixth of that of cow's milk, but the whey-protein content is higher. The amino acid contents of the two milks are similar. However, breast-fed babies 112 days old have a mean serum concentration of albumen significantly higher than that of infants fed on evaporated milk (82). As already mentioned, the fat or lipid content of breast-milk varies from individual to individual, and also in accordance with the time when the milk is taken off. The first milk secreted by the breast is low in fat and for this reason appears rather watery. Unfortunately, in many cultures this suggests to the mother that the milk is watery and therefore unsatisfactory for her baby, and she may not feed it to him. In some areas of South America, this observation of watery milk has led to the belief that cow's milk is stronger and better than human milk. The composition of lipids depends on the diet of the mother, and the fatty acid pattern of human milk resembles that of the maternal diet eaten during the previous few days. The bulk of the lipids is formed by triglycerides. Linoleic acid, the only fatty acid known to be essential for the infant, is considerably higher in human than in cow's milk.

Carbohydrates. – Lactose is the principal carbohydrate in milk. Compared with other disaccharides, it is relatively insoluble, and slowly digested and absorbed from the intestines. Its presence in the intestine stimulates the growth of micro-organisms that produce organic acids and synthesize many of the B-vitamins. Human milk contains 1½ times as much lactose as cow's milk, and also a small amount of nitrogen-containing oligosaccharide. This type of sugar is important, as it stimulates the growth of *Lactobacillus bifidus,* an organism which breaks down lactose into lactic and acetic acids, and produces the acid reaction of the intestinal contents of breast-fed infants. This acidity is believed to interfere with the growth of many pathogenic organisms. Recent studies (34) suggest that the large quantities of iron-binding protein, particularly lactoferrin, have important bacteriostatic functions which may be neutralized by the medicinal use of iron salts.

Mineral contents. – The major mineral contents of human milk are potassium, calcium, phosphorus, chlorine and sodium. The iron and copper required in blood formation are present only in traces, and anaemia is well recognized as a result of children subsisting on a diet of milk for too long. One of the striking differences between human and cow's milk lies in the mineral composition of the two milks. As with protein, this can be linked to the more rapid growth of the calf. The additional nitrogen and mineral in excess of requirements lead to a high load of solutes that have to be disposed of through the infant's kidneys, a serious disadvantage in tropical countries where urinary output may be diminished due to loss by other routes.

Vitamins. – Milk is an important source of vitamins, all of which are present in the milk of a mother consuming a satisfactory diet. The vitamin A level in breast milk is affected by the quality and quantity of the diet, and is generally much lower in tropical than in temperate countries. When the level is unusually low, xerophthalmia can develop in the breast-fed baby, but this is uncommon. Of the other fat-soluble vitamins, vitamin D is present in small amounts, and unless the infant is exposed regularly to sunlight some supplementation with vitamin D is necessary for breast-fed babies if radiological rickets is to be prevented. A poor intake of the water-soluble vitamins in the maternal diet is quickly reflected in the breast milk, and the addition of ascorbic acid, riboflavine and thiamine to the diet results in an increased level of these substances in the milk. Ascorbic acid may be low in breast milk in certain seasons when little fresh vegetable foods are available. This is important, because a severe shortage may lead to scurvy and also increase the liability of a megaloblastic anaemia arising from a deficiency of folic acid. The thiamine content of breast milk in areas with a high incidence of infantile beri-beri has been found to be low, due to insufficient maternal intake. In areas where milled rice, unfortified with thiamine, is the major staple, infantile beri-beri is still not uncommon and unfortunately may go unrecognized.

Volume of breast milk produced

Little information on the volume of milk secreted in tropical countries at different stages of lactation is available. Table 14, taken from work in the Pacific (212) suggests, however, that the volume of

TABLE 14

Volume of Milk in ml Expressed from Papuan Mothers after no Suckling for 10–12 Hours

Area	Age of infants (months)			
	6–11	12–17	18–23	24–35
Waropen	170	140	85	–
Ajamaroe	195	150	130	125
Chimbu	–	–	–	80
Total number of mothers	37	51	44	37

(High individual values were recorded: 400 ml at 12 months, 250 ml at 20 months, 380 ml at 30 months, 105 ml at 51 months)

milk secreted continues higher than was at one time believed, and that towards the end of the second year the child may be getting half as much milk as at the age of 6 months, when it may have been his only source of food. The amounts of milk shown in this table are low for a period of 12 hours but the amount manually expressed is unlikely to reach the quantity that the baby actually can suckle in this period.

The WHO Expert Committee on nutrition in pregnancy and lactation (289) suggested an average yield of 850 ml per day to be adequate, and the adequate suckling could be best judged by satisfactory growth of the infant during the period when he was exclusively breast-fed. This growth can be assessed only by measurement, the only practical method being weighing and plotting the weight on individual weight charts (Chapter 7). A gain of 800 g (± 20 per cent) per month during the first 6 months of life, or a doubling of the birth weight by the end of the fourth month of life, can be regarded as satisfactory, but is a high standard which many infants cannot achieve. A more practical criterion is that babies who gained less than 500 g in any 4-week period in the first 3 months of life, or 250 g in any 4-week period in the second trimester, are likely to be malnourished later (192). Maternal undernutrition does not greatly affect the protein and lactose concentration in the milk, but the fat and other constituents may be considerably lowered and the total volume decreased.

Successful lactation

There is a distinct psychological difference between the unrestricted almost unconscious suckling as practised in traditional cultures in which feeding is freely allowed and encouraged to continue for 1½–3 years, and the 'token' breast-feeding, with usually restricted periods of suckling over a few months, as practised in most countries in Europe and North America. There is ample evidence that the early experience of suckling, particularly in the animal world, will affect later behaviour in a long-term way. How this can be interpreted for man, and its significance, is uncertain.

To understand why breast-feeding is relatively successful in developing countries as compared with the industrialized countries, the attitudes and child-rearing beliefs commonly found in the latter must be considered. Just as strength is considered as a basic attribute of manliness, so fertility linked with an ability to breast-feed successfully are considered basic attributes of the woman. The earliest memory of a girl in a developing country may well include suckling from her mother, and during all her childhood she has been surrounded by relatives and others breast-feeding their infants. These early experiences are likely to be important; they are very different from those of a girl in an industrialized society who will not remember being breast-fed and may well grow up without ever seeing an infant at the breast. When the girl in the developing country has her first baby, she will be surrounded by relatives and friends who have successfully breast-fed their babies, and she herself expects to do the same.

Maternity wards – help or hindrance?

Does the maternity ward, usually situated in an urban hospital, have a major influence against breast-feeding (128)? No one will argue against the need for a greater proportion of births in developing countries being undertaken in hospital. However, there is a real need to study the effect of such deliveries on the attitudes and success of mothers in breast-feeding. In such investigations, assistance from sociologists is required. While the objective of the maternity department is chiefly in the safe delivery of the mother of a healthy child, and little emphasis is put on promoting breast-feeding, these wards may play not a small part in producing marasmus later, due to the mother having difficulties in establishing successful lactation. It may be impossible to overcome the adverse emotions in the mother, produced by the strange environment of a ward compared with her own home. However, these need to be examined, and measures undertaken which will enhance her confidence in her own ability to suckle her infant successfully. Unfortunately, the newborn infant falls between the two specilities of obstetrics and paediatrics, and so often the responsibility for the care of the breast and the instruction of the mother in successful methods of breast-feeding are not clearly defined between the obstetrician and the paediatrician. The crowded, regimented, unprivate atmosphere of the usual maternity ward means that the mother has limited time to receive individual advice and guidance, even if anyone really knows what to advise. Still in many countries her baby is separated from her and put in a nursery – an extraordinary and inhuman travesty of obvious physio-logical and psychological needs. Perhaps it is not surprising that the mother is anxious, apprehensive and uncertain. The difficulties that arise have been summarized in *Figure 31* (128). It will be seen that due to the mother's anxiety, the let-down reflex may be inhibited, and the child responds to his hunger by crying, and in this way further increases his mother's apprehension. Too often the result will be that the over-worked nurse or midwife makes the immediate diagnosis of 'not enough milk' or 'milk does not suit the baby', and either the baby is removed, or at best a temporary bottle-feed is given. The effect of this bottle is to further diminish the mother's confidence and to encourage the baby to accept more easily the milk which is so often over-sweetened.

Breast-feeding at night

In tropical countries, there are almost 12 hours of darkness, and for most rural societies no means of artificial lighting cheap enough to be in general use are available. During most of the hours of darkness, the mother and child are sleeping together, or she may be sitting in front of the embers of a fire with her child. This is a time when she will be resting or sleeping and the baby will have an opportunity to suckle as much as he desires. Her breasts will be frequently emptied and will have

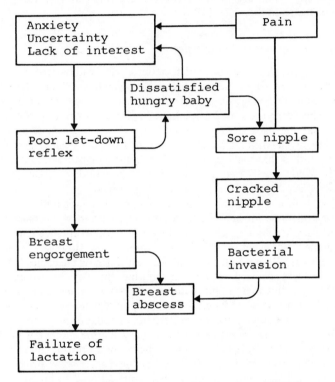

Figure 31. The effect of anxiety on lactation (reproduced from Jelliffe, 1967, by courtesy of the Editor, Journal of Tropical Pediatrics)

ample stimulation from suckling. Even if, as in the Indian village, the child is placed in a hammock, there will still be demand-feeding. In the Western societies, artificial lighting has given the family control of their hours of darkness. The baby will be left in a cot by himself for many hours in the evening, and even during the night is unlikely to sleep close to the mother, who frequently wakes up with distended breasts in the morning. Such distended and perhaps slightly painful breasts will, without the stimulus of suckling through the night, leads to a decline in the amount of milk that she can produce.

In the village of Imesi, analysis of the records showed that mothers who complained that their babies were crying at night were nearly always supplying insufficient breast milk, as indicated by the weight gain of the child thereafter (192).

Breast-feeding during the daytime

During the day in most rural societies a baby will be carried around by the mother, either on her back or her side, and will have abundant opportunities for breast-feeding. The African mother can feed the infant even when carrying a load of perhaps 20–30 kg on her head. When she feels that the baby desires to suckle she swings him round from her back to suckle without removing the load from her head. The mother wears clothes that make access for her infant to her breasts easy at all times. When she is sitting in the home, or working perhaps in the market place, she will be regularly suckling him.

The author attempted to study how much breast milk the baby received in these irregular feeds. A group of mothers was persuaded to spend a day in a primary school building, and arrangements were made to weigh the children before and after each breast-feed. However, the study was a dismal failure, and the difficulty of test-weighing the babies in these societies was realized. Repeatedly during the day he would find mothers suckling their infants without previous weighing, although they had all been instructed carefully on this point. When he remonstrated with them, he soon came to understand that the decision to put the baby to the breast is made subconsciously by the mother while her attention is involved elsewhere. In another study of test-weighing babies before and after feeds in West Africa, the babies were placed in a separate locked room, and the mothers were allowed to breast-feed at regular 3-hourly intervals (245). This 'feeding by the clock' so upset the relationship between mother and baby that the milk supply to the group of babies was clearly inadequate on the first day, but increased on the second, and was still increasing by the seventh day. This experience suggests that the traditional methods of test-feeding of babies are unsatisfactory and misleading in areas where demand-feeding is practised, and reliance has to be placed on a satisfactory weight gain as the best indication of adequate suckling.

The decision to discontinue suckling

Both here and elsewhere, the ambiguous word 'weaning' will be avoided, as the following two meanings are possible.

(1) For some, this word is equivalent to the French *sevrage,* that is cessation of breast-feeding.

(2) Others insist that the word means the time or period in which solid foods, or foods other than milk, are introduced.

Not long ago in the Western society these points in time were close to each other. The child came off the breast and went on to solid food within a matter of a few weeks, and in some societies, such as those in parts of India, this still happens. In these circumstances the difference in meaning is not so important. In rural Africa and many other parts of the world, solid food should be introduced at the age of 4 months, and breast-feeding should continue to around the age of 2 years. The time of offering the first solid food and the time when suckling stops, both described by some as 'weaning', may be separated by 18 months.

However, this confusion is less likely to arise if the term 'weanling period' is used. This has been defined as the period commencing when solids are introduced and continued until 3 months after suckling has been discontinued (242).

In most rural societies, the mother, if asked why she stopped nursing her infant, will say that she stopped because she was pregnant, and in some, as in South America, this seems to be true. The mothers in Imesi, West Africa, said the same, but here, as was shown in *Figure 25,* breast-feeding stopped before conception. Further enquiry elicited that the decision was taken, not by the mother or father, but by some older woman in the household. This decision is made not according to the age of the child, but according to its size and general nutritional state; the less well nourished baby was fed for a longer period (192). Mothers do not stop suckling after so many months but when the child appears healthy and strong. Because mothers whose children are not doing well continue to breast-feed for a long time, some doctors have incorrectly blamed the undernourished state of the child on the long period of breast-feeding.

Medical reasons

The medical reasons for discontinuing breast-feeding are few, if any. With modern therapy, the traditional reasons for discontinuing breast-feeding if the mother has leprosy or tuberculosis are no longer valid. The worry of trying to find the wherewithal to feed a small baby artificially is likely to have a much more serious effect on the mother's health than the possible adverse effects of continued breast-feeding. The danger of infection to the baby can be overcome by the use of chemotherapy. In these countries breast milk remains the best high-quality protein supplement in the nutritionally dangerous second year.

Breast abscess. – The presence of a breast abscess is not a reason for discontinuing breast-feeding. The baby is more efficient at emptying the breast than any other means, so breast-feeding or expression of the milk direct into the baby's mouth is encouraged if the mother can tolerate the pain. Even if some pus is discharged into the lacteal sinuses, it is unlikely that this will harm the baby; he is likely to carry the offending organism in his nose and his digestive tract will not be upset by it.

Puerperal depression. – Puerperal depression may have a harmful effect on breast-feeding, as the mother will lose all interest in suckling her infant, and as a result rapidly lose her breast milk. In several years of caring for many infants in West Africa, the only occasion on which it was necessary to remove the baby from the breast was a baby over 1½ years old whose mother was suffering from severe protein-calorie deficiency, oedema and other signs of kwashiorkor. Clearly, she was unlikely to recover from this condition while she continued to lose protein by breast-feeding. One other reason for discontinuing breast-feeding would be carcinoma of the breast. In a study of breast-feeding in the Gambia total lactation failure occurred only once and that in a mother with severe and widespread tuberculosis from which she did not recover (268).

The law and breast-feeding

The labour laws of a country can do much to facilitate suckling by providing for creches close to where the mother is working, and insisting on the mother having time to feed her infant. Unfortunately, such legislation is frequently not enforced in developing countries, and if stringently enforced, may reduce the number of married women employed. Visiting a cheroot factory in Burma, a mother was seen rolling cheroots with a baby hanging in a shawl at her elbow.

ARTIFICIAL FEEDING

In many countries, artificial feeding has come to stay, not only in the large cities amongst the wealthier members of the population, but also in rural areas. This is largely due to a belief in the 'prestige' of artificial milk developed by the manufacturers of artificial foods determined to sell their particular brand. These beliefs receive support from the 'elite' of the community. To them breast-feeding is time-consuming, tiring and 'messy', while bottle-feeding allows them to return to those interests and occupations for which their education and training have prepared them.

Although the actions of these baby food companies jeopardize the health of many children, few governments have considered it their duty to restrict or in any way influence their activities. Just as the cigarette packet in the UK has to carry a warning on the possible harmful effects of smoking, so also tins of milk sold in developing countries may in the future have to carry a warning on the dangers (far greater than those of cigarette smoking) of artificial feeding by mothers with limited means. One national company in Africa was persuaded to put the following on the label of the food tin:

Breast-feed your child

The best food for your child is the mother's milk. It is better than this or any other kind of artificial food.

Don't feed your child artificially unless you are sure that you have the money to buy enough milk. By the time that your child is four months old, he will want five pounds of milk powder each month. Are you sure that you have enough money to buy this?

Feed your child with a cup and a spoon and not with a feeding bottle.

Ask in the shop where you bought this tin for a paper telling you how to feed your child.

In a country in Asia, the government refuses to import teats for bottles, and these are only available at a high price on the black market. This is a measure that makes bottle-feeding more difficult and encourages the use of cup and spoon, which are probably safer.

Requirements for artificial feeding

In any country, the following are essential for satisfactory artificial feeding.

(1)   A good understanding of the method of making up the milk.

(2)   A method of rapid boiling for sterilizing with adequate fuel.

(3)   A good source of water, not only for preparing the feed but also for cooling it (a feed may take an hour to cool in the tropics).

(4)   Adequate washing facilities for the bottle and hands.

(5)   Sufficient money to buy milk, whether condensed or powder and a reliable supply in the local shops or market.

(6)   Time in the home to prepare feeds.

None of these, not even the last, is available to the mother in developing countries, and this may explain the slim chance an artificially fed child has of surviving. In 1763 in England, of 275 infants accepted into a parish orphanage, 256, or 93 per cent, were dead by the end of one year. In the rural Punjab, an area where cow's or buffalo's milk is available, only one of 21 babies not breast-fed survived beyond his second birthday (242).

Advice when artificial (formula) feeding is essential

With 2–3 per cent of children, the mother may have died or for some other reason, such as insanity, the child cannot be fed by its mother and some form of artificial feeding will be necessary. In the past, many maternal infections, including tuberculosis, leprosy and breast abscesses were considered a reason for the mother to discontinue breast-feeding. The great risks to the infant, and the difficulties and expense for the mother have encouraged most doctors to insist that breast-feeding should now be continued in spite of these or other maternal illnesses. Where the mother has open tuberculosis, the baby can have prophylactic isoniazid (INH). Where this is available, the infant may be given INH-resistant BCG vaccine. In leprosy, sufficient dapsone is secreted in the breast milk to safeguard the infant in the early months. Where the mother has a breast abscess, there is a great need to keep the breast empty of milk, and the infant is better at doing this than any mechanical or other means, nor is he likely to suffer ill-effects from infected breast milk. The main principal of artificial feeding is to give the baby a milk mixture in a quantity of 150 ml/kg (2½–3 oz/lb) body weight. Evaporated tinned milk is slightly more expensive than dried, but it has the advantage that it is more easily prepared and the mother can be instructed to finish a tin in a day; she knows it will 'go off' if kept, and she usually uses it all. Particularly for the older child, a mixture in which the butter fat is replaced by the local cooking oil may be used. The oil and skim milk powder are rubbed together and sugar can be added (skim milk, 10 volumes; oil, 2 volumes; and sugar, 1 volume). This dry mixture will keep satisfactorily in a sealed container for 2–3 weeks.

General rules

A mother has difficulty in understanding what she is taught at a clinic, or what is written on the tin or packet of milk (96). The following points were found to be necessary to teach the less well educated mother.

(1)   The common cause for a crying baby is hunger; the contented baby is a better guide than exact measurement.

(2)   The best food is milk, and if mother's milk is not available, then all other full-cream milks are all equally good.

(3)   Do not be afraid to feed the child. If you are sure he is crying for other reasons, get advice from the doctor or nurse.

(4)   At each feed, give him as many ounces of feed as his weight in kilograms (or half his weight in pounds) – not more than 8 oz in one feed. Frequently offer him boiled water as well.

(5)   At first, put a level teaspoon of milk powder with each ounce. If he is still not content, use a rounded spoonful, and subsequently two or more spoons rounded off.

(6)   Use one teaspoon of sugar to every 4 oz of feed. If the stools are hard, then use a heaped spoon or even two spoons of sugar.

(7)   If you are using cow's milk, put one ounce of boiled water in the bottle, and then add boiled milk, one ounce for each kilogram of weight.

A method of sterilizing utensils that does not involve boiling

In the circumstances in which some form of artificial feeding is necessary, the doctor must see that the mother is taught a method of maintaining her feeding utensils that is simple and inexpensive. The following method proved moderately successful. A set of local utensils consisting of a bowl with a lid, a cup, a small glass and a spoon are shown to the mother, and she is asked to bring similar ones to the clinic. Under the supervision of a competent medical worker, preferably not in a hospital ward, she is taught how to sterilize the utensils and prepare the feeds. Sterilization is achieved by filling the bowl with water, and then adding either Milton Antiseptic or a small quantity of chloride of lime (calx chlorinata). Using the measure, spoon and cup which she picks from the chlorine solution, she is taught to make up the feed, either from tinned liquid milk or dried milk. If no source of milk can be afforded, then the skim milk and oil mixture described above may be used.

Cost of infant-feeding to family

Local workers need to be able to advise the mother on the cost of feeding her child. An example of how these costs may be worked out has been given for Jamaica (173). Mothers need guidance and protection, otherwise they may well buy the most expensive brands of milk, as the producers of these brands have more to spend on subtle persuasion by expert advertising. Table 15 is taken from calculations made

TABLE 15

Weekly Cost of Infant Feeding at Jamaican Prices (173)

Cost of additional food required by mother to supplement her lactation	Cornmeal + skim milk + sugar + vit.*	$0.54	White bread + sweetened condensed milk + vit.	$1.16	Fresh milk + chicken etc. + sweet potatoes, etc. $3.78
Cost of various infant-feeding regimes	Skim milk + vegetable oil + sugar + vit.	$0.76	Evaporated milk + sugar + vit.	$1.18	
	Dried whole milk + vit.	$1.72	Milk-based infant food + fresh orange juice	$2.94	

*Vit. = relevant vitamin preparation

in Jamaica (173) to show the wide range of cost per week. Using skim milk and vegetable oils, the cost of artificial feeding may be reduced to little more than the cost of additional foods required by the mother to support lactation. Problems may arise in low-income families attempting to prepare in their homes these skim milk and oil mixtures. In other communities doctors need to seek assistance from home economists and dietitians so that they can advise the poorer mothers on their local 'best buy'.

CHAPTER 7

The Road-to-health Card

OBJECTIVES

The objective of the 'Ilesha weight chart' or 'road-to-health' card, as it is now called, is to introduce or extend two principles of health care.

(1)   Children need to receive continuing comprehensive health care and not be treated for each illness on what might be called a 'cafeteria' basis. The chart provides a simple visual record that helps in doing this.

(2)   The 'promotion of adequate growth' is a more positive objective than the mere 'prevention of malnutrition' (324), it also reflects a more effective approach to the control of malnutrition in the community.

This chapter attempts to describe the background to these concepts. Other chapters will suggest how this chart may also be used to identify children 'at risk' (Chapter 9), and to promote the achievement of an adequate birth interval (Chapter 18), thereby improving the health of other members of the family.

WEIGHT CHART

Using the weight chart to measure growth

Variables related to growth are being used increasingly as indices of the nutritional status of children. Although there are many possible variables, the most economic and widely used single measurement is that of body weight. But in scientific studies of growth, height is more useful. Height is, however, relatively insensitive to rapid change in nutritional status; also a child can lose weight but not height. In the age group in which malnutrition is most frequent, the measurement of accurate height or length is difficult and requires both expensive equipment and considerable skill, with two workers for each measurement. Measurements of weight do not distinguish between the body content of fat, muscle and water, but this does not matter. In industrialized countries, where childhood obesity is now common, the interpretation of a weight chart is more difficult than in the developing countries. In developing countries the weight of oedema fluid might mislead the health worker. In practice, this is not so, as even 500 g of water is obvious as oedema, and frequently even health workers with quite limited skills do not have difficulty in discerning weight changes due to loss or gain of oedema fluid. Even if measurements of height could be accurately made, a slowing in the rate of growth, as indicated by height, could not be demonstrated in a period much less than 6 months. As long as some allowance can be made for the irregularities of weight gain and loss, a significant slowing of weight gain can be demonstrated in less than a month at the age when malnutrition is likely to occur. Indications of the effect of infections on nutrition can be discerned by the amount of weight loss they cause. No other anthropometric measurement is available which is so sensitive to the effects of infection.

Normal variations of weight gain — concept of centiles

In any community variation in weight of children at all ages is considerable. In Europe, genetics play a great part. In developing countries the nutritional status of the child both before and after birth is of principal importance. These variations need to be expressed in a numerical form and for this 'centiles' are favoured.

The concept of centiles is not always easily grasped, and the following has been found useful in helping medical auxiliaries and others to understand it. Centiles of height are easier to understand at first than those of weight, and for this a diagram *(Figure 32)* represents the height of 100 schoolgirls all aged 7 years.

The girls have been lined up so that the tallest is to the right and the shortest to the left. The fiftieth centile in this group would be the middle child, and the tenth centile the tenth child along from the left, while the ninety-seventh would be the third child from the end on the right. Clearly, to work these out accurately many more than 100 children are needed. When weights are being considered, these are similarly arranged, so that the middle or median weight will be the fiftieth centile.

The weight records of boys in a village in Nigeria (189), shown as smoothed curves, are compared in *Figure 33* with the standards for London boys (263).

The important point to note from this diagram is that although the median weights of Imesi boys and London boys are different, the variation within each group was considerably greater than the difference between them. In *Figure 33* the range of difference between the third and ninety-seventh centile of either London (A) or Imesi boys (B) is much greater than the difference between the medians of both groups. The median for Imesi children followed fairly closely the tenth centile for the London children. Each child has his own growth rate depending on the interaction between his genes and the environment in which he is living.

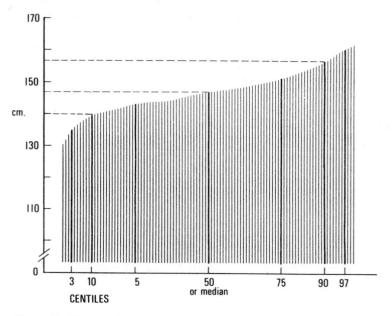

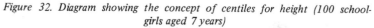

Figure 32. Diagram showing the concept of centiles for height (100 school-girls aged 7 years)

Ever since the earliest descriptions of kwashiorkor and marasmus, emphasis has been placed on the failure of growth as one of their salient features. The growth of children with kwashiorkor and marasmus will now be considered in relation to local standards.

Weight curves of children who develop kwashiorkor

During and after the longitudinal study in the village of Imesi, a number of children developed kwashiorkor (193). Of all the measurements on these children, the weight record was found to be the most valuable. Measurements of height or length were found to be a less sensitive indicator of growth failure. *Figure 34* shows the weight record of a child developing kwashiorkor.

126

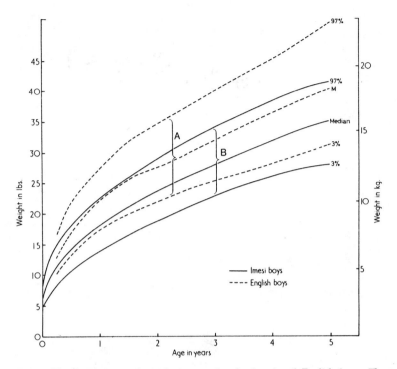

Figure 33. Comparison of weight percentiles for Imesi and English boys. The variation within the English group which is largely genetic is much greater than the variation between the groups which is largely nutritional

The weight records of most children are more complex than this; usually episodes of measles or diarrhoea precede periods of loss or poor gain in weight. The child recorded in *Figure 34* had failed to gain weight satisfactorily ever since his birth, following the third centile until almost the second birthday, when he failed even to achieve this level. At the age of 2 years, the common age for taking children off the breast in this community, breast-feeding stopped. Without breast milk, he lost weight, and developed early kwashiorkor which, however, responded satisfactorily to hospital treatment. The reader examining such a chart will no doubt ask why steps were not taken earlier to give this child some food supplements and teach his mother how to feed him better. This chart is a good example of an important lesson which was only learnt subsequently. He had been weighed, but his weights had not been charted, because the charts had not been introduced for routine use of all children in the clinic. It was found that weighing a child without charting the weight was of relatively little value. In a child such as this it is only too easy to overlook a poor weight gain, which became immediately apparent when it was recorded on a weight chart.

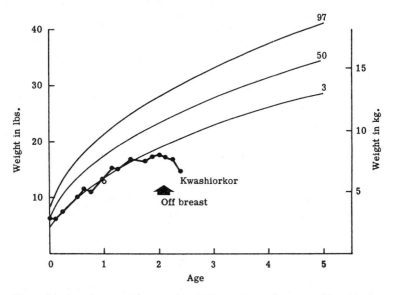

Figure 34. A common weight record in children prior to the onset of kwashiorkor

Although most children with kwashiorkor when, once they have lost their oedema, will be found to be on a low weight centile, there are occasional exceptions, and from these some valuable lessons can be learnt. *Figure 35* is an example of such a child. She was in the Imesi study, and her weight was being regularly charted. She came off the breast at the age of 19 months and within a month of this contracted measles, which in West Africa may lead to severe anorexia and loss of weight. As shown, she lost a quarter of her previous weight within 3 weeks, and instead of being well over the ninety-seventh centile, her weight fell to the fiftieth centile. At this time, when she was admitted to hospital, she was suffering from intractable diarrhoea, oedema and misery, typical signs of a child with clinical kwashiorkor. However, she had normal black hair, because her kwashiorkor was of acute onset and many months of inadequate feeding must elapse before discoloured hair

128

will appear. With treatment she rapidly gained weight and rose to the local ninety-seventh centile once more.

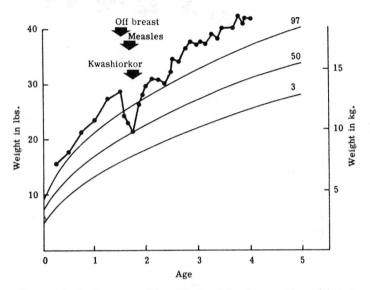

Figure 35. Development of kwashiorkor following cessation of breast-feeding and measles

This child demonstrates the acute form of kwashiorkor that may arise in 2 or 3 weeks following measles and some other acute infections, such as tuberculosis or diarrhoea. These children may be puzzling for unless they have their weight charts it may be difficult to understand how such well-grown children could develop kwashiorkor.

The next child is one with a much less common weight curve which nevertheless demonstrates another important point *(Figure 36)*. He had parents who were well-educated by local standards, and when he was a little over 1½ years old, they both had the opportunity for higher education, and left the child with his grandmother. Probably, because of the psychological upset of being suddenly separated from his parents, and because he received the same food as his grandmother, which was cassava, he failed to gain any further weight. However, since he was well up on the chart and since at the time he first went to his grandmother his weight was on the British ninety-seventh centile, no

129

notice was taken of his failure to gain weight, even though this continued for over 9 months. At the end of this time he was brought to hospital with the misery and oedema of mild kwashiorkor even though he was well grown. Even when he had lost his oedema, his weight was still close to the local ninety-seventh centile.

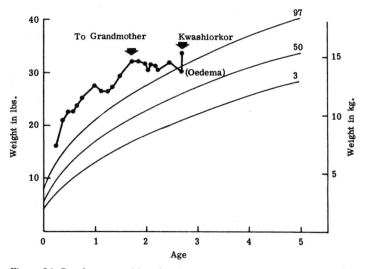

Figure 36. Development of kwashiorkor in a previously well-nourished child

This weight curve demonstrates one of the most difficult points to convey to medical workers, namely the fact that the position on the chart can be misleading. It is the direction in which his weight curve is moving that is most important in assessing the child's nutritional status. The velocity of a child's weight gain is more important than his actual weight at any age. This will be shown by his growing on a curve parallel with those on the chart.

Weight curves of children with marasmus

It is difficult to draw any clear-cut distinction between the appearances of the weight charts of kwashiorkor and marasmus because these syndromes lie at the ends of a spectrum. Children with marasmic kwashiorkor may be more common than children with either pure marasmus or kwashiorkor. Most children with marasmus fail to gain weight satisfactorily even in early life. Their weight gain may often have been unsatisfactory since birth or, as with the child in *Figure 37*, from about the third month of life. When this child was born at Imesi his weight was on the fiftieth centile. He gained weight satisfactorily for the first 3 months. His mother then had some illness which may have been typhoid and on top of this there was a psychosociological problem, namely a difference of opinion between his family and that of the

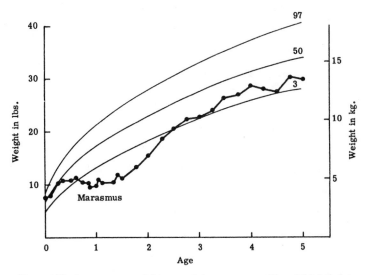

Figure 37. A common weight record in marasmus. The child failed to
gain weight for 15 months

senior nurse. For this reason, communications with his mother and efforts to help him for 15 months were largely unsuccessful. However, after that he was persuaded to eat a mixed diet with supplements, and thereafter he made a steady gain in weight reaching the third centile just before his third birthday, and after that continuing on or above this level.

In *Figure 38* the weight records of two of the children already described have been put together on the same chart. At the age of 2½ years the child who had marasmus was gaining weight well and had just reached the third centile. His mother was being congratulated at the same time that a child of the same age was being admitted to hospital with mild kwashiorkor even though he was on the local ninety-seventh centile.

The records of these two children emphasize the fact that it is not the position of a child's weight curve that is important, but the direction in which it is moving. Unfortunately, too much emphasis is often placed on a child's weight relative to some standard, and decisions are made as regards what treatment he requires on the basis of one weight

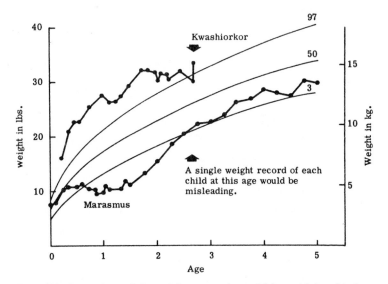

Figure 38. Comparison of the weight curves of two children with kwashiorkor and marasmus. The mother of the marasmic child was being congratulated for a good gain along the third centile while the child on the ninety-seventh centile was being admitted to hospital with kwashiorkor

record only. This should become less frequent as the health services move away from the situation in which they concentrate their resources on a curative service and children receive comprehensive care as in the Under-Fives' Clinic. Such preventively orientated medical service will be established with promotion of adequate growth as their immediate objective. Many others have found a similar poor weight gain; an example is a record from Central America. This is included as it contains bacteriological and other data unavailable in the Imesi study.

Figure 39 shows one of these and the large number of incidents of infection from which such children suffer and, as a result, their failure to gain weight satisfactorily. Only a few centres have been able to document such records and provide practical evidence of the continuing interaction between nutrition and infection.

WEIGHT CHART

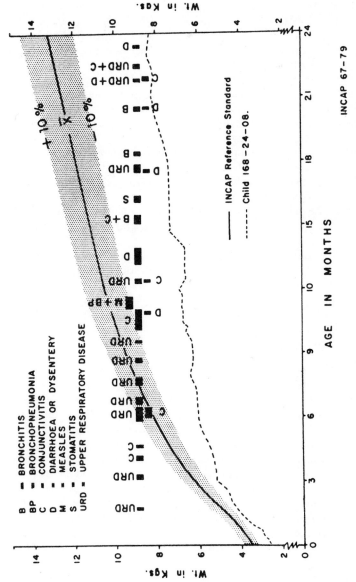

Figure 39. Weight curve and infectious disease in a Guatemalan village child

133

Designing a chart

In children, retardation in the growth rate is the earliest and most sensitive indication of impending malnutrition, and up to the age of 5 years failure to gain in weight is particularly informative. Children can be weighed with sufficient accuracy by members of a medical team recruited locally and trained on the job.

Not only is persistent failure to gain weight (or loss of weight) the earliest sign of malnutrition, but an increase in the rate of weight gain is the earliest evidence of recovery, and hence a valuable measure of the success of treatment. As has been seen, difficulties rarely arise from loss or gain in weight caused by oedema fluid.

Maintaining an adequate* rate of growth has replaced prevention of malnutrition as the goal towards which an Under Fives' Clinic directs its work. Experience has shown that kwashiorkor or marasmus are usually preceded by months or sometimes more than a year of failure to gain weight. The only common exception is when a child develops kwashiorkor suddenly, after illnesses such as measles (as shown in *Figure 35*), whooping cough or diarrhoea.

While maintaining an adequate rate of growth is by present standards a satisfactory objective, eventually some measure of the child activity may be necessary. A study of the activity of African and European children has been made (218) suggesting that deficiency of joules in the diet may lead to a reduction in energy expenditure (Table 16). Reduction of activity will reduce the learning opportunities of the small child and is therefore important.

Objective – maintaining an adequate rate of growth

Maintaining an adequate rate of growth is a positive objective for both the staff of the centre and the child's mother. When a child is seen who has failed to gain weight for several months, the clinic worker will first establish that the child has no obvious symptoms of underlying illness. Once this has been excluded, a mother is encouraged to increase those items of her child's diet which are most needed and the frequency with which he is fed. In some areas a temporary food supplement, such as ground nuts (peanuts) or wheat, may be made available. The gradient of the weight curve can be used to assess the effectiveness of food supplements and nutrition education (255). When, in spite of such measures, failure to gain weight persists, further enquiries need to be

*The term 'adequate' is better than the word 'normal' as still not enough is known about normal human growth

made including, where necessary, laboratory investigations, such as examinations for a chronic urinary infection, or tests for tuberculin conversion which cannot be done on all the children who fail to gain weight.

TABLE 16

Estimated Energy Expenditure of African and European Children Calculated from Observed Activity and Expressed as kcal/kg Body Weight/Day (218)

Activity	African	European
Resting	27.0	29.4
Sitting	12.0	7.6
Standing	18.6	10.0
Walking	14.0	30.4
Running	6.5	20.5
Total	78.1	97.9

The value of weight charts has been appreciated internationally for many years and was suggested by the Joint FAO/WHO Expert Committee on Nutrition over a decade ago (83). This chart, which was first introduced in West Africa in 1959, is perhaps an answer to this recommendation. Over the last 12 years, it has been modified on a number of occasions to make it simpler so that it can readily be used by auxiliaries whose education has not usually included the use of graphs (191). This may be their first experience in the use of any kind of graph. Graphical records involve considerable symbolism, and are probably most easily learnt at school between the ages of 8 and 12 years. Some highly intelligent medical workers have difficulty in grasping the meaning of movements on a chart. This is because their medical training has failed to make good an earlier lack of education in the symbolism involved in such records.

The calendar system

One of the more important ways in which the chart described here has been simplified, and which has made it more widely acceptable, has been the introduction of the calendar system to record the child's age. Four methods of recording the passage of time, or the age of the child, are shown in *Figure 40*.

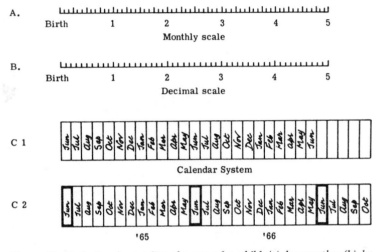

Figure 40. Methods of recording the age of a child (a) by months; (b) by decimal years. C1, the calendar system with in C2 the birth month emphasized; without this emphasis mistakes may occur as can be seen in C1

The traditional method (A) records the age of the child in months and years. In practice, however, this has considerable disadvantages. After the age of one year, the calculation of the child's age in months becomes increasingly difficult, and has to be repeated at each visit. This not only leads to errors, but has been a major deterrent to charting the children's weight in an overworked clinic.

An alternative method (B) is that used in British charts, in which the age of a child is calculated in decimal years (263). This method increases accuracy and allows growth velocity to be calculated more easily. The decimal system has many advantages for research workers but is too complex for general use.

The last method (C1 and C2) which has proved popular and successful in many countries, involves constructing a simple calendar when a child is first seen. This starts with the month of birth, followed by all the months for the first 5 years. Errors may arise because a month is missed out (for example, September in C1), but these can be largely avoided if the month of birth is outlined in darker print (C2); those

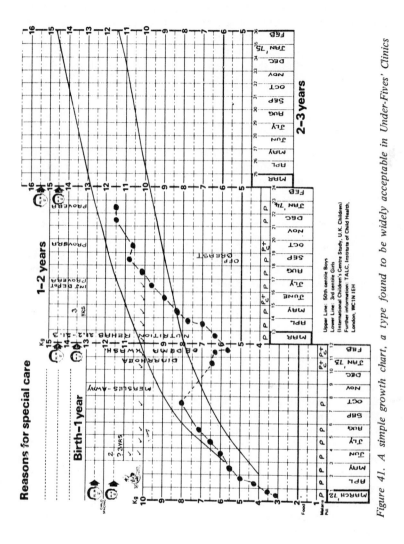

Figure 41. A simple growth chart, a type found to be widely acceptable in Under-Fives' Clinics

137

using the chart are instructed to enter this month in each appropriate space before completing the rest of the chart. In this way, the weight curve can be accurately and quickly recorded on a chart by a worker even with limited education without calculating the age of the child. He can also enter against this curve such incidents as cessation of breast-feeding, the birth of a sibling, or major diseases *(Figure 41)*.

The reference lines on the chart

Reference lines on a growth chart can be of two varieties. They can suggest the limits of normality and could be the third (or tenth) and ninety-seventh (or ninetieth) centile for that community. Alternatively, they can be used to show the 'direction' in which the child's own curve should travel. The curves on the road-to-health chart are of this second type. Reference to *Figure 33* will show the wide distribution of the growth curves of West African village boys and London boys. In both of these, the distribution of weights is so wide that any single line represents no more than a tiny minority of the children. Some comparative reference lines are required but fortunately their exact position on the chart is not important. Some workers have used the Harvard mean (203) as the top line, 80 per cent of this as the second line, and have then put in a third line at 60 per cent of the mean. There are serious disadvantages of using this system based on the percentages of the 'Harvard mean'. It becomes meaningless under 6 months of age, a period now considered of greater significance than in the past. Also there is little evidence that 60 per cent of the 'Harvard mean' at, for example, 9 months has the same meaning in nutritional terms as 60 per cent at 24 months. This system is of more value in undertaking a survey than in measuring the progress of an individual child. Lastly, by introducing 'percentages' great confusion arises in some people's minds between these and 'percentiles' or 'centiles'. Experience of this system on the road-to-health chart has shown that a third (60 per cent) line may be confusing. It may be of interest to doctors to know how many children fall below the 60 per cent line, but the presence of this lower line makes the chart more difficult for auxiliary workers to understand.

Preferably, there should be only two lines, and probably the most meaningful lines to the medical auxiliaries who will be using the charts are the following.

Lower line. – This represents the median (or average) weight for children in the villages of the country concerned. This is the more important of the two lines.

Upper line. — This represents the median (or average) weight for children, such as those living on a university campus, whose parents have both the knowledge and the means to feed them well and are also able to give them good medical care.

Assuming a similar genetic background, the difference between these two lines represents the deficit due to environmental factors, particularly the poor nutrition and frequent infections of village children. These lines have been used on the road-to-health card in the past. Auxiliaries are taught that their objective should be to get the growth curves of all children running parallel to these lines, and as many of them as possible above the lower line. This means that an attempt is made to bring village children of lower weight, likely to be less well nourished, up to the level of the more fortunate children. The upper line is used when a child from more fortunate socio-economic circumstances is being cared for.

At a recent international consultation on weight charts a proposal was made to adopt the fiftieth centile and the third centile of a normally nourished European group (International Children's Centre UK Study). These were found to be similar to the lines suggested above. Where further lower lines were required, the third and fourth standard deviation would be used. In this book the chart shown is that developed and simplified over 15 years with alterations suggested at this consultation. The upper line represents the fiftieth centile for boys, the lower line the third centile for girls. Plastic overlays* are available, the one for boys includes the −3 and −4 standard deviations and is used by placing the fiftieth centile line over the upper line on the chart. The separate plastic sheet for girls is similar and used by placing the third centile over the lower line. With these plastic sheets children's weights can be classified into these new groups which resemble but are not identical with the grouping relying on a percentage of the Harvard mean.

The choice of lines should not be allowed to dominate discussions on the use of a weight chart, as so often happens. Instead, emphasis needs to be placed at all levels of discussion on the direction of a child's own curve — 'Is he growing adequately?'.

Methods of weighing

A satisfactory method of weighing large numbers of children at low cost has still to be found. The ideal machine is one similar to those in the larger food shops in industrialized countries. These use counter-

*These are available with guidance on their use from TALC, Institute of Child Health, 30 Guilford Street, London WC1 1ENH

balanced weights and give a direct and accurate reading. Such scales are available but they may cost as much as $200—300. Moreover, they have to be firmly fixed on a solid base and cannot be moved. While large centres weighing many hundreds of children a day might justify the cost of such a scale, it is clear that they are not suitable for wide use in developing countries.

The next variety of scale widely used is the beam-balance scale. This usually has two movable weights; one moves in kilogrammes, and the other in 10-gramme steps up to one kilogramme. When scales are bought, those with this type of weight are to be preferred. For example, if the larger weight goes up in half-kilogramme movements, more errors are likely to arise due to mistakes in adding the two weights together. Scales of this type are available, and have in some centres been used to weigh 300 children a day for several years without more than minor adjustments *(Figure 42)*.

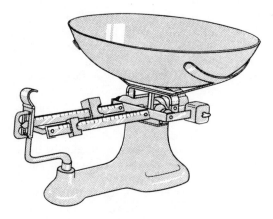

Figure 42. A beam-balance scale

In the past, scales depending on a spring were not considered suitable as older patterns of spring 'tire' with time and varied with climatic conditions. However, the steel used in the modern springs is much improved, and scales made by reliable manufacturers can give years of satisfactory service. Recently, several attempts have been made to use spring scales, and the best system so far has been to use a simple hanging scale on which a child can be suspended in a pair of strong locally-made fabric trousers *(Figure 43)*.

If a number of trousers are available, mothers waiting in a weighing queue at a clinic soon learn to put their own child into them and then to suspend him on the hook of the hanging scales. In this way a child

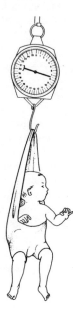

Figure 43. Simple hanging scale. The markings on the face of the scale are similar to those on the weight chart

need not be touched by the operator, and should trousers become wet or soiled, they can be taken away to be washed. This is more easily done when they are made of strong plastic. There are a number of advantages in this type of scale: they are cheap and only cost between $15 and 20 and they are readily transportable. A model has been prepared with markings similar to those on the weight chart*. This makes it easier to transfer a weight from the scale to the chart.

The economy of weighing

Weighing is probably the least costly of all measurements in medicine. In most developing countries 100 children can be weighed, and their weights charted, for less than 20 ¢. Weighing can well be undertaken by

*Details of all the weighing machines mentioned here and the anthropometric equipment available from C.M.S. Weighing Equipment Ltd, 18, Camden High St, London NW1 0JH

minimally trained staff who are taken on for this purpose alone. An efficient clinic may need to employ almost as many clerks to weigh and direct the patients as medical assistants or nurses.

Weighing should be undertaken whenever a child makes contact with the medical service. A recent weighing can be a valuable way of estimating the degree of dehydration if diarrhoea develops.

EVALUATION OF THE ROAD-TO-HEALTH CHART

The road-to-health charts were first introduced in the village of Imesi in Nigeria with a population of 5,000–6,000 in 1959. The staff and local people have had more experience there than any other community. This village was also being used as a location for a long-term study of children growing up, who were offered a higher level of care than in most villages in West Africa. Resident in the village was one expatriate nursing sister, one fully-trained nurse, and four or five nurse—midwives who had received a simple training locally. A doctor visited twice weekly. The figures that follow must be considered against this background although much of the senior staff's time was involved in record-keeping for research purposes. From 1965 to 1967, after the services had been in existence for approximately 10 years, a study was made of the use of the charts and the health of the children, a neighbouring village being taken for purposes of comparison (56, 57).

TABLE 17

Chart-carrying Pre-school Children at Imesi (1966)

	Number	Percentage
Population 0–60 months	1,038	100
Children with charts	1,000	96
Children who acquired chart at birth	856	83
Charts seen during survey	982	95

The proportion of children in Imesi who possessed a chart was high, as is shown in Table 17. Here, as elsewhere, the mother looked on the chart as a sort of 'passport' to health care, and she was proud to possess it. Mothers were sometimes found in tears in the clinic waiting room because someone had picked up their child's road-to-health chart and they thought it was lost.

From Table 18 it can be seen that between the ages of 0–5 years, of 1,038 children in the village the date of birth of 1,002 (96.5 per cent) was known. This information will be valuable to the child as he grows up, as well as being important in assessing his health. In most developing countries only a small proportion of children have records of their date of birth.

TABLE 18

Children with Known Birth Dates at Imesi (1966)

	Number	Percentage of population
Population 0–60 months	1,038	100.0
Children with known birth date	1,002	96.5

A study was also made to discover how often the weight of these children was charted in each year of their life. From Table 19 it is clear that a high proportion of both boys and girls in this village were attending regularly enough to have their weights charted in most months of the year.

TABLE 19

Median Number of Months out of Each Year of Life in which at Least One Weight Was Charted (Imesi, 1966)

Year of life	Boys	Girls
First	12	12
Second	11	10
Third	10	11
Fourth	11	11
Fifth	7	6
Total in first 5 years	51	50

The charts were also used to discover how frequently children attended the clinic. The attendances for 663 or 61 per cent of the children were analysed. The results are shown in Table 20; no explanation can be given for the greater frequency with which girls were brought; this is unusual as in most cultures boys receive more care than girls.

TABLE 20

Approximate Total Visits per Child per Year* to Under-Fives' Clinic (Imesi, 1967)

Year of life	Mean visits/child/year	
	Boys	Girls
Second	23.9	26.3
Third	23.7	27.1
Fourth	17.0	21.2
Fifth	15.7	18.0
Total, years 2–5	80.3	92.6

*Extrapolated from January–August figures to 12 months January–December

The children in Imesi village were attending between 80 and 90 times during their first 5 years of life. The clinic was conveniently situated in the middle of the village, and the mothers were welcome to attend as frequently as they wished. This large number of mothers may be economically too expensive for the society but it has great advantages in the opportunities provided for health education.

Estimations were made of the level of immunization of the children in the village, and the results are shown in Table 21. This high level of immunization was partly due to co-operation between mothers and the staff of the clinic. A system of edged punch cards immediately revealed any child who had not received immunization, and with the use of these it was possible to contact defaulters.

The question was asked whether the mothers in Imesi understood the meaning of the weight chart in terms of growth, and those involved concluded that a satisfactory number had some understanding.

Comparative study of two villages

By comparing Imesi-Ile with the neighbouring village of Oke-Imesi, which are separated by a river passable except in the wet season, the effect of the health service in Imesi on the health of the children could be measured. There were few important differences in the environment and manner of life of the two villages (Table 22).

TABLE 21

Immunization Records from Weight Charts (Imesi, 1966)

Immunization	Number of children	Number immunized	Percentage of sample	Percentage of total population age
Smallpox	939	935	99.7	90.2
DPT (ages 6–60 months)	880	869	98.8	92.8
Measles (ages 6–60 months)	888	729	82.1	77.9
BCG vaccine	982	942	95.9	90.8

TABLE 22

Village Profiles: Imesi-Ile and Oke-Imesi (1967)

Environmental and life style differences	Imesi-Ile (study village)	Oke-Imesi (control)
Population	6,200	7,200
Person/house ratio	7.9	7.9
Percentage of houses cemented	5.7	56
Water supply	Streams	Piped (since December 1966)
Staple foods	Yams, gari, eko, beans, rice	Yams, gari, amala, rice, eko
Cash crops	Yam, cocoa, kola, cotton	Rice, yam, cocoa, tobacco
School students	1,568	1,352
Seamstresses	24	47
Tailors	19	26
Palm wineries	16	29

The people in the two villages were producing and eating much the same foods. The two groups were ethnically related, local history suggesting that the people at Oke-Imesi had moved out from Imesi-Ile towards the end of the nineteenth century.

The staff dealt with over 45,000 visits from children aged under 5 years each year, 90 per cent of whom were from the village, and offered them a well-organized preventive and curative service. Very sick children could at any time be referred to the hospital at Ilesha. During the year of the comparative study, 35 such children were admitted to the Ilesha hospital. Many children were also treated in the dispensary building in Imesi. At Oke-Imesi there were a few private clinics and a local authority 'dispensary—maternity' clinic, which employed one dispenser and two midwives, and during the year under review they had seen just under 4,000 'child welfare' cases. There were 608 children in Oke-Imesi seen during the study year, and of these the doctor had to refer 50 to hospital.

Child mortality and growth in the two villages

Although socio-economically similar, the two villages differed in their health services. Imesi-Ile had an Under-Fives' Clinic, while Oke-Imesi had the traditional welfare centre and dispensary. Against this background Cunningham investigated the health statistics for the year 1966—67 (Table 23).

TABLE 23

August 1966—August 1967 Child Mortality at Imesi-Ile and Oke-Imesi

	Imesi-Ile Under-Fives' Clinic	Oke-Imesi 'welfare' clinic
Live births	302	327
Infant deaths	14	26
Infant mortality rate/1,000 live births	46	80
Child 1—4 population (estimated mid-year)	896	997
Child 1—4 deaths	16	48
Child 1—4 mortality rate/1,000 children 1—4	18	48

Cunningham also demonstrated differences in the survivors, and he illustrated this by expressing the children's weight as a percentage of the standard weight (203) for children of that age and sex (Table 24).

There was a considerable difference in the malaria parasite rate in the villages: in Imesi-Ile it was 15.5 per cent and in Oke-Imesi 55 per cent of the films were positive. In each area malaria is holo-endemic.

TABLE 24

Median Percentage of Standard Weight (203) for Age by Age and Sex Group,
Children 0–4 years, Imesi-Ile and Oke-Imesi, 1966

Age group (months)	Boys			Girls		
	Imesi-Ile (%)	Oke-Imesi (%)	Difference (%)	Imesi-Ile (%)	Oke-Imesi (%)	Difference (%)
0– 5	92.0	92.2	−0.2	90.0	93.4	−3.4
6–11	84.5	84.3	+0.2	85.0	77.8	+7.2
12–23	82.0	78.9	+3.1	80.8	76.2	+4.6
24–35	83.6	81.1	+2.5	83.8	78.9	+4.9
36–47	83.9	81.5	+2.4	79.0	78.6	+0.3
48–60	82.5	80.3	+2.2	80.9	77.6	+3.3

COST OF THE UNDER-FIVES' CLINIC SERVICE IN IMESI-ILE

A full description of the Under-Fives' Clinic is given in Chapter 19. A study of the cost of the under-fives' services, including drugs, supplies, salaries and transport, was undertaken. In the year under study it was 14 ¢ per child visit, and $5.00 per child per year. These figures were similar to those reported in 1963 (184), when the cost per visit was estimated at 15 ¢ and the cost per year was considered to be $7.00. These figures are still many times greater than the national sum available for each child; however, they are considerably less than the sums expended in conventional systems of care.

CHAPTER 8

The 'Home-based' Record and Levels of Care

An assumption is made, and usually accepted by both doctors and nurses, that all medical records must belong to the institution, and, indirectly, to them. Equally it is assumed that all serious disease will be cared for in hospital. In this chapter it will be suggested that some of a child's medical records are best entrusted to his mother. The most important reason for keeping a child's records at home is that it is the only practical place to keep them once the doctor makes himself responsible for all the children in a rural society, and no longer confines himself to those who arrive at the hospitals and clinics. By giving the mother the record, information about past illnesses becomes available to other health workers whose help the mother may seek.

MEDICAL RECORDS

Filing records in developing countries

Filing systems are difficult enough in European hospitals, where the whole community is literate. Here names are seldom ambiguous, and the ratio of medical workers to population is high. Filing clerks are educated and may have been specially trained. Rural societies in the developing world do not have these advantages. Nearly 20 per cent of the population is under five, and the naming system is usually less systematic. Often the majority of names in a country may start with only a few of the letters of the alphabet. For example, in one village 52 per cent of surnames or 'family' names started with one of the three letters A, O or J; in the Amazon all the children's names in one family have the same beginning. Furthermore, a child's name sometimes changes several times in the course of a few years, and in some cultures giving a child a name is considered unpropitious until he has survived the dangerous early years. In Asia one large church-related hospital has been exceptional in achieving a complete record system for both in-

148

patients and out-patients but this has only been accomplished at considerable expense requiring no less than 50 filing clerks.

In the Under-Fives' Clinic there are considerable benefits to be gained by giving the mothers their children's records to keep. More important, experience has shown that once the mothers realize the value of their children's records and the more substantial these are, the better they are likely to be cared for. This is why the weight charts should be printed on strong card and kept in a stout polythene bag so that they are less likely to be damaged. Without this polythene envelope which must be 10 cm longer than the card, the road-to-health chart deteriorates so quickly that the whole system of home-based records breaks down. Losses of around 1 per cent per year have been recorded in many places, and this compares well with losses of over 5–10 per cent in clinic filing systems. It is commonly said that in a particular society the people will be certain to lose them. So far wherever mothers have been allowed to keep their children's weight charts they have kept them safely.

In many clinics where records are filed, the day's work cannot effectively begin until the majority of records have been extracted. An efficient Under-Fives' Clinic can start work as soon as mothers arrive with their cards, and the first children can have been weighed, cared for by the nurse, and be on their way home within 30 minutes of the start of the clinic. A minimum of the mother's valuable time will then have been wasted in waiting.

Analysing records

An advantage of a home-based record system is realized when the records are used to analyse the work of the clinic. Attempts to carry out a survey of most clinic-based records are met by the frustration of finding many records incomplete in basic data. In an analysis of 6,000 in-patient records in a district hospital (260), the following deficiencies were discovered: age, 11.5 per cent; weight, 10.5 per cent; sex, 3 per cent; tribe, 4 per cent. Out-patient records are completed less efficiently, and these deficiencies make analysis hardly worthwhile.

Moreover, analysis of records in a clinic is open to the criticism that it answers only the question 'What does the clinic achieve with the children who come to it?'. By visiting random homes in the community (244) and surveying the records of the children who slept there the previous night, many of their deficiencies can be made good, and a more important and worthwhile question can be answered: 'What does the clinic achieve in the community?'. One can start above all to identify those children, frequently the most needy, who do not come for care (group C in *Figure 12*.

As a significant part of the records is moved out of the hospital and clinic through the Under-Fives' Clinic to the home, at the same time emphasis is shifted from the specialized unit to the home. Greater responsibility is put on the parent for the care of the child, and greater emphasis can be laid on the most important source of care, that within the home.

Responsibility for the child's health

Parents all over the world who are struggling to bring up children under extreme difficulty look to the local hospital and clinic for help, and the doctor and other staff are responsible in part, together with the

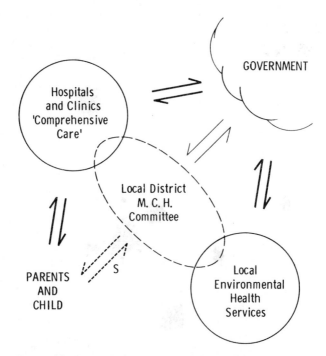

Figure 44. Responsibility for the child's health. Systems of responsibility that rarely exist are dotted

parents, for the health of the child. The doctor is acting as a representative of the government of the country in this, as the final responsibility must rest there, but to the parent this responsibility is too remote to be meaningful. This concept is set out in *Figure 44,* and the need for a further 'body' concerned with the care of the child is suggested.

Committee concerned with the care of children

What form this committee will take will depend on the social and political structure of the community, but it should include a high proportion of mothers with young children in its membership. It may be a sub-committee of the district or village council, a women's association of a religious group, or a women's wing of a political party. Any of these are suitable as long as the aim of the group is to serve the whole community and not give preference to its members. If the clinic or hospital holds all the records of the child, information on the health of the children of the area can be collected only in the clinic or the hospital. Once the records have been taken over by the parent, the local committee can become more effective in improving the health of the children by assuming some of the responsibility. It can encourage the clinic to provide better care, and also encourage the community to make use of this care. This will be possible only if information is provided to the committee on such subjects as the health and 'immunization status' of the children in their area.

The introduction of growth charts into homes allows information on the individual child to move in two directions. As indicated below, the health worker and any other visitor to the home can tell the mother how her child is doing, and what immunizations are needed. At the same time, information on the utilization of health services by the community, and on the health of the children of the area can be obtained for the local committee, and through this committee relayed to the central authorities. This information is collected by visiting random samples of the homes of the community, and it offers means for discovering any improvement in the nutritional status of the children.

The medical personnel in rural societies are already overstretched, and it may hardly be possible for them to undertake additional responsibility. Nor in general is an analysis of a service best undertaken by those offering the service. Some other possible channel should be looked for through which the community can inform itself on the state of its children's health. Currently, the educational policies and services of developing countries are under no less criticism than the medical ones. Writers (119) have shown how irrelevant to social realities is the present system of education. In the future the schools are likely to be more deeply concerned with the society in which they exist, and their objective may well shift to create a better local citizen and parent. A practical step in this direction may be the direct involvement of the senior forms of the schools in studies such as that described above. The senior form of the school could at regular intervals carry out surveys of the records of the young children in their community, the schoolmaster being responsible for preparing them for the committee tables based on these records. The school would be responsible for supplying the information along the dotted line shown by an 'S' in *Figure 44*. This would be a highly educational activity and the school child who has been involved in such a study is likely to ensure that his relatives, and, later, his children are immunized and attend the clinic.

<h2 style="text-align:center">HOME-BASED CARDS AND 'LEVELS OF CARE'</h2>

The concept of home-based cards has been well described (139) under the heading of *Progressive patient care*. This theme is illustrated in *Figure 45*.

Intensive care units in developing countries

The intensive care unit is still a luxury in Western medicine, but it should be standard practice in the developing countries. For all the disadvantages these areas of the world suffer, they are starting with a 'clean slate' and thus can develop a service more appropriate to the real needs of the people than those in the West if only doctors and nurses trained in a European system can discover and develop such new forms of care. This system of patient care originated in North America and has spread elsewhere in the world. It is particularly suited to the needs of developing countries, and parts of it, such as the 'emergency room', the rehydration centre and the nutrition rehabilitation centre, are already part of many health services for children. They are described in this monograph particularly in relation to home-based records and the part that the mother plays at the different levels of care (Table 25).

As one moves from the intensive care unit to the home, the involvement and responsibility of the medical services are reduced, whereas those of the mother and the family increase, as do the volume of sickness and the incidence of disease treated. Clearly, the objectives of different types of care and the relative contribution of the medical worker and the mother need to be examined (256).

Records and home-visiting

Almost all illness starts in the home, and most of it is treated there. Because of the idea that medical records should not be kept in the home, those engaged in home-visiting have either carried records with

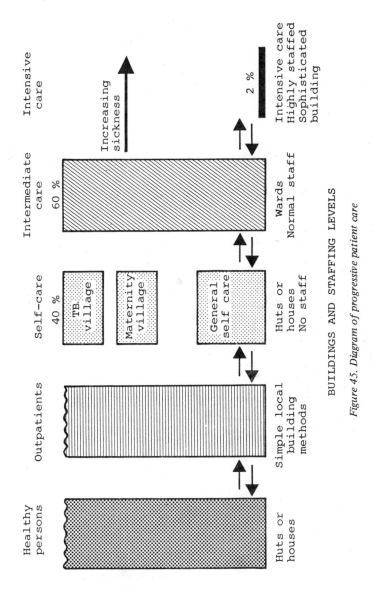

BUILDINGS AND STAFFING LEVELS

Figure 45. Diagram of progressive patient care

TABLE 25

Mother's Role at Different Levels of Medical Care

The levels of care	Mother's responsibility
Intensive care units	
These are the rehydration centres, the emergency rooms, or 'round-the-clock' services which are now being established in many city hospitals, and offer a high, but low-cost, intensity of medical observation, investigation and treatment. Their major objectives are resuscitation and rehydration of the very ill child. Their services are restricted to those living in the large cities and can reach only a small proportion of those in need	The mother has the prime responsibility to bring the child to the unit, but her involvement in the treatment is limited. The records that she brings will show how the acute incident is related to past illness (for example, the interaction of measles, diarrhoea and malnutrition)
Acute children's ward	
This remains the centre of most paediatrician's activities. A greater appreciation of the value of medical care has led to its overcrowding and more emphasis being placed on other levels of care	The mother or a close relative should be present if the child is under five. She will want to take part in the child's feeding and toilet and will participate in health education
Long-stay ward and nutrition rehabilitation centre	
These make less use of traditional medical skills and more of skills in communication and teaching. They are described in Chapter 22	Here the mother should be almost entirely responsible for her child. A major objective of the nutrition rehabilitation centre is her training through her involvement in the recovery of her child in surroundings similar to her home
The Under-Fives' Clinic	
The Under-Fives' Clinic described in Chapter 19 is designed to be able to meet, through the use of medical auxiliaries, the major demands for child health in the rural society	Through the UFC the mother makes the majority of her contacts with the health services. The chart which is her property is maintained by this clinic. She can relate easily with the clinic nurse who is culturally close to her

TABLE 25 *(cont.)*

The levels of care	*Mother's responsibility*
In the home	
Most illnesses are cared for completely in the home. Less than 10−20 per cent of child deaths occur in hospital in most developing countries. Home-visiting undertaken by the staff of the Under-Fives' Clinic will help them to appreciate individual and community problems. Education of the family in better health and nutrition can then be more successful	The mother, the relatives and the recources of the community offer the care that is available at this level. The success of the mother in caring for her child in the home and, with her relatives, making the decision to take the child elsewhere will depend partly on economic and cultural factors, but even more on past experience and 'education' received at other levels of care

them, or studied them and committed them to memory before leaving the clinic. However, the mother and relatives may be suspicious of what is written in the records held in the health worker's hand. Alternatively, if she has left them in the clinic, she may overestimate the accuracy of her memory. If the mother can produce for the visitor her records about her child, this is something that she is proud of, and that the visitor can accept from her graciously. The visit is made more 'human' and valuable, and the medical worker, having examined the records and found something on which to compliment the mother, will hand them back to her for safe keeping before leaving the home. Giving the mother her children's records may be of considerable importance in the context of the general development of women in rural societies.

Records available to non-medical workers

The children's records should not be purely medical. They should also contain relevant material for workers in other fields. For example, if a social worker finds conditions in a house which may be dangerous for the child and lead to an accident, this fact might well be entered on the child's record, so that other visitors in other disciplines coming to the house could encourage the mother to persist in the necessary steps to remedy the situation and praise her if she succeeds.

In the rural societies of most developing countries there are likely to be two agricultural workers for every medical worker. While the medical worker's chief contacts are with the mother, the agricultural extension workers should seek the confidence of the father. As an objective of the agricultural department will be to improve the nutrition of the family, their concern will be with the group most in danger

— the children under 5 years of age. In at least one country the agricultural workers are being taught to understand the growth charts. They can then effectively persuade the fathers to try to ensure that their children are well fed.

Of all home-based records, the growth chart is likely to be of most value to workers in other fields. *Figure 46a* represents those who are concerned with the prevention of malnutrition, or better, with the promotion of adequate growth.

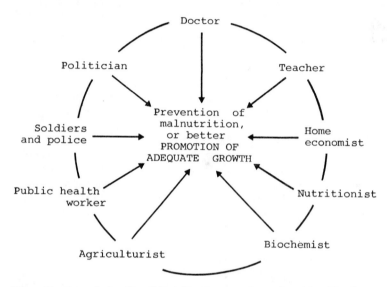

Figure 46a. Interrelationship of disciplines in preventing malnutrition. The doctor has an important place but can only be effective in co-operation with these others

The inclusion of soldiers and police in *Figure 46a* is a reminder that one of the first results of a breakdown of law and order will be an increase in childhood malnutrition. The doctor bears a particular responsibility, as only he can measure the prevalence of malnutrition in the community and the extent to which the policies of other disciplines aggravate or ameliorate this condition. By providing children with their own growth charts, other disciplines may be more easily involved. Representatives of any of these professions and disciplines may be in the home at one time or another. Given a modicum of teaching on the meaning of the growth chart and the importance of the direction of movement of the child's own curve, the chart may provide a useful opening for them in discussions with the mother and the family, remembering at all times that the record belongs to the mother. Just as the growth chart may be a 'passport' through which the mother has confidence to reach the health services when she needs their help, so also in the home the visitor can establish contact and the families confidence through the growth chart.

Other uses of road-to-health card

Those involved in using these growth charts have discovered a number of ways in which they may be used in clinical practice or teaching. For example, they may indicate the volume of fluid required by a dehydrated child (see *Figure 58,* page 190).

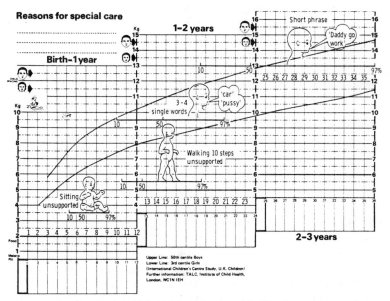

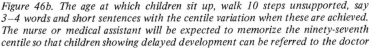

Figure 46b. The age at which children sit up, walk 10 steps unsupported, say 3–4 words and short sentences with the centile variation when these are achieved. The nurse or medical assistant will be expected to memorize the ninety-seventh centile so that children showing delayed development can be referred to the doctor

Four important developmental stages with the span in time in which they take place are given in *Figure 46b.* Copying this out on to their own chart may help the medical assistant to memorize these figures. Another example of the use of these charts is given in *Figure 47.*

CHAPTER 9

The 'At-risk' Child

The theme underlying much of what is written in this book suggests that under the present system of delivering health care the child more in need may be the last to receive it. The reasons may be geographical, racial, cultural or economic. This chapter suggests a method through which the doctor and his team can identify this group of high-risk children. Once identified, a system must be evolved to supply them with the extra care they will need.

On the inside of the 'road-to-health' card, these 'at-risk' factors, or 'reasons for special care', are given a prominent place (*Figure 47*). By this means, whenever the child is seen or visited, the medical worker will be encouraged to give him extra attention and encourage the mother to attend frequently. In this way the child will receive the additional care it may require if he is to survive.

Although considerable effort has been put into methods of identifying high-risk children in industrialized communities (249), it is difficult to find examples where this has been put into practical use. A mathematical model (61) has been designed for 'at-risk children from which the decision can be made as to the optimal division of resources between 'high' and 'low' risk groups. The experienced health nurse in all societies can identify those children, those families and those communities in which malnutrition, accidents, and a high morbidity and mortality are likely to arise in childhood. This chapter will describe one attempt to identify factors that put children 'at risk' in a West African village, details of which have been published elsewhere (189). At the same time, an attempt will be made to see how this and similar methods can be used to improve and maintain the health of children at a disadvantage.

CHILDREN NUTRITIONALLY 'AT RISK' IN A WEST AFRICAN COMMUNITY

This study examined two groups of children. They were identified by their weights at 6, 9 and 12 months, that is in the second 6 months of life, when nutrition is so crucial. Using local centiles for weight (189), the two groups were selected, as shown in *Figure 48.*

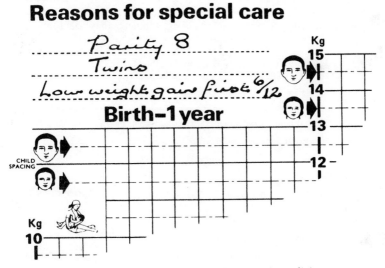

Figure 47. *Identifying at risk children in a busy clinic*

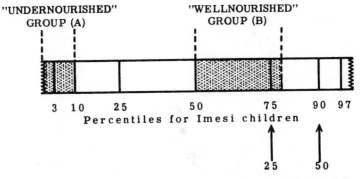

Figure 48. *Selection of groups A and B using percentile figures of children from Imesi, Nigeria*

Examination of the weights of these children at later ages suggested that the two groups remained separate, as did the weights of later born siblings to the two groups.

159

At-risk factors

The following socio-economic and medical factors were considered in this community as being possibly related to the nutritional welfare of the children. An attempt was made to tabulate these factors more

TABLE 26

List of the 17 Parameters Investigated as Possible 'At-risk' Factors. Those in Italics Were Considered to be Significant

Number	Factors
1	Parental heights and weights: *maternal weight below 96 lb (43.5 kg)*
2	Birth order: *all birth orders over 7*
3	The weight of the mother in relation to the birth order of the child
4	Religion of the parents
5	The marital system and parental care: *breakdown of marriage or death of either parent*
6	Occupation of the parents
7	Family size and birth order
8	Stillbirth and death rates among siblings
9	Deaths among older siblings, and family size before the birth of the child: *more than 4 sibling deaths*
10	Seasonal incidence of births
11	Weight changes during pregnancy
12	Birth weight: *a birth weight below the tenth centile (♂ 2.45 kg, ♀ 2.36 kg)*
13	Twinning
14	Monthly weight increments during the first 6 months of life: *failure to gain 1 lb (0.5 kg) a month in the first trimester or ½ lb (0.25 kg) a month in the second trimester of life*
15	Breast-feeding and the introduction of solid foods: *breast infections and difficulties in breast-feeding, particularly those secondary to psychiatric illness in the mother*
16	Influence of disease in the first year of life: *an episode of measles, whooping cough and severe repeated diarrhoea in the early months of life*
17	Influence of malaria prophylaxis on the growth of the child

precisely and investigate their relative importance. In Table 26 these factors are set out, and those that were found to be significant for this community are italicized.

Maternal weight

Nutritional deprivation, particularly soon after birth, and perhaps less so in childhood and adolescence, when the epiphyses unite with the shafts of the long bones, will cause permanent retardation of growth in height. Therefore, the height of the adult is one indication of his nutritional state during childhood. The body weight is more an indication of the adult's contemporary state.

In the author's study, the genetic factors may have played some part, although the community studied was intermarried, and genetic influence was probably less significant than in a more heterogeneous community.

The height and particularly the weight of the mothers of the malnourished group was smaller than that of the mothers of the wellnourished group. The fathers of both groups were similar in their heights and weights. These findings suggest that the mother's nutrition in childhood, and more recently, may have been poor, and that in this community the weight of the mother may be some indication of the future nutrition of her child. In the studied groups of mothers, the individual weights showed great variation in each group. The trend was for mothers in both groups to be heavier with increasing birth order; it is a general finding that women in most societies increase in weight with increasing age and parity. However, the weight of the mothers in the less well nourished group appeared to increase less with parity than did that of the mothers in the better nourished group suggesting that their nutrition may have been unsatisfactory.

No significant correlation between weight gain in pregnancy, birth weight or subsequent weight was shown in the study. This was surprising, as in this community the average weight gain during pregnancy was only 4 kg compared with an average of 11.4 kg for Aberdeen mothers. About 4 per cent of mothers showed no increase in weight during pregnancy.

This small gain in weight during pregnancy in developing countries remains unexplained (118). No satisfactory explanation is available. The 'normal' or optimum pregnancy weight gain is not known. The large weight gain seen in many mothers in Europe is probably excessive. Similarly, the small gain seen in pregnant women in developing countries is presumably related to a deficient calorie intake.

Just as short stature has been used as an indicator of the mother obstetrically 'at risk', so the weight of the mother may in future be used as one of the indicators for special care in the nutrition of the infant.

Birth order over seven

As might be expected, the infant of the older mother is more likely to be malnourished. By the time the mother has given birth to 7 infants in this village, she is likely to have been child-bearing for over 20 years, and her ability to secrete breast milk may be decreasing. *Figure 49* shows an increased incidence of poor nutrition with parities over 7. This was confirmed by another recent study in East Africa, where it was found that the marasmic children were mostly those of older mothers, while kwashiorkor more commonly developed when another sibling was born after only a brief birth interval (79).

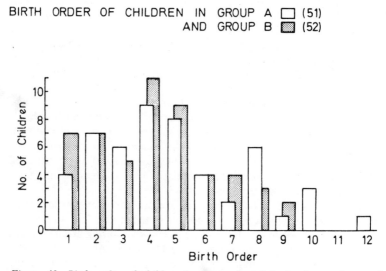

BIRTH ORDER OF CHILDREN IN GROUP A ☐ (51)
AND GROUP B ▨ (52)

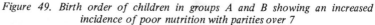

Figure 49. Birth order of children in groups A and B showing an increased incidence of poor nutrition with parities over 7

Breakdown of marriage or death of a parent

In a compound in the village where this study took place, the common family unit is the 'extended family', built on a patrilineal system, where intermarriage within the village is usual. The girl marries at about the age of 17 years, leaving her parents' compound for that of her husband. If the marriage ends in divorce or separation, the wife will return to her parents' family circle with any of her children who are under the age of 7 years. The author's findings as regards the child with separated parents were similar to those of others (280), who examined the environments of children with kwashiorkor in a mixed but mainly rural community in East Africa and concluded that the broken marriage was common in its aetiology. In addition, these families seemed to receive less support from other members of the community. In the community the author had studied, children were not sent to stay with distant relatives when the mother stopped breast-feeding. This takes place in some communities and is believed to precipitate malnutrition in a few children. Polygamy was not associated with malnutrition in the study, nor was it in those of others (162, 280). However, in some studies, such as that in the city of Lagos (89), this factor was important, no doubt associated with the special problems of polygamy in an urban situation.

More than four sibling deaths

As might be expected, the family in which there were a number of previous child deaths was also the family in which children with poor nutrition were more likely to be found.

Birth weight

The babies of low birth weight usually gained well. However, those with birth weights below the local tenth percentile were more likely to be poorly nourished later.

Twinning

Probably in all communities which depend largely on breast-feeding, twinning is a great hazard, in that the infants have to share their mother's breast milk, and twinning is much more frequent in the older mothers of high parity (146) who are likely to have less breast milk. Certainly in West Africa, the chance of twins surviving in the past was poor indeed, and even with improved care it was difficult to bring them successfully through infancy and childhood.

Poor weight gain in the first 6 months of life

Infants who gain little weight in the first few months are those who receive little breast milk. Poor weight gain needs to be sought out carefully in this age group as, if early supplementation can be achieved, much ill-health and difficulty in management in the second year of life can be prevented. This study focused attention on the need for a satisfactory weight gain in the first months of life if the child is to do well later. In the author's experience, a baby who gained less than 0.5 kg (1 lb) in any month of the first 3 months, or 0.25 kg (½ lb) in any of the 3 months of the second trimester was likely to be poorly nourished later, particularly if this poor gain was repeated in a succeeding month (*Figure 50*).

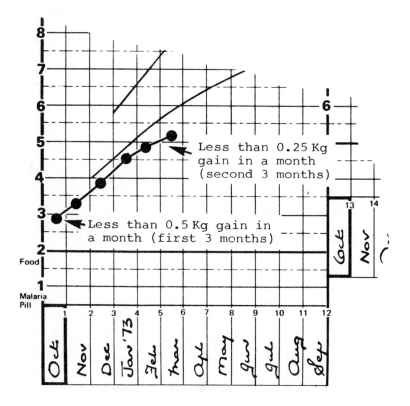

Figure 50. Significant poor weight gain in the early months of life

Such children appear perfectly normal and are overlooked unless weighing is carried out regularly and the weight charted, and even then as shown in *Figure 50* the staff need to be well trained to observe this poor gain in weight. However, there is need to identify them, as steps

164

taken early to increase their food intake will be easier and much more effective than waiting until the first signs of poor growth show clinically.

Poor weight gain in this first 12 months of life is serious. The brain at this time is growing and laying down new cells more quickly than at any other time. If growth is seriously retarded in this period, later intellectual development may be impaired.

Difficulties in breast-feeding

The subject of difficulties in breast-feeding has been fully covered in Chapter 6.

An episode of measles, whooping cough, and severe or repeated diarrhoea in the early months of life

Measles, whooping cough and severe diarrhoea were the three most common infections to be recognized in these children. If the children had been more closely studied, urinary infection might also have been included, and in communities where BCG vaccine has not been used tuberculosis may be important. The tendency for all the respiratory and diarrhoeal infections to concentrate in the early months and years of life in developing countries is repeatedly stressed in this book. The interaction with the child's nutrition is particularly studied in the chapter on measles (Chapter 12).

From experience with the use of 'at-risk' factors, it is clear that many of them are likely to overlap. For example, the mother who was parity 7 + in the studied village was more likely to have a low-weight infant, and also the twinning rate amongst these mothers was as high as 10 per cent (146). These babies would be unlikely to gain weight well in the first 6 months of life, and they would have a clustering of at least three reasons for special care. As more experience is gained in the use of reasons for special care, it may be possible to reduce the number needed and give some an increased 'weighting' as being of greater importance.

OTHER STUDIES OF AT-RISK GROUPS

At-risk groups in developing countries

A study was made in St. Lucia of factors common to a group of 46 children with malnutrition at a time when the incidence of malnutrition had already declined (154). Common factors were (1) illiteracy; (2) the mother who worked out of the home; and (3) a history of a previous child with malnutrition.

Reasons for special care in 5,000 children in the Punjab were studied (153), and in this area they included (1) cessation of breast-feeding before 3 months; (2) serious disease of the mother, or low intelligence; (3) death or blindness in either parent.

In Zambia an arm circumference below 14 cm was found to be more significant than a single weight in predicting children nutritionally at risk (317).

A year's survey of all perinatal deaths occurring in a different rural Punjab population of 30,000 revealed that 74 per cent of these deaths were identifiable as high-risk cases, according to the classification being used there (14).

The effects of season on birth were studied in the Gambia (172) and showed that children born during the early part of the dry season were particularly at risk during the following rains, and suffered more than children born during the wet season.

Many doctors would expect to find congenital abnormalities and haemoglobinopathies placed high on these lists. They have not been included as, although they are frequently seen by paediatricians in hospital practice, they are uncommon at village level, and emphasis has here been placed on those conditions for which help can be effectively given.

At-risk groups in Europe

The at-risk groups defined by a psychologist (135) in England and now generally agreed on are not dissimilar to the groups defined above, and are included here for comparison in order of no particular significance.

(1)   Large families with low incomes.

(2)   Children living in urban conditions with insufficient play space, especially in flats and high-rise housing.

(3)   Families whose cultural conditions and social standards are different from those of the majority, and to which they have not yet become accustomed.

(4)   Families whose personal relationships are impaired.

(5)   One-parent families.

(6)   Those affected by serious or irreversible physical or mental illness, or a disabling handicap.

(7)   Families affected by sudden crises.

(8)   Children who have to live apart from their families for longer or shorter periods.

RUNNING AN AT-RISK CLINIC

A practical method of keeping children 'at risk' under surveillance has been developed (258). The road-to-health chart, made of stiff card and kept by the mother, which is described in Chapter 8 is used. Amongst those attending the Under-Fives' Clinics, the vast majority are either well or have only mild disorders. There are also a number who may be acutely ill and who need immediate therapy or referral to a centre with more facilities. There are always a few children who, with no acute illness, are nevertheless ill — either underweight due to various diseases, or with charts that show a period of failure to gain weight which is significant for that age group. This group of children are at risk, and are particularly liable to succumb to severe infection and chronic diarrhoea, entering a vicious circle of further malnutrition and further infection. The criteria of those at risk may well vary from area to area. The proportion of children attending the clinic who are put in this category should not rise above 5 per cent, as otherwise their management proves difficult. Where possible, they need to be referred to a smaller clinic where more time can be spent on them. A careful note of their address is taken, and a simple copy of their weight record is kept on a chart printed on white paper*.

This 'at-risk' or nutrition clinic in East Africa was run entirely by paramedical staff who had received additional training in a central nutrition rehabilitation centre. In the clinic 10—20 children and their mothers were seen on each occasion, and the weights were carefully recorded both on their own cards and on the duplicate paper record held at the clinic. Those who failed to come would be visited at home, if at all possible. At intervals, those in charge would check the paper weight charts held in the clinic, and those failing to gain would be referred back to be seen by them. These records were useful for teaching, and when the nurses had been particularly successful in treating a child, the paper record would be stuck up on the wall of the clinic as evidence of their success.

Use of local foods

In the management of these children emphasis will be laid on teaching the mothers the better uses of local foods and if possible the prepar-

*A stencil to fit a Gestetner or Roneo type duplicator for duplicating these paper charts may be obtained from TALC, Institute of Child Health, 30, Guilford Street, London W.C.1.

ation of these dishes in a local-type kitchen. Supplements should be limited and consist of local foods with a minimum of imported food if these have to be used. A good example of a successful locally produced food is the Hyderabad Mix. The ingredients for this are shown below.

Wheat 35 g	Skim milk 6 g
Groundnut 6 g	Sugar 11.5 g
Bengal gram 11.5 g	

Total contents: Joules 1,000; protein 10 g

Total cost: $0.03

The first three ingredients are roasted, ground up and mixed with the milk and sugar. The resulting powder is packed in a small polythene bag and sealed. This package supplies a quarter of the calorie and perhaps half of the child's protein requirement.

HOSPITALIZATION FOR MALNUTRITION

Management of malnutrition has been recently well described (141, 254). The advisability of spending resources on admitting children to

TABLE 27
Treatment of Malnutrition In and Out of Hospital (49)

Hospital treatment*	Total cases	Range mortality in hospitals
Central and South America (15)	3,276	11–30%
Asia (7)	980	12–46%
Africa (12)	8,746	8–52%

Further mortality after discharge: Asia 15%, 30%, 37%; Africa 18%; America 34%

Home and nutrition rehabilitation centres	Numbers treated	Mortality (%)
Peru	61	0
Nigeria	346	6
Haiti	56	0
Ghana	44	5
Kampala	112	8
Jordan	72	3

*Figures in brackets refer to the number of studies

hospital with malnutrition has been questioned. The results of treating children in hospital all over the world have been analysed and compared with the results of care provided by a nutrition rehabilitation centre (49) (Table 27).

Assuming that those hospitals which analysed and reported on their results were the best, then the overall hospital care of children with malnutrition may be even worse. Instead, emphasis needs to be placed on Under-Fives' Clinics and nutrition rehabilitation centres. This conclusion may be criticized on the grounds that those admitted to hospital are more severely ill. This is true but those managed in

TABLE 28
Summary of Management of Children Nutritionally At Risk

Grouping of children at risk	Suggested steps to be taken in their care
'At-risk' children	Relevant 'at-risk' factor entered under 'reasons for special care' as early as possible. Regular attendance encouraged to supervise weight, immunize early and treat infections. Special emphasis placed on feeding and giving supplements early if weight gain becomes inadequate
Children showing inadequate growth over a significant period, as indicated by flattening of the curve on the weight chart	A duplicate paper weight chart is kept in the clinic. Attendance at a less busy clinic may be necessary. Home-visiting increased
Continued poor growth. Early signs of malnutrition	Admit to a nutrition rehabilitation centre, or arrange daily attendance
Severe life-threatening malnutrition	Admit to hospital. By now long-term prospects may be poor

nutrition rehabilitation centres if untreated would have deteriorated and required hospital admission. Cook (49) estimated the cost of hospitalization to range from $95 to $950 per child, and for treatment by nutrition rehabilitation to vary from $25 to $70 per child.

The appropriate steps that may be taken with children at various levels of risk from malnutrition have been summarized in Table 28.

CHAPTER 10

Diarrhoea

The understanding and control of diarrhoea have high priority and broad significance, with implications beyond the direct morbidity and mortality this condition causes. In Europe, diarrhoea still ranks as the second most common cause of death in childhood. The same is true in the developing countries for communities where mothers still breast-feed. Where they have taken to bottle-feeding it becomes the first cause of death. Although diarrhoea is so important the wrong priorities are only too commonly accepted in its study and management.

GENERAL CONSIDERATIONS

Definition of diarrhoea

The term diarrhoea shall be used to mean 'an abnormal frequency and liquidity of faecal discharge' as defined in writings of Hippocrates. The term 'gastro-enteritis' is avoided as pre-supposing an inflammatory condition. The major endeavour in research on diarrhoeal disease has been to distinguish the aetiological entities within this syndrome which surely exist. In the developing world, diarrhoeal disease is endemic. The number of cases and deaths is especially high in children under 5 years of age.

Epidemic diarrhoea

Epidemics of acute diarrhoea are common. The reservoir of infection is usually in the prevailing endemic acute diarrhoeal disease of the regions in which these epidemics occur. An example is epidemic diarrhoea in nurseries for the newborn. Fortunately, it is only in industrial countries that newborns suffer by segregation away from their mothers and so these epidemics are largely restricted to these countries. Although the case fatality rate is high in these epidemics, they are sufficiently uncommon to make up only a small proportion of the total deaths from diarrhoea.

The second circumstance in which diarrhoea becomes epidemic arises when people who are largely strangers to each other become aggregated together and exposed to an unfamiliar environment. This situation may arise from natural disasters, man-made disasters largely due to wars, or among migrant or seasonal labourers, holiday makers and their families.

Weanling diarrhoea

An outstanding feature of acute diarrhoeal disease in the developing world is the frequency of cases amongst infants and young children during and after the weaning period. Malnutrition is especially common at this time, and the term 'weanling diarrhoea' (85) pinpoints the synergism that exists between infection and nutrition during this period (100). The weanling has been defined as a child in the course of transition from breast or bottle-feeding to an adult type of diet. The weanling period is the time during which breast-feeding is continuing, but other foods are being added, including also the period of 3 months immediately after discontinuing breast-feeding.

CLINICAL PICTURE AND AETIOLOGY

Clinical characteristics of acute diarrhoeal disease in infants and young children

The diarrhoeal diseases due to different organisms can seldom be clinically distinguished from one another, and in general, those in which an organism can be held responsible are no more severe than those in which no such cause can be found. An important distinction must be made in general clinical behaviour and severity between two groups (107). The first is common in children in Europe and amongst the economically favoured in the developing countries. In this group organisms such as Salmonella and Shigella are quite frequently found. There is usually a mild indisposition and discomfort rather than a serious morbidity. While severe cases arise with occasional mortality these are uncommon. The duration is short, and lasts 1 or 2 days, although loose stools may continue for a week. Deaths are few, although their number is important, as the total number of deaths in this socio-economically favoured group of children is small.

The second type in which recognizable pathogens are less frequently found occurs most frequently in less developed regions. The onset of clinical disease is acute and rapidly progressive, with liquid or semi-liquid stools varying from 3 to as many as 20 a day. A proportion of the children, usually about one-quarter, have blood or mucus in the stools, and frequently pus can be seen. Such diarrhoea is most common in the second year of life or, in some areas, between 6 months and 1 year when the crawling child is first exposed to heavy infection (133). The child's tendency to examine objects by putting them in his mouth, often combined with a poor state of nutrition, make him particularly vulnerable. Low-grade fever is usual, along with malaise, toxaemia, intestinal cramps and tenesmus. Children are usually ill for 4–5 days and often there is a simultaneous onset of respiratory tract infection. In more severely malnourished children, a milder diarrhoea with poor appetite and misery often follows which may last a month or more, and there may be regular recurrences of loose stools. The danger of this intermittent low-grade diarrhoea is that it may lead to less food being offered and further malabsorption of food in a child who is already undernourished. This recurrent form of diarrhoea may amount to 15 per cent of cases, but is usually limited to malnourished children, and is common following measles. In infants with diarrhoea and severe malnutrition, the biochemical disturbance is of a different nature from that in well-nourished infants. Dehydration and electrolyte imbalance are common, have often been prolonged, and are therefore frequently difficult to correct. They are made worse by many mothers restricting their children's already inadequate diet. Too often each succeeding episode of diarrhoea leads to a further decline in the nutrition of a child. As one episode of diarrhoea succeeds another, he progresses from being an under-grown child to become a child with marasmus, marasmic kwashiorkor, or even frank kwashiorkor.

Case fatalities rates for patients in the first and second years of life range from 1 to 4 per cent (100). At a later age, deaths are less frequent. The only other period when the case fatality rate is as high or higher is in small infants when they are of low birth weight. The mortality of hospitalized patients varies greatly. In some studies it has been as high as 30–40 per cent for young children (270), but figures below 1 per cent have been given for Papuan children treated by medical assistants using standardized techniques (18) described later in this chapter.

The mother's attitude to diarrhoea

In the mass of writing on the subject of diarrhoea, little has been said about the attitude of the mother and other relatives. Reference has already been made in Chapter 4 to the beliefs held in parts of Asia that, while mild diarrhoea can be well treated in hospitals, the severe variety is best cared for either at home or at a temple. To the Yoruba mother in Africa the word diarrhoea might on occasion mean constipation (89). As so often, the local term for a particular condition may bear little resemblance to its alleged scientific equivalent (181).

It seems that all communities hold the idea that some degree of 'starvation' is an essential part of the management of diarrhoea. This belief seems to be common to most if not all cultures. A recent example comes from Bangla Desh refugee camps where there were plenty of children running around, but at the back of the tents, lying apathetically, were malnourished, dehydrated children. The mothers said they had developed diarrhoea and were being starved to make them better. One does not have to look far for the origins of this belief. If a child is fed, this in itself is a stimulus to the gastrocolic reflex, increased peristalsis throughout the gut and passage of a stool, whether diarrhoeal or otherwise; this is likely to occur immediately after feeding. Also, if the intestine is considered as a tube, the quantity put in at the top will bear some relation to what appears at the bottom. Complete starvation clearly decreases the amount and volume of diarrhoea stools produced. Unfortunately, mothers – and through them many doctors – are frequently far more concerned with stopping a child's diarrhoea than with the close observation of his condition. Later, a plea will be made for the giving of energy foods in some form even to the child with the most severe diarrhoea, although rehydration is the immediate priority.

Another belief which is held in many communities is that constipation is serious. This probably arises from the fact that it occurs during fever. In many severe illnesses constipation is present, and in the terminal stages of most of them it may be absolute. Deaths, particularly in children, are so common and many mothers have ample opportunity to observe the constipation that so often precedes it. For this reason, many communities know of a variety of aperients, some strong and dangerous, and use them in any illness that leads to constipation. This 'urge to purge' is found in most societies, and medicines and infusions of roots and leaves are commonly given to breast-fed babies. In this instance the desire for such treatment arises because breast-fed babies pass stools infrequently. It is not uncommon for an English baby to remain a whole week without passing a stool and this is not considered abnormal (120).

Because diarrhoea is so common in the period lasting more than 2 years in which a tooth somewhere in the mouth is erupting, cutting of teeth is commonly considered a cause. In parts of South America if a child is cutting teeth the parent delays taking the child to hospital for 3 days; in the same region they believe that if diarrhoea stops suddenly this is dangerous. There is no evidence that eruption of the teeth is related either to diarrhoea or constipation.

There are various reasons why many dehydrated children particularly those in rural areas never reach hospital. A child's condition may deteriorate rapidly and yet his mother may not be able to make the decision to take him to hospital without his father's agreement, and many children die before this family decision is reached. Fear of an autopsy and the desire for the child to die at home, where his spirit may remain, are but two of the many reasons why children are not brought to hospital when they should be. Discovering and dispelling these beliefs is an important part of health teaching.

Causes of diarrhoea

The diarrhoeal stool has been a happy but rather barren hunting ground for microbiologists for many years. The recognized specific infectious diarrhoeas within the diarrhoeal syndrome include shigellosis, salmonellosis, diarrhoea due to enteropathogenic *Escherichia coli,* giardiasis, and amoebiasis. In the UK an aetiological agent can be identified in not more than 15–20 per cent of all diarrhoeas (55). The percentage may be a little higher in hospitals, but any figure over 40 or 50 per cent is unusual.

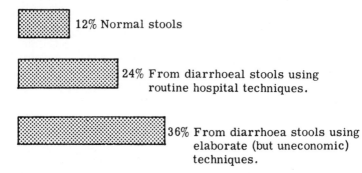

12% Normal stools

24% From diarrhoeal stools using routine hospital techniques.

36% From diarrhoea stools using elaborate (but uneconomic) techniques.

Figure 51. Proportion of children's stools yielding pathogenic bacteria (reproduced from Gordon et al., 1964, by courtesy of the Editor, Bulletin of the World Health Organization)

Only recently have random studies of stools of apparently well children been made in developing countries. Reports from several areas suggest that around 12 per cent of normal children contain one of the bacterial pathogens noted above. From children admitted to hospital 24 per cent or double this number have pathogens. The 24 per cent found by the use of standard bacteriological techniques are not necessarily from those children with the worst diarrhoea. In fact, the frequency with which a pathogen is discovered correlates poorly with the severity of the diarrhoea, and in many children with severe diarrhoea no pathogen can be isolated. A top figure of 36 per cent, 'positive' culture only, comes when several bacteriological methods not available in routine or in most university laboratories are used, including multiple samples and the use of many selective media.

Bacteriological culture of stools should in future be confined to research situations or where an outbreak of epidemic disease such as cholera is suspected. As a routine measure it is a poor use of resources.

The frequency of isolation of diarrhoeal agents is set out in simple, easily memorized terms in *Figure 51*.

Frequency of different infections

Infection with Salmonellae accounts for relatively few cases of early childhood diarrhoea in industrial regions and in many of the developing countries. However, they are more commonly found in some countries such as the Argentine, Tunisia, Costa Rica and countries in West Africa. This may be because Salmonellae, unlike other organisms causing diarrhoea, have a large natural reservoir in birds and reptiles, such as lizards and turtles.

Shigella sonnei predominates in Great Britain and other European countries. In developing countries organisms of the Flexner group are most common. In the Middle East, *Shigella boydi* is common but not before the age of 6 months. Unlike the Salmonellae, Shigellae are found only in man, and are spread by direct contamination with faecal material; they are rarely spread through water.

Serotypes of *Escherichia coli* rival Shigella as the commonest organisms found in bacteriologically differentiated causes of diarrhoea in early childhood. They are recognized more commonly in affluent than in developing countries. This organism is particularly important in the first year of life, and is the most frequently identified cause of epidemic diarrhoea in nurseries. It is easily spread from hospital to hospital by the transfer of children (234) and may remain viable in ward dust for 2 weeks. These apparently pathogenic strains of *Escherichia coli* may be identified in 15–20 per cent of normal toddlers' stools but how they become the predominant organism in almost pure culture in infants with diarrhoea is not yet adequately explained. The presence of the toxin responsible for the diarrhoea described below is unrelated to the antigens through which these strains are identified. The ease with which these strains establish themselves in infants undergoing neonatal surgery for malformations may be related to the nutritional state of these infants.

Viruses

The viruses now known cannot provide the answer to the aetiological enigma of the many children with undifferentiated diarrhoeas. In referring to the possible virological aetiology of diarrhoea, Joan Taylor (265) has written: 'This cloak for ignorance should be abandoned, for from the early days in 1947 to the present day, using modern methods of isolation and investigation, no one in any part of the world has yet produced good evidence of viral aetiology.'

Diarrhoea associated with measles was well recognized in the severe form of the disease in the last century and recently in developing countries (Chapter 12). This diarrhoea develops from the rash which affects the bowel epithelium equally severely as the skin.

Isolation of pathogens before and after diarrhoea

Relatively few workers have investigated the incidence of pathogenic organisms in the community and at the same time examined the incidence of diarrhoea and its relationship to these pathogens. One of the most sophisticated studies of this nature was undertaken in Vellore, India (125) *(Figure 52)*. In this study, routine rectal swabs were taken fortnightly over a period from all the children in the community, and at the same time information on the occurrence of diarrhoea was obtained and culture made from it. The results were analysed, using each child as his own control before and after the episode of diarrhoea. The results are shown diagrammatically in *Figure 52*. The vertical dotted line represents the episode of diarrhoea and the frequency of isolation of various organisms before, during and after this episode is plotted.

In this study the correlation between the presence of pathogens in the stool and the episode of diarrhoea is poor, and could be shown to be statistically significant only in the case of Shigella and poliomyelitis viruses. Even with these, the incidence rose only from around 8 per cent in the case of Shigella to around 15 per cent during the episode of diarrhoea. Experience has shown that when 'carrier states' exist, they can be better identified by giving an aperient to increase the frequency of the stools and make them more liquid. It is possible that some of the increase in the rate of isolation of pathogens from the stool during diarrhoea in this study arose because the diarrhoea has made apparent a pathogen, which was there all the time.

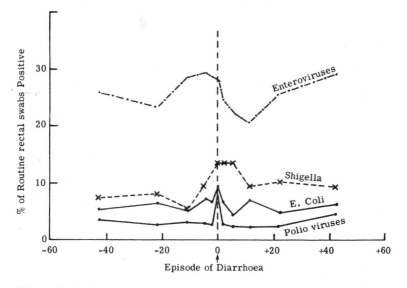

Figure 52. Isolation of pathogens before and after an episode of diarrhoea (reproduced from Jacob, 1968)

The large number of infections from which a child may suffer is well illustrated in the Central American study shown in *Figure 53*.

Other specific microbiological and parasitic causes of diarrhoea

Typhoid. — Many paediatric textbooks suggest that typhoid is neither common nor severe in infants and young children. A recent study suggests that this statement may need revision, and that if *S. typhi* is sought for by blood culture it can be isolated frequently (197). The disease is then found to be common, but presents an unfamiliar clinical picture. This usually includes fever, with or without diarrhoea, convulsions, and particularly anaemia.

Cholera. — El Tor cholera has now spread throughout Asia and to most areas of Africa, and is likely to spread to all other areas of the developing world. It has been said that those who 'wear collars and ties' rarely develop cholera, and that, like other diarrhoeal diseases, it depends on the socio-economic conditions and the nutritional status of the people. Whereas in traditional cholera only one or two carriers exist

177

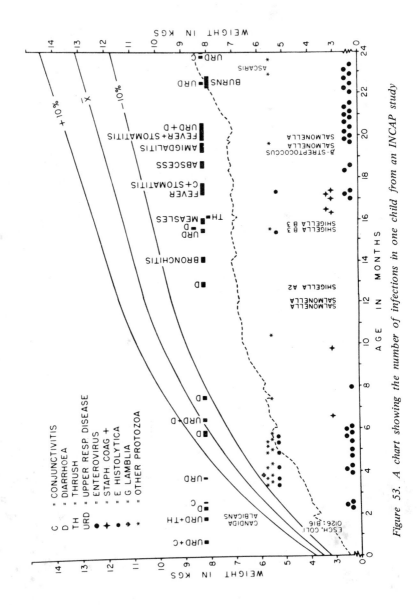

Figure 53. A chart showing the number of infections in one child from an INCAP study

for every infected individual, as many as 20 asymptomatic carriers may exist for every clinical case of El Tor cholera. Young children who are already suffering from malnutrition are those most likely to succumb to the disease. Unless special arrangements are made in cholera epidemics it is likely that the different electrolyte requirements of children will be overlooked. In particular, the standard regimens rely heavily on the drinking of large quantities of 'free' water, in which electrolytes are not present, and the young child may be unable to take this quantity (103).

Proteus morganii. – *Proteus morganii* was believed to be the cause of the 'summer diarrhoea' found in the UK (265) which was common in the early twentieth century and did not finally disappear until about 1947. Before then it was an infection that occurred most commonly in badly nourished infants and young children in poor families living in overcrowded and insanitary dwellings; although not certainly distinguished from other forms of diarrhoea, its disappearance may have been due to improved nutrition of the children through the child welfare movement rather than any dramatic improvement in sanitation.

Amoebiasis and giardiasis. – These are both found in older children but are probably rarely responsible for diarrhoea in the important weanling group in some areas, although giardiasis has been implicated as a cause of diarrhoea in this latter age group. Many doctors have questioned whether helminths are responsible for diarrhoea. In a Southern Indian child population there was no relationship between worm infection and diarrhoea (123).

Epidemiology

In considering their spread, the diarrhoeal diseases will be treated as a group, in spite of the possibility of their being due to such indefinite and diverse infectious agents. Man is the only important reservoir of infectious agents and the carrier state is essential in its spread. In a Guatemalan village, in children under the age of 5 years without diarrhoea, approximately 8 per cent carried Shigella, 0.1 per cent Salmonella and 4 per cent pathogenic strains of *E. coli*. The immediate source of infection in most transmissable diarrhoeas is almost certainly faeces, and spread occurs by direct hand-to-mouth infection. Flies probably do not play such an important part in transmission as was at one time thought, although they may contribute at certain seasons.

The classical picture of epidemic diarrhoea is one of infection derived from a common source, such as water, milk or solid foods, with the outbreak rising and falling abruptly. Such epidemics are not a common feature of diarrhoea in rural societies of developing countries, and in particular weanling diarrhoea does not fit this picture.

Multiple index cases and little
secondary spread

Epidemiological study shows that diarrhoea differs from many other infectious diseases in which the school child frequently carries the infection into the household, and where secondary cases occur particularly in the children under 5 years. In diarrhoea the usual index or primary case is in the young child himself. For example, in a study among 390 family outbreaks during 12 months, 71 per cent occurred first in the pre-school child aged 5 years or under (28). This frequency was out of all proportion to their number in their families. Of these index cases, a third were infants under 1 year. In this study, the appearance of disease in more than one member of a family within a period of 24 hours, that is multiple index cases, was observed in only 1 per cent of family outbreaks. As multiple index cases are characteristic of common source epidemics such as water and milk, this suggests that the latter were not a major cause of transmission. In this study, the incubation period was taken as less than 7 days, and on this basis overall secondary attack rates for the 390 families were only 1.4 per cent, suggesting that most family members were immune, or that the communicability of the agent was low. Even where there were two or more pre-school children within one family, the secondary attack rate among these siblings was only 4.1 per cent. These epidemics of diarrhoea evolve slowly. There is seldom a large number of cases in a short time as would be expected in a common source outbreak. The epidemic may follow a protracted course, sometimes running into years.

There is the characteristic, in rural societies, of a large number of index cases scattered throughout the community developing diarrhoea, secondary cases within the family being the exception rather than the rule. The most likely explanation is that a diarrhoeal agent is spreading throughout the community, that many members are probably infected, not once but many times, and that it is the children in the weanling group, who are particularly susceptible and who develop an actual diarrhoea. If this statement is accepted the present methods of attempting to prevent diarrhoea will have to be considerably modified.

Malnutrition and diarrhoea

Several countries where weanling diarrhoea is a major problem have developed a system of rehydration centres. A visit to one of these centres shows that two problems exist: one is the diarrhoea and dehydration, and the other the poor nutrition of most children who attend them. A statistical relationship between the frequency of a child's diarrhoea and his nutritional state has now been established. Table 29 (242) is a good example. The figures in this table show the tendency for diarrhoea to occur in the undernourished child, but it is

TABLE 29
Nutrition and Diarrhoea

		Normal	'First-degree' malnutrition	'Second-degree' malnutrition	'Third-degree' malnutrition
Number of children		25	74	71	9
Attack rates of diarrhoea cases/year/ 100 children aged 0–4 years	All diarrhoeas	99	164	253	275
	Severe diarrhoea	22	62	73	108

possible that even these striking figures may understate the case, because the system used for measuring poor nutrition is inadequate. The system generally used is the child's 'weight for age' and not his growth rate (that is his velocity of weight gain or his velocity of height change), which is a more accurate indication of nutritional status. As shown in *Figure 36,* children with kwashiorkor may have a weight equal to the local ninety-seventh centile, whereas children who are nutritionally satisfactory and gaining weight may be only on the local third centile. Further evidence for this belief comes from a study of diarrhoea and malnutrition undertaken in South Africa (287). This study also compared the serum albumen levels, as well as the weight of the children. Not only did the 'underweight' children have a low serum albumen, but also a number of the children with diarrhoea, although more than 80 per cent of 'normal' weight, had low serum albumen. Such children may well have failed to gain weight for a number of months, and their nutritional state was worse than a single measurement of weight would indicate. Paediatricians from many countries are now paying great attention to the nutrition of children with diarrhoea. In Iraq the weights of 57 per cent of children with diarrhoea fell into the Gomez III classification and only 20 per cent were breast-fed compared with 63 per cent in a control group who were suckling (301).

Diarrhoea is most common as breast-feeding comes to an end and continues for at least 3 months after its cessation. In the village of Imesi, Nigeria this was the time of the greatest nutritional risk, and many children developed diarrhoea. One study has also shown that while diarrhoea is just as frequent during the early weaning period, when the child is still being breast-fed, it is in the later period, when breast-feeding has just stopped, that the mortality is so high. Malnourished children in New Guinea take longer to rehydrate and they stay longer in hospital (100).

As it has been seen, it is the growth failure which is probably the best indicator of liability to diarrhoea. This may in part be due to a deficiency in cellular immunity arising out of the effects of malnutrition of the thymus. At the cellular level, workers in Chile (29) suggest that in marasmus, in which growth has been slowed or halted for a longer period of time than in kwashiorkor, mitosis may be much reduced in a histologically normal intestinal epithelium (Table 30).

TABLE 30

Mitotic Index in the Intestinal Mucosa of Children with Protein–Energy Deficiency (% of Epithelial Cells Sharing Mitosis) (29)

	Mitotic index	Range	p
Normal infants (8)	3.8	2.6–4.5	–
Kwashiorkor (10)	3.0	1.8–3.7	0.02
Marasmus (8)	1.3	0.7–2.1	0.001

Other studies from Uganda, South Africa and Jamaica have not found a normal mucosa in the children with marasmus. The children in the Chilean study (29) had suffered from severe undernutrition from the first weeks of life, were true nutritional dwarfs and they were not suffering from diarrhoea; the findings of low mitotic counts suggest that the slow production of epithelial cells may be a response to a poor intake of energy. Thus not only has the child stopped growing, but also his intestinal villi of the mucosal lining of the intestine have not been 'growing' and produce fewer new cells on which secretions depend. An early and well-studied change in the intestine is the decrease in lactase leading to lactose intolerance and diarrhoea. While lactase is the most frequently affected, all enzymes may be diminished.

Infection of the small bowel in the
malnourished child

The human small bowel on a Western type diet, unlike that of the rat, is usually sterile. However, in diarrhoea due to enteropathogenic *E. coli* colonization of the small gut takes place. During the incubation period of 4–7 days, or sometimes longer, the organism can be isolated from the stool before the onset of the symptoms, but once the diarrhoea starts it may present in pure culture in the faeces (265). On the diet in developing countries the small intestine is not sterile. It may be that only when stasis occurs or the infecting dose is very large that conditions exist where bacteria can multiply and attach themselves to the mucous membrane of the bowel. Reliance can no longer be placed on isolation of recognizable serological strains of enteropathogenic *E. coli* as non-pathogenic strains have been shown to produce enterotoxin controlled by cytoplasmic DNA ('R' factor or plasmid) and the ability to produce this may be passed to other strains. Perhaps these toxins are more likely to be serious if produced in the small bowel as this is so much more vascular and they may be more readily absorbed. This suggests that many attacks of diarrhoea are of bacterial aetiology, but that stool cultures are of little use because the infecting agents are similar to those in the normal colon (99). The toxin is believed to be similar in its action to cholera toxin, it may have antigenic similarity or be identical (325). The flux of salts and fluid between the blood and intestinal lumen is decreased. The reduction is greater in the flux from lumen to blood so that the volume of fluid in the lumen increases. Recent research suggests that the effect of the toxin may be through prostaglandins.

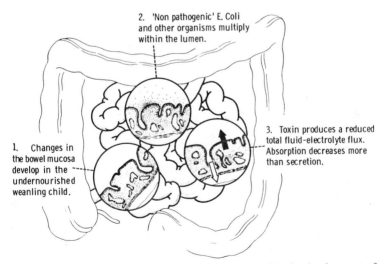

2. 'Non pathogenic' E. Coli and other organisms multiply within the lumen.

1. Changes in the bowel mucosa develop in the undernourished weanling child.

3. Toxin produces a reduced total fluid-electrolyte flux. Absorption decreases more than secretion.

Figure 54. Weanling diarrhoea. Stages in the small bowel in the development of this diarrhoea which is commonly unrelated to recognized pathogens

The train of events suggested here is given in *Figure 54*. This diagram offers a possible explanation to fit observations made on weanling diarrhoea in developing countries.

183

Summary

In summary, the new knowledge suggests that young poorly nourished children are much more susceptible to diarrhoea than older children and adults who may be equally exposed. They have to develop an immunity to many common organisms at a time of rapid growth and large food intake. If the dose of organisms is small, they may cope, if it is large, they may develop diarrhoea. This fact fits in with the knowledge that it is the volume of water used in the home rather than its purity which is important. The malnourished child has a shrunken thymus and his cellular immunity is depleted. His ability to develop a non-specific immunity embracing several similar organisms appears to be reduced.

PREVENTION OF DIARRHOEA

Health education

In health education in many countries, considerable attention is given to those aspects of hygiene believed to reduce the incidence of diarrhoea. Unfortunately, it is likely that much of this is ineffective. For example, stress may be laid on the boiling of water, although it is

TABLE 31

Annual Case Rates of Acute Diarrhoeal Disease by Age in Households With and Without Privies in Four Guatemalan Villages (Population 4,311)

Age (years)	With privies (rate/100 persons)	Without privies (rate/100 persons)
< 1	81	53
< 5	60	80
<14	8	12
>15	5	7

unlikely that diarrhoea is water-borne. Secondly, persuading people in rural societies to boil their water may in some communities be extraordinarily difficult, due to their beliefs about boiled and unboiled water (220, 189), and the effort and expense involved in carrying wood and in heating and cooling water with local utensils. Great emphasis has also been placed on persuading people to dig and use latrines. However, here again the evidence so far produced (28) showed that in children under 1 year of age, the diarrhoea rate in a village with privies was certainly no lower than that in an otherwise similar village without them (Table 31).

In improving hygiene, the step that seems to be of greatest importance is bringing piped water not only to the village but through a pipe and tap into the home. As long as water has to be carried from a central stand-pipe, it is little used, and only when there is a tap within the house is sufficient water used to reduce the diarrhoea rate. This step has proved to be particularly effective in reducing Shigella infections. A possible explanation is that the dose of bacilli received by the child is diluted by the use of larger quantities of water in the house. The health education of the mother should concentrate on the natural history of diarrhoea and the signs and symptoms of dehydration and salt loss. This training should have a high priority in the prevention of serious morbidity and mortality. Mothers will already be familiar with these changes, but they need to be able to express them and relate them to the action that they should take, and realize when it is urgent that the child should be referred to a health centre where parenteral fluid can be given if required.

Mother's observations

The mother needs encouragement in observation and in the recognition of dehydration and its significance. Remarks such as 'his eyes don't close properly when he sleeps' suggest, as is well recognized, the capacity for acute observation by the mother. Teach her their significance.

It may well be that the most effective teaching for reducing diarrhoea will not be concerned with diarrhoea but with improving the child's nutrition and maintaining his growth as shown on a weight chart. If a child is growing well, it is likely that his intestinal mucosa will be healthy, thus making him less prone to diarrhoea.

Finally, it is essential that mothers should learn how they can in their own homes improve the hydration of their child with diarrhoea.

TREATMENT OF DIARRHOEA

General principles

In most books on the management and treatment of diarrhoea, little reference will be found on how this can be managed at home, although in practice the vast majority of children with diarrhoea can well be treated in this way. Nor are the methods taught usually practical. Recently, particular emphasis has been laid on the need to examine more closely this essential level of health care in the home (256). In the developed countries the tradition as to what conditions should be treated in hospital or home is questioned and being made the subject of scientific enquiry. In the treatment of dehydration simple but practical methods of rehydrating their children need to be taught to the mothers (44). Mothers should use a rehydration kit which they can make up in

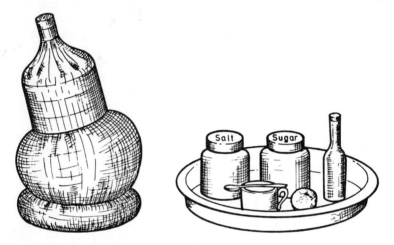

Figure 55. The rehydration kit consisting of a calabash and lid to hold water, a mug, spoon and tins of salt and sugar (reproduced from Church, 1972, by courtesy of the Editor, Tropical Doctor)

their own homes. The only essential pieces of equipment are some covered utensils in which to maintain water for the baby as clean as possible, salt and sugar containers with tight-fitting lids and a pint mug and a spoon *(Figure 55)*. Mothers are taught to measure 1.5 grammes of salt, using a 'three-finger pinch' *(Figure 56)* twice into the pint mug of clean water.*

Church (44) has shown that as long as the salt is a dry powder, a three-finger pinch is a more accurate measure than the wide variety of spoons suggested in the past. The mother is also taught to add to the solution about 30 g of sugar which can be most easily done using a 'four-finger scoop' *(Figure 57);* experience suggests that 30 g may be more sugar than dehydrated children can cope with at first and only a three-finger scoop should be used. In this way the use of 'spoonfuls' 'cupfulls' or 'ounces' can be entirely avoided. The sugar is important because not only is it a source of much-needed energy, but also a source

*In the original article two pinches of salt are suggested but this will lead to a slightly hypertonic solution and probably one pinch is safer.

of glucose. The most practical source of potassium in the home is an orange, the juice of which may be added. The success of oral rehydration with a sugar-electrolyte solution is based on the knowledge that glucose absorption by the small bowel remains intact during cholera,

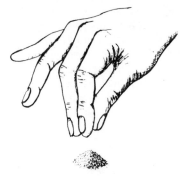

Figure 56. The thumb and two-finger pinch equals 1.5 g (reproduced from Church, 1972, by courtesy of the Editor, Tropical Doctor)

and presumably also in *E. coli* and other diarrhoeas in which a similar toxin may be at work. The glucose is linked to sodium absorption in such a way that a molecule of sodium and chloride, and with it water,

Figure 57. The four-finger scoop of sugar equals 30 g, a three-finger scoop may be sufficient (reproduced from Church, 1972, by courtesy of the Editor, Tropical Doctor)

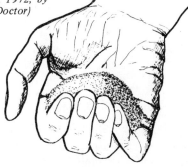

are absorbed by a mechanism which is independent of the electrolyte secretory process stimulated by cholera toxin (222). Adding glucose will enhance the speed of absorption of water in the child with diarrhoea (127). Thirty grammes of sugar will produce a 5½ per cent solution. In the severer stages of a diarrhoea perhaps only half this quantity will be more suitable.

Mothers with dehydrated children should sit down with a set of this equipment in the clinic, prepare the solution, and then with cup and spoon rehydrate their children under the supervision of the nursing staff. The quantities the child requires are given on page 191. The frequency of feeding is particularly emphasized and should at first be continuous and later hourly using small volumes of the solution. The mother is persuaded to do the same thing in her own home whenever the child develops diarrhoea or if there is any other cause for the child to become dehydrated, for example with a high fever. Emphasis is made to the mother that not all of what is taken by mouth ever comes out as a stool — a lesson she will understand best when she has seen one of her children recover through her own efforts.

Treatment of the dehydrated child

From many methods and regimens for the management of the dehydrated child, the one recommended was chosen because it has stood up to the test of time. The method described here has been used extensively by medical assistants and nurses in Papua New Guinea. In their hands there has been a mortality around 1 per cent. In one hospital a mortality under 1 per cent was achieved in treating 4,000 consecutive cases (18). The standardized treatment regimen is based on the following five points, each of which begins with 'D' — the initial letter of diarrhoea.

      (1)   Dehydration
      (2)   Diagnosis
      (3)   Drugs
      (4)   Diet
      (5)   Disaccharidase deficiency

Dehydration

Emphasis is placed on early rapid rehydration as it is the loss of fluids and electrolytes, with resultant acid—base disturbance, that causes death. Rehydration is obtained simultaneously in the following ways.

(1)   Early intravenous rehydration, as soon as dehydration is detected clinically.

(2)   Continuing breast-feeding.

(3)   Oral or intragastric fluids with sugar (glucose if possible) and electrolytes.

Intravenous rehydration. – Only one type of intravenous fluid is used, namely 2.5 per cent dextrose in half-strength Darrow's solution. The electrolyte composition of this fluid is as follows.

Sodium	–	61 mEq/l
Potassium	–	17 mEq/l
Chloride	–	52 mEq/l
Lactate*	–	26 mEq/l

Intravenous fluid is given by means of a scalp vein needle inserted into a vein on the dorsum of the wrist or ankle. Only occasionally does the medical assistant or nurse find it necessary to shave the scalp to find a vein, and cut-downs are rarely necessary. Auxiliary staff readily learn to insert scalp vein needles under supervision following adequate training.

Intravenous fluid rates are given as follows.

(1)   The child's weight in kg × 20 equals number of ml of fluid given fast (in about 4 hours).

(2)   If the child's weight is under 5 kg, 25 ml per hour is given.

(3)   If the child's weight is 5–9 kg, 50 ml per hour is given.

(4)   If the child's weight is 10–14 kg, 75 ml per hour is given.

(5)   If the child's weight is 15 kg or over, 100 ml per hour is given.

These instructions may be further simplified by the use of a weight chart on which the amounts are set out. The medical assistant knows the weight of the child and where this goes on the chart and can deduce from this the amount required *(Figure 58).*

The initial amount of fluid equivalent to the child's weight in kg × 20 ml is repeated as necessary every few hours if the child continues to appear dehydrated clinically. The child's state should be frequently reassessed.

The intravenous fluid is obtained in non-collapsible plastic or glass containers, so that the amount of fluid given can be readily measured. A strip of paper is gummed down the outside of the container on which the times that the fluid level should have reached each hour are written. The nurse, who with the mother watches the drips, ensures that they do not stop and regulates them so that the fluid levels in the containers keep up to time. Overhydration is uncommon. Oedema of the eyelids is the earliest sign of this and is readily recognizable by the nurse. Should this occur, she stops the drip and notifies the doctor. No other treatment beyond ceasing the intravenous fluid has been found necessary.

*Lactate is not an easy substance to handle in modest pharmacies, and acetate may be used to replace it (326)

DIARRHOEA

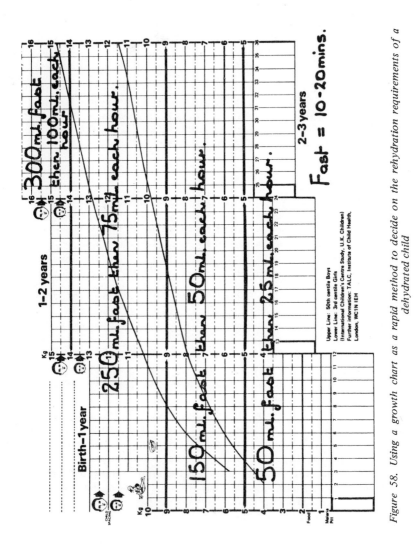

Figure 58. Using a growth chart as a rapid method to decide on the rehydration requirements of a dehydrated child

190

The intravenous fluids should be stopped when the child is drinking well, vomiting has stopped and the stools are no longer watery and frequent.

If the child shows evidence of vitamin A deficiency, this should be given by injection as a water-soluble solution. At other times vitamin A is better absorbed if given orally in oil but after diarrhoea all the bile salts are washed out and absorption is poor.

Oral fluids. — A sugar—salt solution is made by dissolving 2 level tablespoons of sugar, 1 salt tablet (2.6 g) and 2 potassium chloride tablets (1 g) in 1 litre (1,000 ml) of previously boiled water (or the method suggested on page 186) can be used. Oral fluid, either as a sugar—salt solution or as sweetened condensed milk diluted 1 in 8, is fed to the child by the mother every 2—3 hours throughout the day and night, using a cup and spoon or an intragastric tube. Calculate the amount of oral fluid to be given at each feed as 1 ounce (30 ml) for every kg of the child's weight, every 3 hours, with a maximum of 8 ounces (240 ml).

Recent work on the treatment of cholera, which resembles acute non-specific diarrhoea in young children, has shown that oral or intragastric sugar—electrolyte solution can replace continuing stool losses in most patients. It cannot substitute for intravenous fluids in the initial correction of dehydration, but by replacing fluid losses in the stool it reduces total intravenous fluid requirements and lowers the cost of treatment.

If a child is vomiting, the oral fluids should be stopped for a few hours and a single small dose of intramuscular chlorpromazine is given, no larger dose than 5 mg being needed.

Diagnosis

Each child should be checked for other illness besides the diarrhoea. As mentioned earlier, the frequency of a concomitant respiratory infection with diarrhoea is high in many epidemics, so look for evidence of such infection or its sequelae, such as, otitis media or bacterial pneumonia. It is probably better to consider these as having a similar cause than to use the term 'parenteral diarrhoea' which suggests that infection in a middle ear or elsewhere can be responsible for the diarrhoea.

Drugs

Minimal use of drugs is advised. In countries where malaria is still endemic antimalarials are routinely given for most illnesses. The general trend is to move away from the use of antibiotics in diarrhoea, and the majority of large children's hospitals no longer use them for this purpose. Laboratory reports which include antibiotic sensitivities play some part in encouraging and maintaining the use of antibiotics (75). Most studies have shown that antibiotics play little part in reducing the period of diarrhoea or stay in hospital. Another reason for giving them has been in an attempt to reduce the infectivity of the child for other children, and through this the spread of the diarrhoea. However, studies on the use of antibiotics in carrier states have shown how ineffective these are, and investigations even suggest that the duration of the carrier state may be prolonged by the administration of antibiotics, and person-to-person spread encouraged (8, 66). Paediatricians who limit the use of antibiotics for most diarrhoeas will frequently wish to give antibiotics to severely ill children with fever, toxaemia, convulsions and a bloody diarrhoea. Which antibiotics will be used will depend on investigations and local availability. There is little justification in using other preparations, such as kaolin, pectin, or Lomotil; although these may alter the frequency and consistency of stools evidence does not exist that they alter the mortality. Their use focuses the attention of the staff on the diarrhoeal stools and distracts from the urgent need to rehydrate the child and restore his intake of nutrients.

Diet

Children should be encouraged to eat as soon as they are willing — the child's mother who should be sitting beside him ought to persuade him to eat what she knows he likes. If a child fails to take any of the 4 megajoules he requires in one day, he will clearly be unable to take 8 the following day. Calculations show that to make good the energy and protein lost through even one day of starvation requires many days or even a week of refeeding. Except in the period of acute and severe dehydration those caring for the child should be encouraged to give him food. Few studies have been undertaken on the degree to which children absorb various nutrients during episodes of diarrhoea but those that have been done suggest that most nutrients are more than 60 per cent absorbed, and that for this reason every effort should be made to feed the child. Even if this does prolong the number and frequency of the child's stools, he will improve more rapidly.

Disaccharidase deficiency

Temporary lactase deficiency has already been mentioned as playing an important part in causing diarrhoea. The practical application of this is that the stools of all malnourished children who have diarrhoea should be tested for sugar. The simplest test in use is the Clinitest Reagent Tablet. Liquid stools are collected on a plastic sheet, because bed linen or napkins will absorb the sugar contained in the watery part of the stool. Five drops of liquid stool are then pipetted into a test tube and 10 drops of water and 1 Clinitest Reagent Tablet are added. The colour of the solution is observed after 1 minute. If the colour goes beyond that indicating 0.5 per cent of sugar in the stool, then it is definitely positive. Alternatively, Benedict's solution can be used (8 drops of liquid stool are added to 5 ml of Benedict's solution which is then boiled). Tests, such as Clinistix, which only test for glucose cannot be used as the usual offending sugar is the disaccharide lactose. If lactose is present in the stool, milk should be reduced or withdrawn from the diet. Feeding mixtures can be used containing some other carbohydrate which will usually be glucose, or failing that the more expensive fructose.

The significance of widespread lactose intolerance with an early decline of lactose in the small child is still uncertain. However, milk will probably be unsuitable as a basis of diet in many parts of the world and substitute protein-rich foods are likely to be developed.

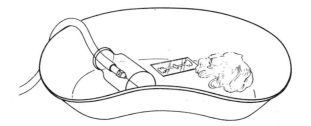

Figure 59. Total equipment used in Brazilian rehydration centre

Rehydration centres

Rehydration centres are well established in South America. The author had the privilege of visiting some in Brazil that had been in existence for 10 years. The intravenous transfusions were given by women who in the early days had been illiterate; by now those employed had some basic education, but no specific training other than in the techniques they were using. There were over 30 infusions in progress in the centre. The equipment consisted of a No. 20 needle mounted in the rubber tubing of the infusion set, and a razor blade when it was necessary to shave the scalp *(Figure 59)*. No special scalp-vein needles were used. The results were highly successful with an overall mortality of only 2 per cent in spite of the poor nutritional state of many of the children.

Other methods of rehydration

The widespread availability of intravenous methods makes other methods less satisfactory. However, fluid can be given intraperitoneally, or by clysis (subcutaneously) using the thigh without hyalase, which can be satisfactory in the less severely dehydrated children and may have to be used if the local staff are not yet familiar with intravenous methods.

Another route for rehydration that has been used successfully in children with a collapsed peripheral circulation is the internal jugular vein (166). This method has also been used on a larger scale by workers in other studies.

Link between rehydration and nutrition rehabilitation

The emphasis in this chapter has been on malnutrition as a major factor in childhood diarrhoea. So far in most countries rehydration centres and nutrition rehabilitation centres have developed separately. The newer understanding of diarrhoea suggests that in the future these two services should be linked or even amalgamated.

PRIORITIES

If the mortality from severe diarrhoea is to be reduced, the following points should be put forward as priorities.

(1) Improving the nutrition of the children.

(2) Improving the community's water supply.

(3) Teaching the mother how to recognize and care for a mildly dehydrated child at home, and how to recognize when to take him to a health centre or hospital.

(4) Providing all health centres and hospitals with a standardized and auxiliary-based method of intravenous rehydration.

CHAPTER 11

Acute Respiratory Infections

GENERAL CONSIDERATIONS

Respiratory infections are the most common cause of death in childhood, both in industrialized countries and in those in the developing world. In the latter countries the greater frequency of respiratory infection in the young children leads to a high mortality probably associated with the greater danger of obstructive inflammatory changes in their small air passages. This chapter will also emphasize the need to educate both medical and auxiliary staff and the general public in their better understanding, so that the limited resources especially of antibiotics can be better used (37).

In the search for a working classification, that from Newcastle (52) has been chosen as the simplest and most suitable for general use. This classification groups acute respiratory infections such as colds, tonsillitis sometimes with pharyngitis and otitis media, croup, bronchitis and pneumonia.

In the temperate climates, colds, bronchitis and pneumonia are usually thought of as a connected group with a high incidence in the winter months. On the other hand, tonsillitis and otitis media which are put separately in the Newcastle classification have much less of a seasonal incidence. Their causal agents also show little tendency to spread to the lower respiratory tract. A serological survey (290) of severe respiratory infections in many developing countries suggests a similar pattern of causal organisms as in temperate zones with the respiratory syncytial virus (RS) being most common, those in which bacteria were isolated also showed similar organisms.

If auxiliaries are to be taught how to care for these conditions, a clear definition is necessary, and the following categorization is suggested.

Clinical categories in acute respiratory infections

Colds

The main feature of colds is nasal discharge — watery, mucoid or purulent. In more severe colds there is malaise and moderate fever.

Tonsillitis and pharyngitis

Tonsillitis and pharyngitis are illnesses with sore throat in older children and a range of fever and malaise. The tonsils and pharynx are 'red', sometimes with yellow exudate.

Otitis media

Otitis media is an illness with fever, malaise and variable ear pain. There is redness or swelling of the drum, or purulent discharge.

Croup (laryngitis or laryngotracheitis)

Croup is an illness with varying degrees of fever, coryza, hoarseness, croaking cough and stridor. Increasing respiratory obstruction and cyanosis are present in the severe forms.

Bronchitis

Bronchitis is a febrile illness with moderate constitutional disturbance, cough and, in younger children, wheezing. Widespread rhonchi and râles are heard in the lungs.

Bronchiolitis

Bronchiolitis is an acute illness affecting infants and young children. After a cold for one or more days, there is the swift development of rapid respiration, expiratory wheeze and distressing cough. Fever varies in degree or may not be present. The excessive pulmonary distension may be visible and there is lower chest recession. Radiographs show air trapping, peribronchial thickening and sometimes subsegmental collapse.

Pneumonia

Pneumonia presents in two forms. It can present as an acute illness with fever, pallor or cyanosis, restlessness, cough and rapid respiration.

The main signs in the lungs are diminished air entry and localized or widespread crepitations and fine râles. Radiographs show lobar, segmental or lobular consolidation.

Pneumonia can also present as an illness in which the onset is insidious and the constitutional disturbance less intense. The degree of fever is more variable and lassitude, cough and localized râles may persist for several weeks. Radiographs show segmental or subsegmental more commonly than lobar shadows.

Unclassified respiratory infections

Illnesses which are regarded as respiratory infections but which do not fit satisfactorily the above definitions are grouped together under the term unclassified respiratory infections.

Malnutrition and respiratory infections

In writing on measles, a strong correlation between nutrition and infection was postulated. In general respiratory infections, such interactions are more difficult to define. Clearly, respiratory infections do have a place in the nutritional state of children. This is particularly so in the child who is dependent on one or two meals a day of a large and bulky staple which may have to be taken in competition with other children from a communal dish. If in such a child an upper respiratory infection reduces the intake for even as little as 2 days, the child may have considerable difficulty in making up for this period of poor intake over the succeeding days and possibly weeks. Similarly, the baby who has chronic nasal obstruction may have difficulty in breast-feeding resulting in poor growth and maramus. The mothers need to be taught that during respiratory infections the child requires even more frequent meals if the energy and protein intake is to be maintained.

When writing about measles it was suggested that this disease might be as much as 400 times as severe in some populations, and that this difference was largely due to the nutritional state of the child. To what extent respiratory infections are worse in the malnourished child is still unknown. Clearly, the child with kwashiorkor who, if undisturbed, will lie immobile for hours at a time, is highly susceptible to bronchopneumonia, and a terminal pneumonia due to staphylococci, pseudomonas, or coliform organisms is common.

In milder degrees of malnutrition the evidence that the child is more liable to a severe respiratory infection is still lacking. If cases of more severe malnutrition are excluded, poor nutrition is not a major cause for the high mortality from respiratory infections in developing countries. The cause for this high mortality is more likely to be found in the increased incidence of droplet infections in younger children, and in the absence of facilities to treat these infections with antibacterial drugs, with a lack of adequate oxygen and other supportive therapy in the early stages. Malnutrition is more likely to develop in the child living in poor surroundings with a mother who is unable to cope well. As these are known in temperate climates to be also conditions in which respiratory infections are more dangerous, then clearly similar factors are operating, and it can be expected that malnutrition and respiratory infections will frequent the same families.

Seasonal and age incidence of respiratory infections

In the village of Imesi the incidence of measles was seasonal. A peak incidence developed in the months of January, February or March. All respiratory infections also seemed to be at their lowest level in the months of June and July, and to have a high level in the months of November and December and the first few months of the year. The high rate of respiratory infection in December would correlate well with the tendency for the population to gather for celebrations at this time of year. These were due to festivities associated with Christmas, and even more to the fact that the ground had by this month become too hard and dry to farm, while the scrub was not yet ready to be cut down and burnt off.

June and July were months when fewer children were brought in with respiratory infections. However, this may well have been due to a proportion of the families living out on their farms during the whole of the week in these months, and only returning to the village at the weekend. This dispersion would reduce the spread of droplet infection.

There is no direct relationship between low environmental temperature and respiratory infection. The association that has been noticed between these two is more likely to be due to the tendency for the population to live indoors, associated with reduced ventilation, during cold and wet periods, increasing the opportunities for the spread of droplet infections. In Nigeria, the mean daily temperature shows only slight variation and respiratory infections were most common in some of the hottest months of the year. Here, the environmental temperature is not the main influence that decides the level of droplet infection. Instead, it is the season of celebrations that is responsible for a high level of droplet spread. In this, as in most communities, there is a strong belief in the association of environmental temperature and respiratory disease. In some countries, particularly those of Western Asia, this belief results in the children wearing excessive clothing, which may cover almost all of their bodies, and may be in part responsible for the high incidence of rickets found in some communities bathed in sunshine. Fortunately, this was not found in Nigeria and the majority of infants and toddlers wore few, if any, clothes.

The increased incidence of all droplet infections in younger infants in Imesi was found also in another study carried out in East Africa (217). The figures are compared with a previous Newcastle study in Table 32 (the same definitions are used in the two studies). This table

TABLE 32

Respiratory Illnesses During the Second Year of Life

$$\left(\frac{\text{Total Number of Illnesses Recorded in 1 Year}}{\text{Number of Children at Risk}} \times 100 \right)$$

Illness	Namulonge (217) (Uganda, 1969–70)	Thousand family survey (303) (Newcastle upon Tyne, 1948)
Colds	167	109
Bronchitis	62	12
Pneumonia	29	3
Tonsillitis Pharyngitis Otitis media	74	13
Unclassified	29	11
Number of children at risk	42	847

demonstrates the much greater risk of children aged 2 years suffering from pneumonia, which as already suggested is responsible for much mortality.

Health education

Emphasis in health education is largely placed on prevention, but the mother can do little or nothing to prevent respiratory infection except perhaps to keep her small infant away from crowded places, advice she may be unwilling to accept. However, she needs guidance in the management of respiratory infections in the home. She should learn the need to maintain the child's fluid intake and encourage him to eat as much as possible. In dry areas of the world she should know how to raise the humidity round the child by hanging clothes rung out in water. The greater danger and fast progress of infections in the first year of life must be known to her as well as the urgency to bring children with rapidly moving alae nasi, grunting respiration, listlessness and loss of appetite.

INDIVIDUAL CONDITIONS AND THEIR MANAGEMENT

Colds

Two forms of colds may be recognized, the mild and the severe. Mild colds are afebrile with watery nasal discharge and little obstruction or cough, and do not lead to much loss of appetite or alteration in behaviour. Only in the infant do they need treatment if they are associated with any difficulty in breast-feeding. Under these circumstances the mother may be supplied with 0.25 per cent ephedrine nasal drops in saline. These need to be introduced with the infant's head dropped well back over the mother's knee, so that they pass upwards into the nasal cavity and not straight back into the throat.

Severe colds are often febrile with malaise and loss of appetite. The nasal discharge may be purulent and there is likely to be a cough, probably associated with a postnasal discharge. Such a cold may upset an infant and may be associated with abdominal pain and diarrhoea. Certainly, if the nasal discharge continues for more than 10 days, there is a need for antibiotic treatment, as there is a likelihood of chronic sinusitis developing.

Bronchitis

Bronchitis is a febrile illness with cough as the main symptom. The child is not severely ill and rhonchi are found in the chest. Usually it lasts for only 7–10 days, but it may continue with persistent cough and malaise for a month or more.

Bronchitis in the older child does not require antibiotic treatment. However, if there is any doubt, it is better to treat it as pneumonia. In most communities mothers have come to expect some form of cough medicine for their toddlers with bronchitis. If this is not supplied by the doctor, the majority of mothers will obtain a cough medicine from other sources in developing countries.

Medical auxiliaries as well as doctors need to bear in mind at all times the possibility of an inhaled foreign body as a cause of unexpected wheezing attack or bronchitis. Groundnut or maize seeds in the respiratory tract are one of the most hazardous surgical emergencies in infancy, indicating transfer to a centre well equipped for removal of the obstruction in a bronchus (278). There may be physical signs in the form of diminished breath sounds over one are of the lung, or a radiograph, particularly if taken in expiration as well as in inspiration, may reveal the diagnostic tension emphysema.

Pneumonia

Pneumonia is an acute respiratory infection with fever, cough, pallor or cyanosis, restlessness and rapid respiration, often with movement of the alae nasi. It is recognized above all by the severity of the illness rather than x-ray changes or signs discovered by auscultation.

In developing countries, the priority is that this condition should be recognized for what it is by first of all the mother and relatives, and secondly by the medical personnel available at village and clinic level. This recognition will be of avail only if adequate supplies of suitable low-cost drugs of the sulphonamide range are available at the periphery, backed up where possible by an antibiotic. The blame for these not being sufficiently widely available can frequently be laid at the door of the physicians' organizations, usually based in the large cities, who have no appreciation of the difficulty of bringing a child with pneumonia to a hospital and create legislation limiting the availability of these substances to use by doctors.

Pneumonia in the older child

Frequently, pneumonia in the older child can be treated on an out-patient basis, particularly if the child lives in the environs of the hospital, or can remain there for 2–3 days. If there is no improvement within 48 hours, or if there are indications for the use of oxygen, such as restlessness or cyanosis, then the patient clearly needs to be admitted. The presence of other diseases, such as malaria must also be considered. Among other parasites special mention should be made of tropical eosinophilia and its association with filarial infection (278).

Pneumonia in children under the age of 3 years

In Europe, pneumonia remains the chief cause of death in the first year of life after the hazards of birth have been passed. The failure of the parents and the medical attendants, even in the UK, to appreciate the severity of this illness is shown by the fact that in the early 1960s, more than one-half of those who died from pneumonia died in the home. Health education has almost certainly failed in the past in this field. Health education on the early recognition of severe respiratory infection already described is particularly necessary. Pneumonia may be 10 times as common in the first year of life (see Table 32) in developing countries.

The younger the child, the less capable the mother and the greater the danger. The respiratory infection which is a cold in the adult may be a bronchitis in the toddler and fatal pneumonia in the small infant. The virus that gives symptoms in the nose and throat is also likely to be present in the lower respiratory tract, and the small diameter of the infant's bronchus may be one reason why pneumonia is so frequently fatal in this age group.

The majority of infants who develop infections of the lower respiratory tract respond satisfactorily to standard methods of treatment with antibiotics, oxygen, humidity and when necessary tube-feeding. This is not true of around 5 per cent of infants, and if x-ray changes are present of around 10 per cent, or of those who present with circulatory or respiratory failure, or with a staphylococcal pneumonia. Among these children, even in expert hands, the mortality may be as high as 50 per cent. To save even this 50 per cent, in a large proportion such measures as intubation, control of blood carbonate level, and positive pressure ventilation may be required, and management is only possible in the few major centres in developing countries. In assessing the child's condition, the evidence of hypoxia, dehydration and heart failure is sought as all of these conditions are commonly associated with respiratory infections. Irritability and cyanosis indicate hypoxia which requires oxygen if available. Dehydration may be corrected with oral fluids or an indwelling catheter. Restlessness, if it fails to respond to oxygen, may respond to the cautious use of sedatives; Phenergan (promethazine hydrochloride) 1–1.5 mg/kg per day, divided into three 8-hourly doses or chloral hydrate 30 mg/kg also in 8-hourly doses can be used. Congestive cardiac failure is a common complication and should be suspected in the presence of a raised jugular pressure and an enlarging tender liver. As well as propping up in bed and receiving oxygen, the child should be digitalized. Digoxin 0.08 mg/kg body weight, one-half at once and the rest 8 and 16 hours later, should be given. A maintenance dose of 0.02 mg/kg of digoxin daily will be required as long as evidence of congestive failure exists.

Principle methods of treatment

The following are the four principle methods of treatment on which emphasis needs to be laid.

Antibiotics. – Sulphonamides, such as sulphadimidine, need to be widely available in rural areas of developing countries. Given in appropriate dosage they have a safe margin against toxicity and have a major part to play in overcoming respiratory infections. Penicillin will remain the second antibiotic to be used in many countries, and its low cost justifies this position. Chloramphenicol, because of its low cost and because it is the antibiotic most suitable for whooping cough, has many advantages. Those using it must understand the dangers of this antibiotic in the small baby, unless it is given in a suitably reduced and carefully controlled dosage. The medical auxiliary will of necessity be taught that where there is no improvement in 24 or 48 hours, the child must be referred to a doctor.

Humidity. – Due to the dramatic effects of antibiotics, many practitioners in developing countries do not place sufficient emphasis on other measures in the management of children with lower respiratory infections. Adequate humidity is one of the more important measures, particularly in dry climates. The humidity can be most satisfactorily raised by hanging round the cot or the room cloth which has been wrung out in water with a fan blowing if electricity is available. Steam kettles are unsuitable in a hot climate, as well as being dangerous, and other methods of raising the humidity by mechanical means are not generally available. This is part of the nursing that the mother can satisfactorily undertake herself.

Tube-feeding. – The child who has respiratory embarrassment may have difficulty in swallowing, particularly if only a few months old. For these infants, feeding through a nasogastric tube may be of considerable help in their recovery. Once passed, the polythene tubing may be left, *in situ*, for a week or more. Expressed breast milk is preferable for the young infant or one of the fluid diets mentioned in Chapter 12 on the treatment of measles may be satisfactorily used.

Oxygen. – Although the use of oxygen can be of enormous benefit, it is frequently not available outside a few large hospitals in developing countries. Where it is available, lack of equipment or an adequate knowledge of the use of the equipment reduces its value.

The small infant can be placed in a box with a transparent lid; the bottom of the box can rest on a plastic sheet on which the infant lies. In this way effective levels of oxygen can be reached without the danger of the child becoming overheated. Oxygen therapy for the older child is usually less satisfactory. The expense of purchase and maintenance of oxygen tents and the steps that need to be taken to keep them cool are not easily resolved.

Treatment near the home

In common with diarrhoea the vast majority of children with respiratory infection still receive no treatment other than in the home or in what facilities there are available in their village. For this reason local availability of antibiotics and personnel with a relatively simple understanding of their use appears to be the priority in reducing mortality from pneumonia. The medical assistant or nurse must be able to recognize which are severe cases, or when, because of the age of the child, specific therapy is required. For the remainder, a liquid that smells and tastes like a cough mixture but from which expectorants and sedatives are excluded may be essential, if the parents are to be satisfied and return with future respiratory infection in their children.

Indirect evidence for the priority of treatment in the home comes from a breakdown of health expenditure in the UK (211) (Table 33). While diseases of circulatory and digestive systems required much heavier hospital expenditure, those of the respiratory system involved larger expenditure in the home

TABLE 33
Distribution of Expenditure, UK National Health Service,
between Hospital and Domiciliary Service, 1961–1962
(Total Expenditure £ 665 million) (211)

	Home (£ million)		Hospital (£ million)	
Respiratory system	33.0	(5.3%)	22.1	(3.7%)
Circulatory system	14.5	(2.3%)	37.4	(6.2%)
Digestive system	10.5	(1.8%)	28.0	(5.4%)

Acute bronchiolitis

Acute bronchiolitis can be best considered a variant of pneumonia in infancy, although in an epidemic form it can be considered a distinctive clinical entity. In a high proportion of cases it is not due to a bacterial infection but rather to a virus infection, and probably well over two-thirds are due either to the respiratory syncytial virus, the influenzal virus or the adenovirus type 7 or 3. Some paediatricians oppose the routine use of antibiotics in bronchiolitis and keep these for those children who showed radiological evidence of pneumonia (115). Their practice is to give penicillin for 48 hours and then discontinue all antibiotics, and in 80 successive cases it was not necessary to give any further antibiotics. However, whether or not antibiotics are used in this

204

condition, it is clear that in the majority of children with bronchiolitis antibiotic treatment is of only minor importance. In the management of the child with bronchiolitis, maintaining the child's fluid and electrolyte balance, if necessary by intravenous therapy, is important. In severe cases digoxin, corticosteroids, humidity and where possible oxygen are required.

In summary, the management of pneumonia in childhood must depend largely on the early referral of these children to the best medical facilities available. At village level at least sulphonamide, and if possible some antibiotic, should be provided. Even the most junior members of the medical team need to have a simple effective regime for managing this conditon that can be so fatal.

Sore throat and otitis media

The incidence of streptococcal sore throat and streptococcal infection in general seems to show a wide variation in different parts of the world. In rural areas in West Africa, streptococcal throat infection is uncommon, and acute tonsillitis is rarely seen. However, this is not true of all hot areas, and in many acute rheumatic fever is a major problem. As with other diseases in developing countries, it may develop at a much younger age and for this reason be more difficult to diagnose and manage. No satisfactory explanation has been given for this difference in incidence of streptococcal disease. It is certainly not purely climatic, as there are regions such as Singapore, with a similar climate to West Africa in which streptococcal infection is important, and its complications, acute rheumatic fever and nephritis, are frequently met.

Of all acute sore throats, only approximately half will be due to haemolytic streptococcal infections, and not all children with acute episodes will require antibiotics. They should be given to the child who is ill, or where there is evidence of spread to the middle ear. The antibiotic of choice is penicillin. If the child has had a history of a previous discharging ear, or has evidence of a perforation, then antibiotics are required with each sore throat. Hyperpyrexia is particularly common with sore throats and any child whose temperature rises above 39.9°C (103°F) must be cooled by wetting the skin and fanning. As described in Chapter 14 aspirin may have a dual action in preventing fits and lowering the temperature.

Croup

Croup is a febrile disease, probably due to *H. influenzae*, although it may also by due to staphylococcal or streptococcal infection. Starting as a mild cold, it spreads down to the larynx, and the child very often

CHAPTER 12

'Severe' Measles

Measles will be described in detail for the three following reasons.

(1) Measles is an excellent demonstration of the interaction of nutrition and infection in the child.

(2) Severe measles is limited geographically to the developing countries, in some of which it is the most serious of the common infectious diseases of childhood. As a result of the strong beliefs held by the majority of peoples, doctors until recently have remained both ignorant of the severity of the disease and unable to guide parents in its management.

(3) Measles immunization is the most cost-effective public health measure now available to improve the health of children, if certain logistic problems can be solved.

INTERACTION OF NUTRITION AND INFECTION

Two separate forces are working to the detriment of the child who is both malnourished and suffering from an infection, and measles exemplifies this well.

In the malnourished child measles is more severe. A greater difference in severity is found in measles than in any other common disease. The malnourished child may have a mortality 400 times higher than his well-nourished counterpart with measles.

Measles has a deleterious effect on the nutritional status of the child more serious than any other common childhood infection. The evidence for this statement comes from records of children's weight loss and the finding that protein–energy malnutrition supervenes more frequently after measles than any other infection.

EPIDEMIOLOGY OF SEVERE MEASLES

Knowledge of measles built up during the last century suggests that densely populated countries can expect a measles epidemic every year,

207

with a peak incidence every second year, and only a few of the unimmunized will escape measles in childhood. In areas with smaller populations and poor communications, epidemics are likely to occur less frequently – at 7-year or perhaps 12-year intervals. Such areas are now experiencing epidemics more frequently, since with improvement in transport young children visit other communites more often. Island communities, or those which due to their geographical position could be reached only after a long journey, have in the past remained free of measles for long periods. Such places have experienced catastrophic attacks of measles. Good examples are the Fiji Islands and Terra del Fuego (114). In such epidemics, a considerable fraction of the population has died. However, the circumstances in these regions were different from those that exist at the present time anywhere in the world. In these isolated communities, when measles struck, whole families would be infected at the same time. There would be no one to fetch or carry even water, let alone carry out the tasks of gathering and bringing in food from the farm and preparing it. For this reason, there is little doubt that starvation would follow in the wake of the disease, as described in the *Lancet* (1875) (150) record of the Fijian outbreak in that year. ' . . . the great mortality has been in large measure due to the fact that the sick were exposed to the most unfavourable conditions. Unprotected from exposure, untended and untreated chiefly because of their unhappy prejudices . . . . '.

In Africa, records are available which show that measles has been a disease of young children for at least 120 years, and there is evidence that it has existed in the communities of Africa and Asia for many centuries. There is no reason to believe that the severity of the disease in these communities arises because it is to them a new or recently imported disease.

In most communities, there appears to be a seasonal prevalence of measles, although the nearer to the equator the community lies, the less marked is the seasonal increase. This seasonal variation in the incidence of measles may be related to humidity or temperature. In West Africa the relationship seems to be indirect; the land becomes too dry and hard to cultivate in December, and it is at this time of year that the people gather together for community celebrations. The young child attends these on his mother's back, offering excellent opportunities for droplet spread of infections. The epidemic will decline with the onset of the rains, and the dispersion of the people back to their farms.

The age incidence of measles in developing countries is unlike that of Europe. In *Figure 60* measles among over 13,000 African children is compared with the disease in England and Wales during

1965–66, before the widespread use of immunization. During the first 4 or 5 months of life, the child is spared recognizable infection by the presence of maternal antibodies. However, from the fifth month

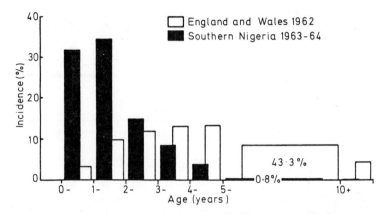

Figure 60. Comparison of age distribution in England and Nigeria. In Nigeria most children develop measles before the age of 3 years, in England many escape measles until after the age of 5 years

TABLE 34
Age of Measles in Developing Countries Compared with the United Kingdom

	Median age (months)	No. of cases reported
Jordan	18.0	2,038
Ghana	24.7	5,059
W. Nigeria	16.5	6,759
E. Nigeria	21.5	3,799
Uganda, Kenya, Malawi	18.5	2,997
Zambia, Tanzania and Rhodesia	29.7	2,801
S. Africa	29.4	1,364
England and Wales (1966)	51.7	343,525

onwards, the disease becomes increasingly frequent, and in urban communities, by the age of 1 year around a third of all the children will have suffered from the disease, while before the third birthday three-quarters are likely to have become infected. The median age for children with measles in Nigeria was 17 months. In Table 34 this is compared with other countries and with English children in whom it was 52 months.

Adequate information has now been collected to show that measles is associated with a high mortality. Few figures are available from community surveys. An exception to this is the study in the isolated village of Jali in Gambia (171) *(Figure 61)*. The epidemic of measles not

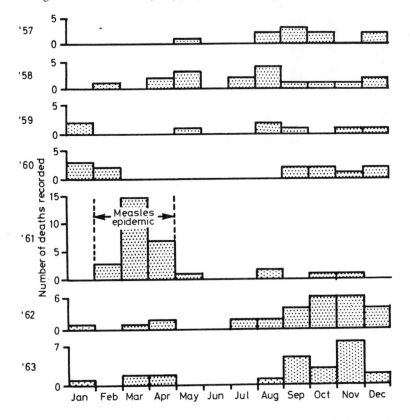

Figure 61. Mortality in the village of Jali, Gambi, from 1957 to 1963

only caused twice as many deaths in one month as in any other period but also reversed the pattern of mortality in that year. The highest mortality recorded in West Africa is from the records of an epidemic in Mali (121) where there were 78 deaths among 213 cases of measles – a 38 per cent mortality. This high mortality was in part due to food and fluid being withheld from those with measles.

A survey of the information available in West Africa suggested a case mortality of 3–5 per cent, but this may be a conservative estimate. In the village of Imesi, 15 (7 per cent) of 222 children died with the disease (163). The mortality in those admitted to hospital is higher. In West Africa, where figures are more complete than in other areas, the overall mortality was just over 12 per cent (188). However, in some hospitals, which only admitted children with the more severe forms of the disease, a mortality of between 20 per cent to over 40 per cent has been recorded. Mortality in other areas of Africa is perhaps not quite so high. For example, in East Africa the overall hospital mortality was found to be in the region of 5.5 per cent (190).

Outside Africa the severity of measles has been well recognized in South America. In Chile recently a 6.5 per cent case fatality in measles was reported and it was considered the most severe infectious disease of children in that country (232). In Brazil, a decline in overall case fatality, has been reported (182) but a recent combined study from PAHO *(Figure 62)* suggests that in the impoverished areas such as Recife mortality from measles is unrivalled by any other disease (226).

MEASLES IN CENTRAL AND SOUTH AMERICA 1972

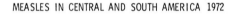

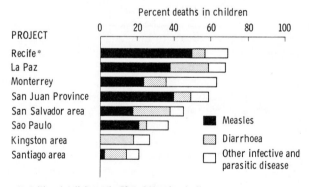

* Nutritional deficiency in 72% of Measles deaths

Figure 62. Mortality from measles in Central and South America in 1972. A high mortality is related to areas of poor nutrition

BELIEFS AND ATTITUDES TO MEASLES

No account of measles in the developing countries would be complete without reference to the beliefs about the disease, and how this affects the course of the disease, and whether children with measles are brought to the doctor.

In rural India, measles is believed to be due to a goddess, Matta. The child is likely to be kept in the dark at the back of the house. As even the neighbours are unlikely to be informed of the illness, the child is most unlikely to be seen by a doctor, and if measles develops while the child is in hospital, he may be taken home. In some areas of Africa the diet may be restricted, the fluid intake reduced and injections avoided. Overwrapping and consequent hyperpyrexia is another danger found in West Asian countries. For over a thousand years in Europe measles was thought to be due to the 'bad blood' of menstruation, which did not escape during pregnancy, went into the foetus, and came out later in the form of the rash of measles. A universal belief is that the rash must be allowed or encouraged 'to come out'.

Three proverbs collected from West Asia suggest the respect in which measles is held in developing countries:

A child that gets out of measles is a child that is reborn (Arabic)
Count your children after the measles has passed (Arabic)
Smallpox will make your child blind, measles will send him to his grave (Farsee)

The doctor's knowledge of the disease will be influenced by the attitude of his own culture to the disease, and if the traditional villagers do not bring the disease to him, and his experience is limited to his own children and those of his private patients, he is unlikely to realize its severity. The doctor's own training may have been influenced by teachers trained in the West and by textbooks written in Europe or America describing the mild disease. The delay in the appreciation of the severity and peculiarities of measles in the developing world arises from these strong beliefs about the disease which are found in rural societies.

Up to quite recently, the majority of doctors felt their responsibility did not stretch much further than the child patients in their wards and those who came to clinics. This attitude is now changing, and many doctors accept that their responsibility is to the whole community, and appreciate that what they experience in hospital (and private) practice is a one-sided view of ill-health in the community. Persuading the villagers of Asia to bring their children with measles for medical care against their local cultural beliefs could be an enormous task. Fortunately, this difficult piece of health education may be unnecessary. The introduction of measles vaccination should bring to an end this drama in which the measles virus, poor nutrition, and men's beliefs, have all played their parts.

CLINICAL MANIFESTATIONS

Skin changes

The progress of the rash and subsequent changes in the skin are different in severe measles. In the early stages of measles, the rash is similar and is preceded by the appearance of Koplik's spots in the mouth. In a proportion of children, however, the rash becomes confluent. In some it darkens to a deep red colour which may even progress to a violet or purple hue, a change rarely seen in European children. A few days after the appearance of this darkened rash an intense desquamation begins. Some desquamation develops in every child who has measles, the degree being apparently related to the extent to which the rash darkens in colour. When the rash acquires a purple hue, large scales of skin are likely to separate. The desquamation is more extensive than the mild and superficial desquamation now seen in European and North American children. There are two additional reasons for the rash being more apparent: (1) the scales are white and show up against a more pigmented skin; and (2) — as mentioned above — the parents believe that the child should not be washed during the illness, and washing might clear away an accumulation of scales. After the desquamation, there is a variable and patchy depigmentation which lasts for several weeks, and during this time the child is prone to develop a troublesome pyodermia.

The skin changes in the child with severe measles are similar to those which have been described in a number of historical accounts of the disease in England and elsewhere. The pride of place must surely go to the Arabian physician Rhazes (230) who, in his original classic description of measles in the year 850 A.D. said, 'Measles which are of a deep red and violet colour are of a bad and fatal kind.' A more recent and perhaps typical description of the same phenomenon is given in an eighteenth century textbook of medicine (33).

The changes in the skin deserve particular study and attention on the part of both the clinician and the pathologist. Variations in the type and appearance of the skin rash may well be correlated with changes in other epithelial surfaces, which in turn may account for the so-called 'complications' which have rightly been regarded as the cause of the majority of fatalities from the disease.

Probable results of equivalent changes on other epithelial surfaces

The possible association between the severity of the rash and the manifestation of the disease in other epithelial surfaces is summarized in *Figure 63*.

At the bottom of *Figure 63* are listed the stages of the rash seen on the skin and on the right the probable results of equivalent changes on other epithelial surfaces.

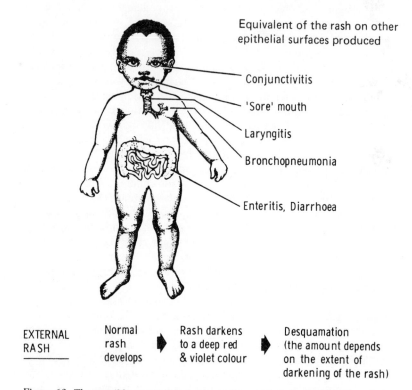

Equivalent of the rash on other epithelial surfaces produced

Conjunctivitis

'Sore' mouth

Laryngitis

Bronchopneumonia

Enteritis, Diarrhoea

EXTERNAL RASH	Normal rash develops	▶	Rash darkens to a deep red & violet colour	▶	Desquamation (the amount depends on the extent of darkening of the rash)

Figure 63. The possible association between the severity of measles rash and the manifestation of the disease in other epithelial surfaces

Changes in the mouth

Except for the discovery of Koplik's spots, the clinician in Western countries is seldom further concerned with the changes in the mouth. The mother who is accustomed to prolonged breast-feeding is alert to the occurrence of a sore mouth in her child, and often comments on the fact. Sixteen per cent of the mothers of a group of children in hospital in Nigeria said that this soreness was sufficient to prevent the child sucking for more than a day. In a few cases breast-feeding had ceased for long periods or altogether. On occasion the sore mouth and failure to suck led to engorgement of the breasts; damage to the nipple from attempts to feed is succeeded by infection in a cracked nipple with spread to the breast, causing a deep breast abscess. A sore mouth in measles was well recognized in England in the past; it was reported that the tongue and mouth become dry and ulcerated or covered with sores, and rapid emaciation took place (97). Cancrum oris or noma is a condition that has virtually disappeared from Europe, but it still occurs in some developing countries, where – as in the past in England and America – the sore mouth of measles is the common precipitating cause (266).

A sore mouth after the initial 3 days may be due to Monilia infection which is perhaps not unexpected in a child with an acute deficiency in cellular immunity. A 'slimy' mouth has also been recognized as sometimes being due to a concomitant infection with herpes simplex virus.

Laryngotracheobronchitis

If the epithelium of the mouth is affected, that of the larynx may also be involved. Laryngitis is frequent in children with severe measles, just as it was 60 years ago in England, when it was present in 8 per cent of children with measles.

If tracheostomy is required it carries a high mortality. In London in 1911 there were 248 deaths due to laryngitis associated with measles (229). The laryngitis may come on late, 1–2 weeks after the rash has appeared.

Bronchopneumonia

If the epithelial changes in the bronchus are similar in severity to those described for the skin, the frequency and severity of bronchopneumonia in children might be predicted. In Ilesha, of 604 children admitted with bronchopneumonia, 169 (28 per cent) died (183). In the village study, in which it was possible to follow up various stages of the disease, the bronchopneumonia developed at about the same time as the desquamation of the skin.

There are many accounts of the severity of bronchopneumonia associated with measles in the past. In an epidemic at the Necker Hospital, Paris, in 1845 22 out of 24 children with measles died from pneumonia (271). In England today, however, bronchopneumonia is no longer a frequent cause of death following measles. In a recent survey, measles bronchopneumonia was observed in only 3 per cent of previously healthy children (277).

Recent investigation of the infecting organisms in Nairobi showed a high incidence of Klebsiella and resistant staphylococcal infection, and kanamycin or gentamycin have been found to be required if many of these infections are to respond satisfactorily (84).

It appears that mortality from this condition in England was declining before the 1930s − that is, before the introduction of sulphonamides and antibiotics. Experience in Nigeria shows that these drugs are valuable in the treatment of measles bronchopneumonia and will prevent some deaths from this cause, but they can have been only partly responsible for the decline in the incidence of measles bronchopneumonia and the mortality associated with it in England during recent decades.

Diarrhoea

Changes in the epithelium of the gut are known to take place in measles. The diarrhoea so frequently associated with measles in developing countries may well be a manifestation of these changes in the intestinal epithelium. The more dramatic changes observed in the skin may well have a counterpart in the changes in the epithelium of the gut.

In an early account of measles in Africa dysentery and diarrhoea were considered more severe and fatal than pneumonia amongst children (60). The doctor who has received his training in the industrial societies of the Western world will be surprised by the prevalence of diarrhoea following severe measles. However, in the past it was important in England and America. In an account of measles in 1904, 28 per cent of the children attending a clinic for the London poor had diarrhoea (12). In earlier writings on measles in England, diarrhoea is frequently mentioned and, as in Africa, it was noted that the diarrhoea following measles tended to be chronic and to relapse over several weeks or months (60). Apparently the damage to the epithelium took some time to repair and recovery could be delayed by the poor nutritional status of the child. The severity of the diarrhoea may be worsened by purges in those areas where the bowel is believed to be the seat of the disease.

Effects on the eye

Microscopic section of the cornea during the acute stage has demonstrated the presence of corneal lesions of measles. As a loss of sight following measles is relatively common in some developing countries, the relationship between this sequel and a vitamin A deficiency has been explored in Rhodesia, where measles is a common cause of blindness. Serum vitamin A levels were reduced in kwashiorkor, but were even lower in children after measles (9). This fall may be in part due to the period of fever.

Encephalitis

The encephalitis and the frequent electro-encephalographic changes associated with measles have recently been made the subject of intensive studies in Europe and America. As facilities for autopsy and EEG studies are not widely available in Africa and Asia, the relative importance of encephalitis in the high mortality from measles remains unknown, although convulsive episodes and coma are frequent in children with severe measles.

SEVERE MEASLES: A RESULT OF POOR NUTRITION

Traditional factors of severe measles
The nutritional state of the child before and during the attack of measles appears to be the dominant factor in producing the severe form of the disease described above. However, some traditional reasons for this variation, such as virus virulence and host immunity, will be considered first.

Variation in virus virulence

While this possibility cannot be excluded at present, it seems unlikely that a virulent strain would remain confined to Africa and Central America and never, in these days of overnight transport, spread to Europe and America, where the disease is so consistently mild, except in the occasional malnourished child.

Variation in host immunity

Measles is not a new disease in Africa. The evidence for this statement, which has been given elsewhere (186), includes the following reasons: (1) measles was present in Accra in 1852; (2) there is a name for the disease in most of the local languages; and (3) in a relatively small community of about 200,000 around Ilesha, there were sufficient births to maintain measles as an endemic infection over an observation period of 9 years.

Experience from the United States of America suggests that racial factors are unlikely to be important. The mortality rates from measles in those with an African ancestry in the United States of America between 1921 and 1940 were similar and declined at the same rate as those derived from Europe.

Lastly, if there has been a change in 'herd immunity' in countries such as England, it is difficult to understand how it could have happened so quickly. In 1908 there was an epidemic in Glasgow with a case mortality of 5 per cent (41). Between 1961 and 1965 the case mortality rate in that city was only 0.13 per cent. In the early 1960s a review of measles in England and Wales estimated the case mortality to be around 0.02 per cent (10).

Variation in age specificity

The frequency with which measles is encountered in children under 1 year of age in Nigeria has already been stressed. The greater severity of the disease in infants compared with older children has been recorded by many writers. The report on recent mortality in England confirms that this trend in age mortality is still present today (10). In Nigeria, observation from Ibadan suggested that measles was more severe in the second and third years of life than in the second half of the first year (111). However, even if the age-specific mortality found in the UK is applied to the age distribution of the disease as recorded for Nigeria, the overall case mortality would be 0.6 per cent, whereas in fact it is in the region of 3–5 per cent.

Variation in the child's environment

This would go far to explain the variation between different regions and different socio-economic groups. In a poor environment the child may be open to more cross-infection. However, it could hardly explain the difference in the type of rash associated with the severe form of measles. The likely explanation is a deficiency of some as yet unspecified nutrient or nutrients.

Evidence connecting nutrition with severity

The evidence connecting nutrition with the severity of measles arises from historical records and from recently obtained knowledge of the variation of measles in differing present-day communities.

Historical evidence

This can only be indirect. In the detailed analysis of measles mortality in Glasgow (41), the mortality in children from families

SEVERE MEASLES: A RESULT OF POOR NUTRITION

which could afford to live in a house with more than four rooms was a quarter of that among children from families confined to one room *(Figure 64).* In this figure a four-fold difference is shown in mortality depending on the rooms available to the family.

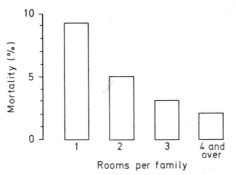

Figure 64. The relationship between mortality and socio-economic circumstances in 22,000 cases of measles in Glasgow for the year 1908

This extreme difference in mortality, depending on socio-economic circumstances is probably greater than in any other disease. The only group in which it was higher was in orphanages, where the mortality was over 10 per cent. In 1908 the difference in medical care available to the different groups is unlikely to have been responsible for the difference in mortality, but the variation in the nutritional status of children living under these two conditions is likely to have been considerable.

A severe epidemic of measles occurred in Sunderland, England, during a period of industrial depression accompanied by semi-starvation (71). There was an 8 per cent mortality among children with measles. In half the children the rash was darker than had been noticed in previous years.

The frequency of exfoliation, diarrhoea and other characteristics of severe measles in the past in England have been recorded in more detail elsewhere (183). The decline in the severity of measles was well established early in the twentieth century at a time when little improvement in the medical care of children had taken place and long before the advent of antibiotics.

Geographical evidence

As a result of the findings in West Africa a world-wide postal survey of measles was undertaken. From this survey a strong correlation was

219

discovered between the distribution of kwashiorkor and measles in different countries (186). There was also evidence that the mortality was higher in the under-weight children (190) (188).

In Lagos groups of children from differing socio-economic groups were studied (228). Those in the higher socio-economic groups were heavier and taller than those in less privileged groups, and developed a less severe form of measles with few 'complications'.

Recent research

Recent research in Africa (247) has given a possible explanation for this greater severity of the disease in the malnourished child. The immunity in measles is largely cellular and the rash is probably evidence that sufficient lymphoid cells have been produced to neutralize the virus by attacking and destroying the virus containing cells wherever they may be. In the child with malnutrition the reproduction of these lymphoid cells is delayed due to the lack of protein and other material required for cell multiplication. This delay allows the virus to increase in a logarithmic phase. As a result when sufficient lymphocytes are produced the destruction of cells is much greater; evidence of this is the endothelial damage leading to more extravasation of blood, or the rash and desquamation, or the bloody diarrhoea. Giant cells are present in the acute stages of all children with measles; in the well-nourished child they disappear in 1–3 days, but in severe measles they last for an average of 10 with a range of 7–29 days, and they have also been recovered from a blood diarrhoea for 28 days. It is possible that these children may continue to be infectious while secreting these giant cells.

DETRIMENTAL EFFECT OF MEASLES ON THE NUTRITIONAL STATE OF THE CHILD

Experience of many thousands of weight records plotted on the 'road-to-health-chart' (Chapter 7) has made it possible to determine which of the common infections of children were most likely to have an effect on the child's regular weight gain. Of these, measles was pre-eminently important as a disease causing loss of weight. The weight changes occurring after measles in 220 children in the village of Imesi were analysed and expressed as a percentage of the child's weight immediately prior to the measles infection. The results are shown in Table 35.

Almost 1 in 4 of these children lost more that 10 per cent of their former weight as a result of this infection. So much weight loss is serious among children who should be gaining weight regularly.

Information was also available on the time that a proportion of the children took to regain their weight. This is given in Table 36.

TABLE 35

Weight Lost During Measles by 220 Imesi Village Children

	Percentage of previous weight					
	None	Under 5%	5% +	10% +	15% +	20% and over
Number of children	24	71	72	34	16	3
Percentage of all children	11	32	32.7	15.5	7.3	1.5

TABLE 36

Time Taken to Regain Former Weight after Measles in Imesi Village Children

	0–4 weeks	5–8 weeks	9–12 weeks	Over 12 weeks
Number of children	77 (40%)	70 (36.5%)	16 (8.3%)	29 (15.1%)
	Mean period = 7.2 ± 0.45 weeks			

The time taken to recover former weight gives some indication of the duration of the disability; 15 per cent took more than 3 months, and the average child took 7 weeks. Children with diarrhoea took an average of 8.1 weeks to recover their previous weight, compared with 4.5 weeks for those with no diarrhoea.

The reasons for this loss of weight are multiple. There is a tendency to restrict the child's diet during measles, which accentuates protein-energy depletion. The foods given to a child are already predominantly starchy foods, and during an infection such as measles the few foods in the diet which are good sources of protein are less frequently given. The starchy pap or other simple staple diet is preferred as the only food for the sick child, partly because it is watery and easily fed to the child, and also because in some societies the traditional soups and sauces contain peppers and are unacceptable to a child with a sore mouth. In view of this weight loss, it is not surprising that measles has been implicated more frequently than other acute infections in precipitating acute malnutrition in many countries (21). A recent survey among better nourished children attending a welfare centre in Bombay showed only slight loss of weight.

MANAGEMENT OF MEASLES

If the children who are seen with measles are to be helped, the medical worker must have a detailed knowledge of local beliefs about the disease and about child feeding. Probably in few other diseases are local beliefs likely to affect the outcome to such a large extent. Measles is one of the so-called immunizing diseases of childhood, and except for 5–15 per cent of children who may undergo infection during the first 5 or 6 months, while still partly protected by their maternal antibodies (147), it is likely that all children will develop measles at some time. Assuming therefore a birth rate of 40 per 1,000, and making allowances for an increase in alternate years when the disease is more epidemic, there will be 30 cases of measles for every thousand of the population. From this figure, the doctor can calculate what proportion of children with measles are being attended to. Whether those who are brought to the doctor are a cross-section of the disease is problematical. Only too often the mother who is least willing to bring her child to seek medical care is also the mother who comes from the more impoverished family and is therefore least able to care for the children in whom measles is likely to be more severe.

Management of measles in the out-patient clinic

A number of other viruses may give a picture transiently similar to that of florid measles, and this has led most mothers and many doctors to believe incorrectly that the child can have measles twice. However, antibody studies suggest that this is unlikely. The diagnosis can be made with greater confidence if the child is seen on several occasions.

A difficult decision is which of the children require admission to hospital. An analysis of 4,500 records collected in West and East Africa (188) (190) suggests that the following clinical features are associated with a high mortality and can be used as criteria in deciding on admissions.

At all ages

The clinical features indicating the necessity of hospital admission are as follows.

(1) A rash that darkens or desquamates in large plaques.

(2) Hoarseness, particularly if there is any suggestion of laryngeal obstruction.

(3) Dehydration, blood and mucus in the stool, or more than five stools a day.

(4) Convulsion, or loss of consciousness.

(5) Underweight, particularly if below the local tenth centile. To help in identifying these children, it may be as well to have a spare weight chart kept beside the doctor in the Under-Fives' Clinic, on which the tenth centile line has been marked. The tenth centile for African village children runs as follows: 3 months, 4.2 kg; 6 months, 5.3 kg; 12months, 6.7 kg; 18 months, 8.1 kg; 2 years, 9.0 kg; 2½ years, 10.0 kg; 3 years, 10.9 kg; 3½ years, 11.8 kg; 4 years, 12.4 kg; 4½ years, 13.0 kg; 5 years, 13.5 kg.

Under the age of 3 years

The clinical features indicating the necessity of hospital admission are as follows.

(1) Soreness of the mouth, particularly if it interferes with suckling.

(2) Dyspnoea, particularly movement of the alae nasae, and increased respiration or other signs of pneumonia.

These are the children most likely to die, and they should presumably be hospitalized. Some doctors doubt whether hospitalization of these children, with its inherent dangers of cross-infection, does reduce the mortality, and is therefore justified (261).

No drug is known which influences the course of the virus disease. As the severity of measles depends on the state of nutrition, and the disease is so likely to be followed by weight loss precipitating the child into malnutrition, the maintenance of his intake of food and fluid at a satisfactory level must be a priority in treatment.

The importance of continuing breast-feeding for at least 2 months after measles should be emphasized. Unfortunately some mothers and even health workers see measles as a reason to stop breast feed and accordingly give disastrous advice to this effect.

If milk is available, it is frequently the food most acceptable. If skimmed milk only is available, then this should if possible, be converted into a 'filled' milk by mixing with oil (139). The best way to prepare this mixture will be to find a suitable small tin and mix together 10 volumes of skimmed milk, 2 volumes of a suitable locally used cooking oil, and one of sugar, to form a dry powder. This can be stored without going rancid for a week or two. The volume of oil may be increased, and any vegetable oil used in cooking is suitable. The resultant powder readily dissolves in cold water.

When mothers report that diarrhoea repeatedly develops with skimmed milk, this may be evidence of a lactase deficiency which may be congenital, or the acquired variety due to the poor nutrition of the child. The mother should be encouraged to persist, but if the diarrhoea continues some other form of animal protein should be made available; egg whipped up in boiling water, scraped meat, or meat powder are possibilities.

Attention must be given to the diarrhoea. A strong saline mixture containing a gramme of sodium chloride and a gramme of potassium chloride to the half-ounce may be available for the mother to dilute (half an ounce to the pint) and used for the child's drinks (see also Chapter 10).

In a disease as severe as measles, many doctors will find it difficult not to give the child routine antibiotics. However, the few controlled studies suggest that these do not prevent bacterial complications, and one of these studies suggested that those receiving a broad-spectrum antibiotic suffered more, as many became infected with Gram-negative and other resistant bacteria (279). In Africa, the author has used 5-day courses of sulphadimidine routinely, but no satisfactory evidence of its value is available. When the child's condition suggests secondary bacterial invasion, antibiotic therapy is essential. A combination of long-acting penicillin and streptomycin (10 mg/lb, or 20 mg/kg) is economical.

The immediate illness of measles will be followed by a period of ill-health lasting sometimes for several months — a period in which much of the mortality occurs. The child is in danger of a recurrence of diarrhoea, a breakdown of a previous primary tuberculosis, further respiratory involvement, or frank kwashiorkor, any of which may be fatal. This is a period when nutritional rehabilitation is essential, a testing time for the out-patient staff, and one when the simple weight chart will show whether the child's nutrition is improving.

Caring for children with measles in hospital

Measles is highly infective in the catarrhal stage, and in the well-nourished child excretion of virus declines within 24 hours after the appearance of the rash. As suggested already in the malnourished child this may not be so. Until further information is available on this point, these children must be considered as potentially infective.

Maintaining the child's hydration and supporting his nutrition will be given priority. For such children, the intake of protein and calories must be prescribed just as accurately as the intake of a drug. Techniques that have been developed in the feeding of children with kwashiorkor may well be used for the child severely ill with measles. Table 37 gives a diet that may be fed by tube. If there is still diarrhoea from malabsorption on this diet, the skimmed milk can be dropped for a few days and the Casilan increased to 45 g and the sugar to 40 g. If this diet is fed for more than a few days, special mineral and vitamin supplements must be added. Full details of these diets are recorded in the literature (254).

TABLE 37

The Ingredients and Nutritional Value of the Routine Casilan–Dried Skimmed Milk–Sucrose Diet (CaDSu)*

Ingredients of the 'dry' mixture (g)		Nutritional value per 100 g of reconstituted diet	
Casilan	33	Protein g	4.0
Dried skimmed milk	30	Fat g	6.1
Sucrose	30	Carbohydrate g	4.6
Cottonseed oil	60	Calories	90
Potassium chloride	2.7	Potassium mEq	4.7
Magnesium hydroxide	0.3	Magnesium mEq	1.3
Sodium chloride	None	Sodium mEq	0.9
Total	156		

*(1) The mixture of 'dry' ingredients is prepared for use by taking 156 g of this mixture and making it into a paste with a little cold boiled water, in scalded equipment, and then adding, gradually, enough cold sterile water to make a total of 1,000 g.
(2) The reconstituted diet is fed at the rate of 100 ml per kg of body weight per day.
(3) At present the cost of this diet is under 10p ($0.30) for a 10 kg child per day.
(4) For areas where weighing may be difficult, this diet may be prepared using volumes (for example, a cigarette tin): skimmed milk, 27 volumes; Casilan 10 volumes; sugar 10 volumes; oil 10 volumes and mineral mixture 1 volume.
A supply of mineral mixture from 4 volumes of potassium chloride to one volume of magnesium chloride should be prepared and marked Mineral Mixture, with the ingredients.
(5) Oral Abidec (Parke Davis), 0.6 ml and 5 mg of folic acid are given on alternate days and an injection of 1,000 μg of Vitamin B$_{12}$ is given on admission. These expensive vitamin supplements may not be necessary in all areas, but supplements of Vitamin A (5,000 IU daily) and folic acid (1 mg daily) are recommended in most centres. If clinical signs of Vitamin A deficiency are apparent (for example, xerophthalmia), then more intensive therapy is required.

MEASLES VACCINATION

Well-tried measles vaccines are now available, and in some developing countries their widespread use will do much to lower mortality and reduce malnutrition. A large body of experience from the use of over 50 million doses of this vaccine in Europe and North America has confirmed its safety, and in some countries measles is now uncommon. A large study has been undertaken using this vaccine in West Africa, and from this considerable experience in the use of the vaccine in the circumstances of developing countries has become available (176) (204). The young age of infection in developing countries makes effective control more difficult. With their high birth rate the unprotected population grows rapidly, and vaccination should be undertaken as far as possible in the ninth month, or soon after. If vaccination is carried out in campaigns, these will have to follow each other at not less than 6-monthly intervals. The necessity for a continuing or at least frequent vaccination is shown in *Figure 65*.

In *Figure 65* only limited vaccine had been available up to 1962. From the middle of 1962 vaccine became available except for periods towards the end of 1963 and 1964. Some recurrence of the disease developed in the epidemic seasons when vaccine supplies ran out, but was controlled when they again became available.

Questions that arise over measles vaccine

What vaccine should be used in a developing country?

Any of the further attenuated vaccines can be used, and as there is considerable price range it is worth discovering which of the reliable firms can supply at the most competitive price (194). Killed vaccine should not be used.

Can developing countries afford measles vaccine?

The cost of preventing measles in the United States of America has shown to be only a fraction of the cost of treatment (202). However, this argument will not apply to most developing countries, as the majority of children with measles go untreated. The principal cost of a new vaccine lies in its development, testing and initial production. The price of vaccines should fall in the next few years (194). Economy in the cost of syringes and personnel to give the vaccines is difficult. The wider use of jet injectors by staff specifically trained to use them offers scope for economy (153). Meanwhile, as it is a living vaccine, one dose, if its strength has been maintained by careful storage, may be divided effectively amongst several children. The 1 cc ampoule can be safely given in one-fifth doses to five children, as long as extra precautions are taken once the vaccine has been reconstituted. These include having all the children ready before diluting the vaccine, and not using anything other than soap and water to clean the skin, and wiping it dry. The vaccine and syringes should be kept cool, and this may most easily be achieved by preparing a box lined with polystyrene in which is placed a 'cold dog' that has been frozen overnight in the ice-box. Such a box can be easily made, is cheap, and effectively replaces a vacuum flask, which is so easily broken.

Can convulsions or encephalitis occur after measles vaccination?

A small proportion of children develop a convulsion when their temperature rises above 103°F, whatever the cause of the fever. Only 5–10 per cent of children receiving the further attenuated vaccine will develop fever of this level. For this reason, convulsions following its use are infrequent (1/1,000); convulsions with measles will be both more severe and more frequent (at least 10/1,000).

Abnormal EEG tracings are seen in over 50 per cent of children with measles but in less than 5 per cent of children with measles vaccination (94). In the United States of America in 1966 it was estimated that encephalitic illness occurred at a rate of 0.9 cases per million doses of measles vaccine distributed, and on detailed enquiry it was discovered that other agents were probably responsible for a number of these. For comparison, the incidence of encephalitis of unknown aetiology was 37 per million per year (202).

How long will protection from measles last?

As the first measles vaccination was given only 17 years ago, no answer can be given to this question. However, the evidence suggests that protection is prolonged and may be lifelong. The decline of antibody level following measles vaccination is similar to that seen following measles. The level in vaccinated children no longer exposed to measles falls below that which can be measured. If these children are re-vaccinated (or exposed to measles), a proportion will become 'infected' and show a rise in antibody level without any clinical manifestations (147). An account (215) of measles in the Faroe Isles in 1846 suggests that complete immunity established 65 years previously still existed among those who had not been in contact with the disease during that time.

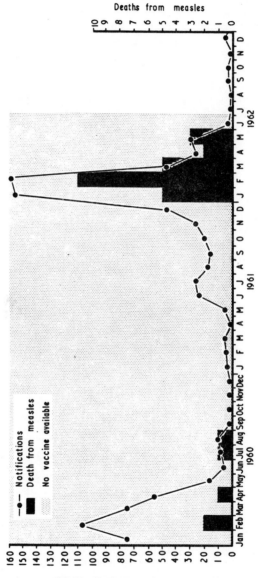

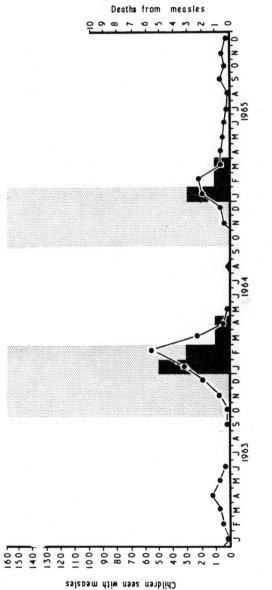

Figure 65. The effect of vaccination on morbidity and mortality from measles in Imesi, Western Nigeria, from 1960 to 1965

229

At what age should measles vaccine be given?

In countries such as Britain, where measles in infancy accounted for only 4 per cent of all notifications in 1966, the vaccine can be given after the first birthday. In the developing countries, where more than 30 per cent of children in urban areas may develop measles in the first year, the correct age presents some difficulties. A proportion of children given vaccine before the ninth month will not be protected, as the residual antibody they received from their mother will prevent the vaccine virus from multiplying. If, however, the vaccination is left till after nine months, a proportion of children will already have developed measles, and by the age of 1 year as much as a third of the children may have become infected. If possible, vaccination should be given between the ninth and tenth month of life, and vaccination programmes must be undertaken at least every 6 months or be continuously available.

What contra-indications are there to giving measles vaccine?

In the developing countries these are few, if any. The condition of the children with malnutrition may be made a little worse by giving them vaccine. On the other hand, if they get measles, many of them will die. If possible, children with malnutrition or with known primary tuberculosis should be under treatment for a period before the vaccine is given. If hyperimmune measles sera (gamma globulin) is available, 0.2 mg/lb given simultaneously with the further attentuated vaccine, but in a different site, will further decrease the reaction, but not interfere with the level of immunity developed. If a child has leukaemia, do not give him measles vaccine.

To prevent outbreaks of measles in a children's ward, vaccine may be used routinely on admission for all except the tuberculous or severely malnourished children.

CHAPTER 13

Whooping Cough

The whooping cough syndrome will be considered at some length for the following two reasons.

(1) It illustrates a disease which develops at a younger age, with a clinical presentation different from that taught in most medical schools.

(2) In the young infant it is rarely recognized, and its significance as a cause of mortality is underestimated throughout the developing world.

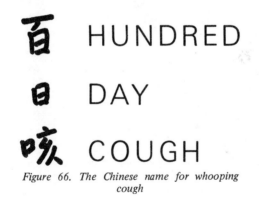

百　HUNDRED

日　DAY

咳　COUGH

Figure 66. The Chinese name for whooping cough

In the name given by the Chinese *(Figure 66)*, emphasis is laid on the long duration of this disease, which may be so debilitating to the child. In developing countries where illness is concentrated in the early years of life, whooping cough may overlap and aggravate many other infections.

EPIDEMIOLOGY

'The whooping cough is exquisitely communicable' (144).

Several workers in developing countries have suggested that the incidence of whooping cough follows the pattern found in industrialized countries 50 years ago (273) (187) (7) (36). The opportunities for infection at an early age are higher in developing countries, due to earlier exposure. This is brought out by the median age of infection, that is, the age when half the children are likely to have had whooping cough, and which is given for a number of countries in Table 38.

TABLE 38

Median Ages in Months
Based on the Number of Notifications Given in Brackets

	Measles		Whooping cough	
West Africa	20.0	(17,580)	24.4	(2,569)
East Africa	22.8	(5,798)	35.1	(2,778)
Congo and South Africa	29.3	(2,198)	23.6	(860)
Jordan	18.0	(2,038)	23.5	(942)
Lebanon and North Africa	30.9	(422)	35.6	(554)
England and Wales (1945)	53.0	(306,721)	45.6	(92,266)
Aberdeen (1890–1900)			38.4	(15,094)
Massachusetts (1945)			62.4	
Glasgow (1908)	49.0			

There are probably two prinicipal reasons for the earlier age of whooping cough and many other infectious diseases; (1) because the child is carried around more, and (2) because he comes from an 'extended' or 'joint' family. In the developing countries, infants are carried on their mothers' backs or sides as they go visiting, make their way to market, church, temple or other places of worship, and attend family and other reunions. In these circumstances, the chances of droplet infection by other sick children are greater than in industrialized countries. In rural societies of developing countries, 'extended' or 'joint' families are common, in which infants who are cousins or otherwise related may share a common home. In the industrialized countries, with their 'nuclear' families, the young infants are now largely isolated from other young children. The opportunities for droplet infection which existed in the past through overcrowding, and were so well described in Aberdeen (149), have now largely been overcome.

MORTALITY FROM WHOOPING COUGH AT DIFFERENT AGES

The frequency of death in whooping cough is closely related to the age at which the child is infected, and this makes the low age incidence found in the developing world of considerable significance. This relationship between age of infection and mortality has been brought out in most accounts of the disease, and is illustrated in *Figure 67,* which compares the age distribution of deaths from whooping cough in a hospital in Ilesha, Nigeria (187) with the city of Aberdeen, Scotland (149) in the nineteenth century.

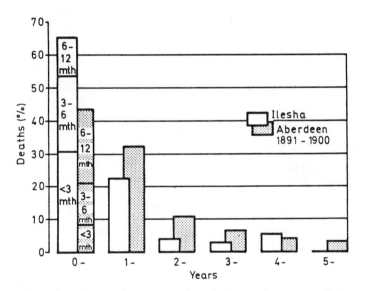

Figure 67. The age distribution of deaths from whooping cough in Ilesha, Nigeria, compared with Aberdeen before the turn of the century

The mortality in different age groups in the Ilesha hospital from whooping cough is similar to that recorded in Aberdeen in the past. There is a difference in the greater incidence of deaths in the first 6 months of life in the African children. In Ilesha the disease was particularly sought for in this age group, and all suspected children were admitted to hospital.

More girls die from severe whooping cough than boys. In this whooping cough is exceptional. In other common childhood infections, deaths among boys predominate. There is no satisfactory explanation for this difference, although there has been a suggestion from Scotland in the past and from the Ilesha study that some of this greater mortality may be due to the convulsions associated with whooping cough being more lethal to girls.

AETIOLOGY OF WHOOPING COUGH

In countries where immunization has not been undertaken, a large proportion of children with the whooping cough syndrome have been infected by *Bordetella pertussis* (1). *Bordetella parapertussis* is probably responsible for less than 5 per cent of cases, and virus infections are also responsible for only a small proportion of children with this syndrome. Viruses have received particular attention recently in industrialized countries, where the immunization programmes have made infection with *B. pertussis* infrequent. Unfortunately, the identification of *B. pertussis* by bacteriological culture has not been undertaken in studies in developing countries. Isolation of the organism by pernasal swab early in the disease, with immediate bedside plating (224) has made this a technique that should be available to clinicians where reasonable bacteriological facilities exist.

Bacteriological investigations show that the highest infective period is in the catarrhal stage in the first week. *B. pertussis* may be isolated from 100 per cent of patients in the first week, 95 per cent in the second and 94 per cent in the third, but by the fourth and fifth weeks this is reduced to only 44 per cent and 2 per cent respectively (68). *B. pertussis* can also be recovered from contacts who do not develop clinical whooping cough.

CLINICAL DIAGNOSIS OF WHOOPING COUGH

As the vast majority of children with whooping cough will have to be diagnosed, particularly at village level, by a knowledge of the clinical presentation, a better understanding of this is important. In some centres the diagnosis may at times be supported by a high lymphocyte count, and as the disease advances fairly specific changes may be found on x-ray.

Whooping cough should be considered as an acute respiratory disease, starting with a slight cough, usually accompanied by a coryza; the cough then assumes a frequency which is out of proportion with the thin nasal discharge, and comes in bursts. Unlike the child with bronchitis, the child with whooping cough does not take a breath in anticipation of a burst of coughing. At the end of the second week the coughing spasms increase in speed, rise in pitch, and the paroxysms become longer and more intense. The rapid spasmodic cough is at this stage generally associated with choking and vomiting, with the production of sticky, stringy sputum. In spite of the disturbing cough, auscultatory signs may be absent from the lungs and in the early stages the effect on the child's health may be surprisingly small (51). Oedema of the eyelids is more common in undernourished children and its presence is useful in aiding diagnosis (187).

In view of the universal practice of breast-feeding in most developing countries, the mother has an intimate knowledge of the state of her child's mouth, and the presence of whooping cough may be indicated by the way she picks the stringy sputum from the child's mouth. In small infants, in whom the disease is so dangerous, the diagnosis is more difficult; in these, the march of events outlined above provide valuable diagnostic criteria (51). The mother's knowledge of older children suffering from the disease in her area may help in reaching the diagnosis. A proportion of small infants may die of a 'suffocating' bronchospasm with their lungs full of tenuous viscid secretion without developing a characteristic cough.

Development of whooping cough

Periods of the disease

The classical description of whooping cough divides it up into a number of periods.

Incubation period.– The incubation period is between 6 and 12 days (224). At the end of this asymptomatic period a positive culture may be found.

Catarrhal period. – The catarrhal period lasts for 7–14 days. Cough and nasal discharge are present, and cannot easily be differentiated from any other upper respiratory infection, except sometimes by the march of symptoms as described above. In the younger infant the nasopharyngeal discharge in this period may be scanty.

Paroxysmal period. – The bronchitic cough becomes more and more severe until the typical paroxysms develop. There are bursts of coughing not preceded by inspiration, producing cyanosis, choking spells and vomiting, and ending with the typical whoop. This whoop is uncommon in children under 6 months, and is acquired in older children in order to replace the expired air rapidly by a forceful inspiration that causes a sharp blast through a half-opened glottis. During this stage, thick tenacious secretions are produced, and the child becomes exhausted. These attacks are brought on by attempts to feed the child, or by other disturbances, but can develop without any stimulus.

The violence of the paroxysms is often suggested by subconjunctival haemorrhages, epistaxis, haemoptysis and punctate cerebral haemorrhages, which may cause convulsions and coma. There may also be mediastinal emphysema, pneumothorax, or subcutaneous emphysema.

Convalescence. – The paroxysms of coughing tend to diminish from the sixth to eighth week, and usually around the ninth or tenth week the period of convalescence has started.

Period of recrudescence. – The period of recrudescence may last for at least a year, and in this period the child may develop an apparent relapse of the whooping cough. Various suggestions have been made as to the reason for this outbreak of what may appear to be typical whooping cough. Probably the most likely is that areas of lung remain collapsed, and these have been shown on x-ray for up to 10 months (81). These areas may become infected with an organism causing an upper respiratory infection, and lead to a fresh outbreak of the disease almost identical with that seen at the height of the paroxysmal stage. These are of course neither reinfections nor relapses of the original infection, and *B. pertussis* cannot be isolated.

Whooping cough in immunized children

A mild or modified illness is not uncommon in previously immunized children. It is usually so mild as to be of no more than nuisance value. This is not evidence of a failure of an immunization policy, as the primary objective of immunization is to prevent deaths and severe disease with complications.

Whooping cough in the very young child

The development of whooping cough is set out in *Figure 68.* This figure shows the relationship of the various symptoms, signs and laboratory findings in the average case, although there are likely to be wide variations in the timing (238). If this picture is now compared with that seen in the young baby under 3 months of age, the differences will become apparent *(Figure 69).*

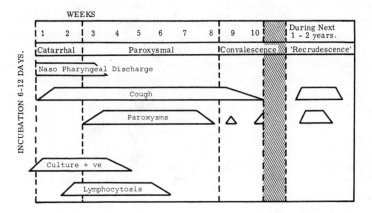

Figure 68. The natural history of whooping cough in the child

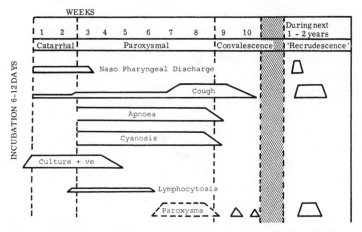

Figure 69. The natural history of whooping cough in infants under three months old

In the small baby, the nasopharyngeal discharge is less marked, as is the cough, and only too frequently attacks of apnoea and cyanosis may be the first sign of the disease. If the paroxysms appear, they may not be seen until fairly late in the course of the disease, from the sixth week onwards. The child may therefore die with very little cough in apnoeic or cyanotic attacks, and these are unlikely to be recognized as

237

whooping cough. Another difficulty arises in the apparent well-being of the child between the attacks of spasm. Whereas the child with measles bronchopneumonia is brought to the doctor breathing rapidly and with obvious auscultatory signs in the chest, the child with whooping cough may have a chest free of physical signs and be quietly sleeping on his mother's knee. With the pressure for admission that exists in all children's wards in developing countries, the small baby with whooping cough is unlikely to gain a cot, and may subsequently die in acute spasm at home, and the cause of death is likely to remain unrecognized and unrecorded. In the study village of Imesi, 367 children were at risk to the disease, and 206 were known to develop whooping cough before their fifth birthday. Among these there were 13 deaths for which whooping cough was considered to be at least partly responsible. Of these deaths, at least 5 were sudden and occurred in convulsive or apnoeic episodes.

WHOOPING COUGH AND MALNUTRITION

Although the malnourished child will clearly not stand up so well to the rigours of a severe attack of whooping cough, the disease does not seem to be so much more severe in the less well-nourished child. If we examine figures for whooping cough in Aberdeen (similar to those for measles in Glasgow — see *Figure 64*), we find that there was a socio-economic difference, although not so striking as in measles *(Figure 70)*.

Although whooping cough may not be so much more severe in the malnourished child, there is considerable evidence that whooping cough may cause malnutrition. Records of the loss of weight of a group of children are given in Table 39.

As will be seen from this table, the weight loss in children following whooping cough is less than that in the same village study following measles (compare with Tables 35 and 36). Weight loss may also be due to dehydration if the vomiting has been severe. However, when the time taken to recover from the weight loss is examined (Table 40), it will be seen that the recovery of weight lost is just as slow as after measles.

In the village study, the small child who developed whooping cough was particularly liable to a prolonged period of poor gain in weight, and whooping cough appeared to be a common cause of marasmus *(Figure 71)*. No doubt this could be related to the result of the baby being unable to suck during the severe part of the illness, which leads to a retention of milk in the mothers breasts and a reduction in the supply of breast-milk. Because whooping cough can occur in the first few weeks of life, and lead to a period of failure of growth in the important

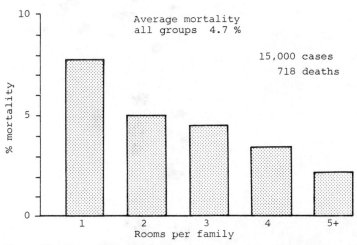

Figure 70. The relationship between socio-economic circumstances and mortality in 15,000 cases of whooping cough in Aberdeen, for the year 1882. Recorded deaths total 718

first year, it may have a considerable long-term significance in that these children are likely to grow up short in stature and possibly with an impaired intellectual potential. Even if these children showing

TABLE 39

Study of the Proportion of Weight Lost during Whooping Cough by 232 Imesi Village Children

	None	Under 5%	5%	10%	15%
Number of children after whooping cough	114 (49)	67 (29)	43 (18)	7 (3)	1 (1)
(figures in brackets refer to the percentage of children)					

marasmus following whooping cough are treated with antibiotics and dietary supplements, there may be difficulty in establishing satisfactory weight gain for some time. This difficulty almost certainly arises due to an inadequate calorie intake, which should be in excess of 150 cal/kg. In the older child who develops whooping cough, kwashiorkor is more likely to arise, and these children appear to be particularly prone to develop oedema and not the darkening and desquamation commonly associated with kwashiorkor after measles.

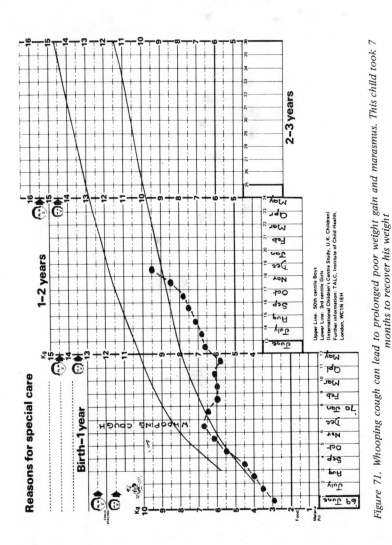

Figure 71. Whooping cough can lead to prolonged poor weight gain and marasmus. This child took 7 months to recover his weight

TABLE 40
Time Taken to Regain Weight after Whooping Cough

	0–4 weeks	5–8 weeks	9–12 weeks	Over 12 weeks
Number of children after whooping cough	50	37	14	17
Proportion	43%	31%	12%	14%

Other complications

A common complaint in Africa in the older child with whooping cough was haemoptysis. This was particularly seen in school children who developed whooping cough. Nose bleeding and the vomiting of blood are also common complaints.

Of the more serious complications, the neurological are the most important, and may be very varied; after prolonged convulsions the child may be left hemiplegic.

Other complications that may arise are a subcutaneous emphysema and a flare-up of a primary tuberculous lesion.

TREATMENT OF WHOOPING COUGH

In the hands of the author and his colleagues chloramphenicol palmitate (25 mg/lb, 50 mg/kg) was effective in alleviating or aborting the disease when used within the first week from the start of symptoms. Other workers have used erythromycin or tetracycline (15). The author and his colleagues were particularly concerned to treat the young infant, in whom the disease is both so dangerous and so difficult to diagnose in its early stages. To achieve this, the staff of the Under-Fives' Clinic, whenever they saw an older child with whooping cough, advised the mother to bring any infants in the same compound who developed even mild catarrhal symptoms or the slightest cough. Treatment was continued for 7 days if possible, although many infants received only 5 days' treatment and recovered. The cost of chloramphenicol for a 15 lb (6.7 kg) infant is about $0.14 a day in Africa. Prophylactic treatment of young infants in contact with known cases may be undertaken. This allows time for immunity to be achieved with triple antigen.

Late bronchopneumonia was treated with penicillin and sulphadimidine. This combination proved satisfactory for the majority of children.

While antibiotics have a most important part to play in the first week of the disease, and when a bronchopneumonia develops, the major part of the management of the established disease and its successful outcome will depend on the standard of nursing and maternal care. The persistence or recurrence of the cough is *not* evidence of persisting infection, and chloramphenicol should not be used except in the early stages. The mother will need advice and support, and if available, food supplements which contain protein and are also a rich source of calories in a low bulk. The mother must be encouraged to refeed the child if vomiting occurs, and to spend a great deal of trouble in maintaining the nutrition of her child. For the children who can be kept in a ward, their nutrition is again highly relevant. Oxygen and moisture may also be of assistance in the paroxysmal stage.

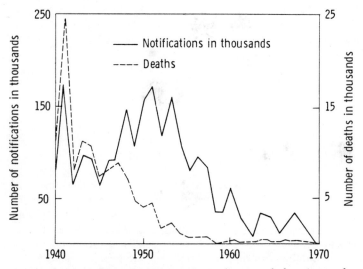

Figure 72. The decline in incidence and mortality rate of whooping cough in England and Wales from 1940 to 1970

PREVENTION OF WHOOPING COUGH

In Czechoslovakia in 1951 there were 400 cases per 100,000 of the population, but in 1961 the incidence had fallen to 34 per 100,000. Similar falls have been recorded in England (1) and elsewhere in Europe, and in the USA. The decline is shown in *Figure 72.*

It is noteworthy that even in a highly protected population, it is the younger children who suffer from the disease and in whom the high mortality can be expected.

A detailed study of deaths from whooping cough in the UK in 1960 and 1961, produced support for the importance of immunization in preventing deaths from whooping cough (88). Their results are summarized in *Figure 73*.

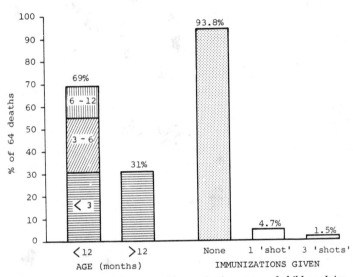

Figure 73. A study of the age and immunization states of children dying from whooping cough in the UK, between 1960 and 1961

Again two-thirds of the deaths occurred in children under a year old, and a high proportion in those under 6 months. Over 90 per cent of deaths were among children who had received no immunization, and of particular interest was the small number of deaths that occurred in children who received only one injection, suggesting that even one inoculation may offer some protection. Some difficulty has developed over the last decade in providing vaccines with adequate amounts of the three agglutinigens that are needed for adequate protection. However, those who are responsible for the production of vaccines are now likely to maintain adequate antigen effectiveness, even if further changes in the organism develop.

The other concern in the developed country is the toxicity of the vaccine and the frequency of severe reactions. The most serious reaction is the encephalopathy following pertussis immunization. In one study it was found that following encephalopathy 50 per cent recovered, 17 per cent died and about 30 per cent survived with sequelae (136). Large unexplained variations in the frequency of this complication have been given, but all figures suggest that it is fairly small, either between 1 in 6,000 or 1 in 50,000 vaccinations. In a 7-year period in the UK, there were only 7 fatal cases reported.

Timing of immunization

Recent studies (281) suggest that the previous rigid timing is unnecessary; that longer intervals than 1 month between the first and second doses of vaccine may lead to a higher level of immunity as measured by the agglutinin response, and that two widely-spaced inoculation of 0.5 cc will give as good a protection as three doses at monthly intervals. This regimen is now suggested by the World Health Organization. As a result it is unnecessary to restart a course if a child is brought back late for the second dose. In developing countries where immunization at an early age is so important, three injections at approximately monthly intervals early in life might be preferred to a two-dose, widely-spaced schedule.

Immunization in developing countries

In the study village of Imesi, immunization against whooping cough was not undertaken at the start of the study, as at that time little information was available either locally or in Africa as a whole on the severity of whooping cough. However, as the experience of the 1960 epidemic in the village unfolded, the author and his colleagues began to appreciate what a dramatic and severe disease whooping cough could be particularly among young infants. Fortunately, it was possible to make triple antigen available, and its routine use in the village since then has led to only a small number of children with the whooping cough syndrome *(Figure 74)*.

No official figures are available on the number of children in the pre-industrialized countries who are protected against whooping cough. However, some estimation of the amount of vaccine being used to various developing countries was attempted in 1964 (187), and at that time no country was immunizing more than 40 per cent of its children, and a majority of the countries investigated were immunizing less than

10 per cent of their children. Since 1964, some countries have improved their levels of immunization, but it is known that in some there has even been a reduction in the amount of whooping cough immunization undertaken.

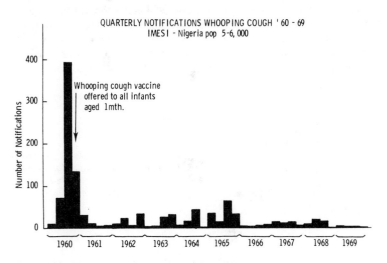

Figure 74. The effect of immunization on the number of quarterly notifications of whooping cough between 1960 and 1969 in the study village of Imesi, Nigeria (population 5–6,000)

Local circumstances must decide the age at which children should be vaccinated in each region. However, in the developing world, where whooping cough appears to be so severe in infancy, there are strong arguments for early immunization. The earlier that immunization can be given, the sooner some protection may be available, and for this reason in the village of Imesi immunization was given largely at 1 month of age, followed by further immunization in the second and third months. As a result, in the first 5 years the protection was perhaps not too satisfactory, but with improved supervision and better vaccines after 1966 the vast majority of illness was prevented, the few remaining cases probably representing the whooping cough syndrome that arises from infection with *Bordetella parapertussis* and certain viruses. A booster dose of triple antigen should probably be low in the priorities, unless required to increase the level of protection against diphtheria. Efforts should be concentrated on achieving a high level of immunization to protect against whooping cough in the early years when it is a killing disease; whooping cough after the age of five is not much more than a nuisance.

In the past, on immunological grounds, experts have advised against giving triple antigen at birth. However, the circulating antibodies are probably not a satisfactory measure of whooping cough immunity, and for this reason a trial was undertaken in 1964 and 1965 in the village of Imesi, in which children born on alternate days were given triple antigen at birth or at 1 month. In the follow-up, the number of children with whooping cough, and the severity of the disease were the same in the two groups, with slightly more children getting whooping cough

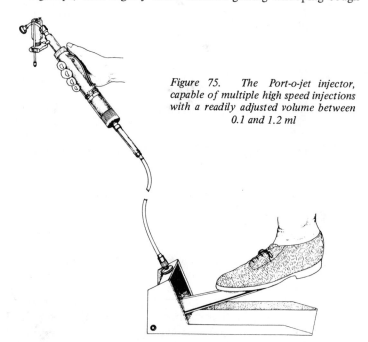

Figure 75.   The   Port-o-jet   injector, capable of multiple high speed injections with a readily adjusted volume between 0.1 and 1.2 ml

who had the immunization at 1 month. This result would suggest the need for further trials to discover whether whooping cough immunization can be satisfactorily given at birth, with all the advantages of early immunity in a disease so lethal among small infants (319).

Methods used in immunizing

The last decade has seen a rapid increase in the use of jet injectors in large immunization campaigns. These machines will inject a varying quantity of fluid, depending on their size, through the skin as a fine jet of fluid. Experience of these injectors *(Figure 75)* has now reached the stage when they may be used more routinely in hospital practice, and

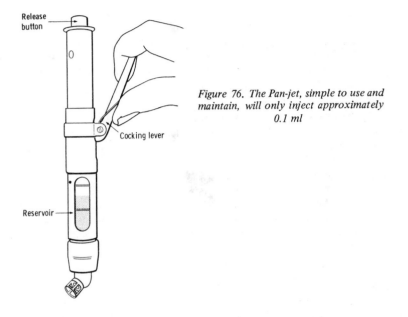

Release button

Cocking lever

Reservoir

Figure 76. The Pan-jet, simple to use and maintain, will only inject approximately 0.1 ml

already some early reports of their routine use are available. Their use has been extended by reducing the volume of triple antigen and acetone freeze dried preparations of *Salmonella typhosa* to around 0.1 ml, when smaller and less expensive machines such as the Pan-jet can be successfully used *(Figure 76)*. The Port-o-jet and Pan-jet can be obtained from Schuco International, Halliwick Court Place, Woodhouse Road, London, N.12. In India it has been possible to obtain locally prepared vaccine which cost only about $0.01 for each immunization (153). One study using this machine with triple antigen gave a satisfactory result in the levels of tetanus antitoxin (309, 308).

CHAPTER 14

Malaria in Children

Many people have studied malaria, but few have studied its effect on children, who are certainly the chief sufferers from it, particularly between the ages of 6 months and 5 years. The evidence for severity in this age group comes from India (275), West Africa (26) and South Africa (159). A pathologist (73), in almost 30 years' experience in West Africa, has not observed a single death which could be attributed solely to malaria in any child over the age of 4 years.

Recent years have seen a progressive decline in the areas affected by malaria. The situation at the end of 1968 is shown in Table 41. However, since then malaria has been reported to have returned to a number of areas from which it was hoped that it had been eradicated.

TABLE 41

The Population of Adults and Children Protected and Still Unprotected in 1968

	Protected areas	Unprotected areas
Population living in malarious areas (millions)	1,733	380
Children under 5 years of age in these areas (millions)	325	68

Although there has been a remarkable improvement, there are still probably 68 million children below the age of 5 years who are seriously at risk from malaria. Two-thirds of these children are in Africa. This chapter is particularly concerned with children in this age group, wherever they live.

MORTALITY FROM MALARIA

Mortality rates are difficult to determine, because the presence of a doctor or even a shop or general store in an area usually means that

248

antimalarials are available. Even the occasional dose of one antimalarial may considerably lower the mortality. In holo-endemic areas it has been suggested that as many as 10 per cent of all deaths in children may be due to malaria (27).

A long-term investigation in the Pare Taveta area on the border between Kenya and Tanzania in East Africa produced interesting results (225). Records of mortality in various age groups were available during three periods: (1) before any changes were brought in; (2) a period of both rapid economic development and malaria control; (3) a period when economic development was maintained but malaria returned to the area. The results are set out in *Figure 77.*

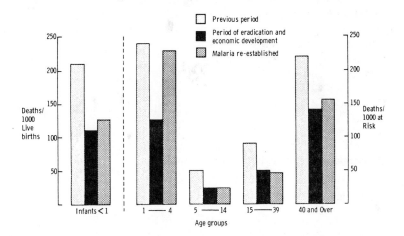

Figure 77. Mortality of different age groups before eradication, during eradication and after the re-establishment of malaria (after Pringle et al., 1969)

In each age group the mortality fell during the second period in which there was economic development and control of malaria. In the third period, however, when economic development was maintained but malaria returned, the mortality returned to almost the pre-control level in the 1—4 years age group, while in the infants under 1 year and in those over 5 years it remained low.

After the child, the next most seriously affected person is the pregnant woman. Some of the immunity to falciparum malaria developed in childhood seems to be lost during pregnancy, making pregnant women more liable to overt attacks of malaria and particularly to an anaemia that is often accentuated by a concurrent folic acid deficiency. The placenta is no barrier to infection in non-immune mothers, and their children may be born with congenital malaria. If, however, a mother has some degree of immunity, her child is almost never infected, even though her placenta is often heavily parasitized. In holo-endemic areas of malaria over 60 per cent of placentae of primiparous mothers may be so affected (38). Babies born to mothers with infected placentae are smaller than otherwise would be. However, in parities over three, placental infection rates may fall to 10 per cent, and it appears that with repeated pregnancies the placenta becomes less susceptible to infection.

Where malaria is endemic it is the major cause of low birth weight, and accounts for the large number of 'small for date' babies, particularly those born to primiparous mothers. This reduction in growth comes towards the end of pregnancy, when the cells of the brain are multiplying rapidly, so that the prevention of this maternal infection may improve a child's potential for intellectual development.

CLINICAL PICTURE OF MALARIA IN THE CHILD

In the past, clinical descriptions of malaria have been taken from non-immune and usually expatriate patients. There are few satisfactory descriptions of malaria in indigenous children.

Main clinical features

The main clinical features in West Africa are fever, convulsions, hepatosplenomegaly and anaemia (170) (110).

Fever

The child with malaria has repeated attacks of fever, which do not follow any regular pattern. Mothers notice this fever (185), as well as its reduction by regular antimalarials. Children with many parasites in their blood may appear to be quite normal and be afebrile.

Convulsions

Until recently the term 'febrile convulsion' was well accepted, and it was supposed that the convulsion was a direct result of the fever. However, closer examination suggests that in many children the convulsion precedes any rise in temperature. The extreme muscular activity of the convulsion may be partly responsible for the rise in

250

temperature. It is more likely that both the pyrogen and the convulsion are the direct effect of the infection (286) *(Figure 78)*. This theoretical relationship between fever and convulsions has a practical application in the prevention of convulsions and is discussed later in this chapter.

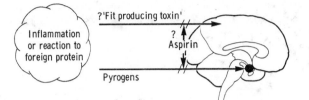

Figure 78. The possible similarity between agents that cause fever and those that lead to convulsions

Hepatosplenomegaly

Malaria infection leads to an enlargement of both the liver and the spleen. Since enlargement of the liver is more difficult to measure and has many other causes, splenic enlargement is more significant. Although in childhood there are other causes of splenic enlargement, few produce such enlargement as malaria.

Anaemia

The child with malaria suffers from chronic anaemia, usually has a haemoglobin between 7 and 10 g/100 ml, and is liable to episodes of acute haemolysis in which the haemoglobin may fall to well below 5 g per cent, and he may die from heart failure. Parasitaemia may be light in these children, so a low parasite count or a negative film does not exclude malaria as a cause of anaemia (110). Children receiving regular antimalarials do not suffer from this anaemia.

Cerebral malaria

This extremely dangerous complication of falciparum malaria is difficult to diagnose where coma and convulsions are common. The presence of coma between convulsions may be suggestive of cerebral anaemia. It arises due to a blockage of the capillaries with sludging and destruction of red cells. In one hospital study (110) the deaths of about half the children in which malaria was the primary cause were thought to be due to cerebral malaria. All these children had strongly positive blood films.

Diarrhoea and malnutrition

Most authorities suggest that malaria is causally associated with both diarrhoea and malnutrition. This belief has arisen out of the finding that children with these conditions frequently have high parasite counts. However, since in holo-endemic areas parasites are present in about 90 per cent of all small children, a positive blood film may have little causal relationship with a child's illness. In the experience of the author and his colleagues diarrhoea is not a symptom of malaria, and malaria plays a small part in the production of malnutrition. In the Imesi study diarrhoea was equally common in the children who were given antimalarial drugs and those who were not. Diarrhoea was found to be highly correlated with measles, and less so with whooping cough, but no association could be shown with either malaria or otitis media (183). In one hospital study (112), the incidence of diarrhoea was slightly lower in children in whom malaria parasites were found than in the group without them. In the Gambia acute malaria would temporarely interrupt the growth of children (171). However, those in whom the disease had not been suppressed eventually caught up with the protected group. The Imesi findings were similar and showed that malarial suppression made little difference to the height and weight of children. In the Ibadan study more severe malaria was seen in the well-nourished children that in those who were poorly nourished in the same community (112). Severe malaria was most uncommon at post-mortem in children dying from either marasmus or kwashiorkor (73).

Haemoglobinopathies

There is now good evidence that children with haemoglobin type AS suffer less from malaria than those with haemoglobin types AA and AC. In 50 autopsies on children who had died of cerebral malaria (73) none had haemoglobin AS, although these make up 18 per cent of the population. The evidence for the protective influence of glucose-6-phosphate-dehydrogenase (G-6-PD) deficient subjects being protected is less certain.

REDUCING MORBIDITY BY MONTHLY PROPHYLAXIS

Effectiveness of pyrimethamine

Children born into the Imesi study were allocated alternately into two groups on the following regimens: (1) pyrimethamine 25 mg monthly, plus chloroquine for any episode of fever, the dosage being 15–20 mg chloroquine base per kg body weight; and (2) a lactose tablet monthly, plus chloroquine for any episode of fever.

Both groups of children grew identically in height and weight, but those receiving pyrimethamine had a slightly higher haemoglobin level at all ages, showed a lower incidence of splenomegaly and had convulsions much less often, as shown in Table 42.

TABLE 42

The Incidence of Convulsions in Two Groups of Children Aged 6 Months to 4 Years, Both Given Chloroquine for Fever

	Monthly pyrimethamine (25 mg)	Lactose placebo
Number of children	128	149
Number of 'febrile' convulsions related to recognizable infections (for example, measles, pertussis, respiratory infections)	20 (3.5)*	24 (3.6)*
Number of 'febrile' convulsions unrelated to any recognizable infection	18† (3.1)*	41† (6.1)*

*Figures in brackets represent rate/100 child years
†χ^2 = 7.453 p > 0.01

The children receiving pyrimethamine came with fever in only 24 per cent of months, while those on the lactose placebo were brought with fever in 46 per cent of months.

As a result of this study, and because of strong clinical impressions of the value of pyrimethamine, this drug was used routinely for a number of years in the Under-Fives' Clinic at Ilesha. It was popular with the mothers, who noticed that it decreased the incidence of 'fever' in their children. The children were also given chloroquine whenever they were feverish.

Arguments in favour of routine use of pyrimethamine

The arguments in favour of this regimen for routine use in Under-Fives' Clinics in holo-endemics areas are summarized as follows.

Cost. — Chloroquine is both more expensive for each tablet and has to be given more often. A weekly chloroquine tablet is required, whereas a tablet of pyrimethamine provides some protection for two or three weeks, and can be given monthly.

Acceptabilitty. – Pyrimethamine is almost tasteless. A monthly bitter tablet such as chloroquine will be difficult for many mothers to accept. Even when the giving of chloroquine has been closely supervised by a nurse, there has been considerable difficulty, particularly as vomiting may occur (170), a complication not experienced with pyrimethamine. As long as individually wrapped pyrimethamine tablets are used, a dangerous accidental overdose is unlikely.

Immunity. – As the protection does not persist throughout the month, some parasitaemia does occur and the child develops at least partial immunity.

Resistance. – Fears of a widespread resistance to pyrimethamine have been given as a reason for not using this drug. There is little evidence for this. Resistance in Ibadan school children receiving pyrimethamine 25 mg weekly was found to be no more than 15–20 per cent (157). There is no cross-resistance between chloroquine and pyrimethamine and if pyrimethamine-resistant strains do arise, they are not necessarily permanent. Any fever that could be due to a resistant strain can readily be treated with chloroquine.

If pyrimethamine is used in this way, chloroquine can be reserved for treatment of febrile episodes and the appearance of strains resistant to chloroquine may be delayed.

Arguments in favour of regular antimalarials

There are several arguments in favour of giving regular antimalarials. The more important are the following.

(1) Convulsions and anaemia are common in severe malarial infections. Children between the ages of 6 months and 4 years are particularly prone to these; in children over 5 years of age they are less common.

(2) Protection from the effects of malaria up to the age of 5 years is particularly helpful to the overall health of the child. During this period the child experiences many respiratory infections, frequent diarrhoea, measles, whooping cough, and other childhood infections. Further, he is passing through the period when the interaction of these infections and malnutrition is a serious health threat.

After the age of 5 years the child can often make his way to the clinic independently if he develops fever and headache. In the older child the parents do not so easily accept illness as in the child under 5 years, and they are more likely to seek treatment.

TREATMENT OF MALARIA IN CHILDREN

Malaria should be treated with chloroquine; there is no satisfactory evidence that the more expensive amodiaquine is more effective. The most economical form should be used. The dosage is set out in Table 43.

TABLE 43
Dosage of Chloroquine or Amodiaquine Base Used for Children (mg)

Age (years)	up to 1	1–3	4–6	7–12	13–15
Initial dose	75	150	300	300	450
After 6 hours	75	112.5	150	150	300
Once daily for 4 days	75	75	75	150	150

In areas where the population has a relatively high immunity, only the initial dose should be given, as this appears to be satisfactory. A dose of chloroquine at this level should also be given at the start of suppressive therapy with pyrimethamine, as suggested above. If for any reason the pyrimethamine is allowed to lapse for more than a month, the dose should be repeated.

Treatment of severe malaria in children

Evidence of cerebral involvement demands urgent treatment, and the choice is between intravenous chloroquine or quinine. If chloroquine is used, the dose should not exceed 5 mg base/kg body weight, and should be diluted in 150 cc of glucose saline. Repeat once if necessary, but not until after 12 hours. Quinine dihydrochloride has a more rapid schizonticidal reaction and there are strong advocates of its use. The dosage to be given is 10 mg/kg body weight, and it may also be repeated after 12 hours, but the total dose should not exceed 20 mg/kg. Intramuscular therapy may also be used, and in some areas suppositories of chloroquine have been successfully used. Both chloroquine and mepacrine, when given intravenously in larger doses than stated above, and also if given undiluted, have been followed by sudden death, and for this reason they must be used with great caution.

In the adult, steroid therapy (dexamethazone 10 mg) has been considered to be life-saving (288). It can be given intravenously; the steroids help to diminish the transudation across the cerebral capillaries which develops in cerebral malaria.

Management of convulsions

The treatment of choice in the immediate management of convulsions due to any cause is paraldehyde, which is usually given intramuscularly, or can be given effectively intravenously. Diazepam may be used, but is more expensive. The use of phenobarbitone is now questioned, and the present evidence is that aspirin is more satisfactory in preventing children with malaria, or any other fever, from developing convulsions (286). The suitable dose of aspirin is 150 mg under 1 year of age, and this may be repeated 6-hourly. Between 1 and 4 years, 300 mg, and over 4 years 600 mg may be used. Those using this regime must be familar with the signs of aspirin poisoning.

Phenobarbitone will be used only when the child has developed convulsions on two or more occasions, and then should be considered only if the doctor is confident that a regular dose can be maintained for a period of at least a year, and the possible disadvantages are considered.

Phenobarbitone is widely used in short courses, and so the disadvantages of these, which are summarized below, need to be considered.

(1) Effective therapeutic levels of phenobarbitone can only be produced over 48 hours or more. Oral tablets given at the beginning of the majority of short febrile illnesses will be of no value.

(2) If short courses of anticonvulsants are given intermittently, usually lasting only for a few days, there is a real danger of encouraging withdrawal fits.

(3) The better appreciation of the profound effect of phenobarbitone on behaviour, mood and learning in a majority of children is so adverse that even short periods on this treatment may be worse than the disease.

If a long-term anticonvulsant is to be used, then phenytoin in a dose of 5 mg/kg body weight/day seems to be largely devoid of the unfavourable effects of phenobarbitone mentioned above. However, as it costs five times as much as phenobarbitone, its use for long periods on a wide scale may not be feasible.

CHAPTER 15

Tuberculosis

Tuberculosis as seen in developing countries has many differences from that seen in Europe or North America. These differences arise from the nutritional state, intercurrent infections in the children, the age of infection, genetic inheritance, and possibly the size of the infective dose. Nutrition, intercurrent infection, and the age of infection are emphasized in this chapter as the three most important factors. Identification of the relative importance of each of these is necessary, both to understand the disease better and to decide the steps necessary to reduce its severity and, where possible, prevent it altogether.

TUBERCULOSIS IN DEVELOPING AND INDUSTRIALIZED COUNTRIES

In Table 44 a comparison is made between tuberculosis towards the end of the nineteenth century in Europe with the disease in developing countries and in Europe now (178). The higher prevalence of tuberculosis in the under-five group must be expected in relation to the greater frequency of droplet infections in infants and very young children in developing countries. This arises from greater opportunities of exposure as they are being carried about, or living in joint or extended families as has been discussed elsewhere (see Chapter 13).

The high mortality from tuberculosis in Europe in the nineteenth century continued into the beginning of this century, and even in 1914 in Edinburgh one-third of children dying from all causes had tuberculosis lesions at autopsy (248). In those developing countries in which autopsies on deaths in children can be undertaken, tuberculosis is a frequent and sometimes unexpected finding. The difference in pathology is also summarized in Table 44. Progress of the primary lesion to caseation and cavitation and the liability of the regional nodes to form large caseating masses are relatively more frequent now in developing countries, as they were in Europe towards the end of the last century. Records of tuberculin sensitivity at different ages only exist after 1920,

257

TABLE 44

Comparison of Tuberculosis in Developing Countries with Europe in the Nineteenth Century and Now*

	Nineteenth century Europe	Developing countries	Europe now
Tuberculosis < 5 years autopsy	++	++	Rare (in 1969 only 0.1% tuberculin +ve at 5)
Incidence of the disease at	'One-third of all child autopsies'	++	Almost nil
Progress of primary lesions to caseation and cavitation	+	+	–
Regional nodes caseating	++	++	–
Tuberculosis with negative tuberculin reaction	?	++	–
Sensitivity phenomena: Erythema nodosum, phlyctenulae, pleural effusion, ascites	Uncommon	±	±
Tuberculous meningitis	+	+	Most rare
Tuberculomata	50% Intracranial tumours Encephalopathy	30% Intracranial tumours Encephalopathy	No tuberculomata
Association with malnutrition and vitamin A deficiency	+	++	–

*Approximate frequency: ++, seen about once a month; +, seen at least yearly by a doctor serving a community of 10,000

when the tuberculin test became widely used. Tuberculous erythema nodosum, phlyctenular conjunctivitis and pleural effusions or ascites are all associated with a strong tuberculin reaction and are probably evidence of a high degree of sensitivity. Absence of a high level of tuberculin sensitivity, which is now known to be a cellular rather than an antibody response, may be explained by malnutrition. This will lead to an inability to multiply lymphocytes, just as there is an inability to produce cells and show adequate growth. These sensitivity phenomena were less common in the nineteenth century than 20–30 years ago, when childhood tuberculosis was still common in Europe, but the overall nutrition of children had improved. Erythema nodosum is particularly uncommon in many developing countries, and probably the other sensitivity reactions are not so frequent. In tuberculosis of the central nervous system, tuberculomata are common in developing countries but are now rare in Europe.

The widely-held view that the problem of tuberculosis is largely one of cities may be partially true in some areas, but in India it has been known for many years to be almost equally severe in the rural areas.

INTERACTION OF NUTRITION AND INFECTION

This interaction includes two quite separate reactions.

Poor child nutrition allows rapid spread of tuberculous lesions

The severity of tuberculosis in the malnourished individual is well documented (242). One study (153) demonstrated a reduced incidence of progressive disease by an improved diet and was of particular significance, because improved housing in a previous study had not reduced the incidence of progressive disease (155). Protein–energy as well as vitamin A, D and C deficiencies have all been shown to increase the severity by reducing the resistance to tuberculous infections both in men and experimental animals (242).

Tuberculosis makes the child's nutrition worse

An association with protein–energy malnutrition and vitamin A deficiency in childhood tuberculosis was reported in the older European literature and is of major concern to health workers in developing countries. This association is by no means simple. Tuberculosis may present as kwashiorkor or marasmus following a slow deterioration of the child's nutrition over many months. When kwashiorkor appears to be resistant to improvement by diet, unsuspected tuberculosis is a frequent cause and improvement is prompt once treatment is started. As described later, a suspicion of

259

tuberculosis in a malnourished child will justify the use of anti-tuberculous drugs in a therapeutic trial.

Interaction of nutrition and infection in the infant

In early infancy a state of undernutrition develops in 2 or 3 weeks after infection, so that poor nutrition due to tuberculosis leads to a more rapid spread of the tuberculous disease. This interaction can still be seen in the first months of life in well-nourished children, and is particularly important during the first few years of life among those from undernourished societies.

Variable opinion on the problem of childhood tuberculosis

The seriousness of the problem of childhood tuberculosis is viewed differently by different groups of health workers. Adult physicians and those concerned with community health place childhood tuberculosis low in their priorities, because it is non-infectious and goes largely unrecognized. In community health surveys, almost total reliance has been placed on the tuberculin test, and findings such as those of recent studies (227) (101) may be misleading. In these it was found that the overall mortality amongst children with positive tuberculin reactions was not much higher than in those with a negative reaction. These results may underestimate mortality, as those who succumb to childhood tuberculosis in a poorly nourished community will develop a strong reaction to tuberculin for only a short period of time, if at all, and are unlikely to be identified in the tuberculin survey.

The paediatrician may for different reasons develop a distorted picture of childhood tuberculosis. His attitude to this disease may be imbalanced by the experience of caring for children with tuberculous meningitis — one of the most chronic and disturbing diseases of childhood that he will meet — for whom treatment has only partially succeeded. A child who develops tuberculous meningitis is likely to be taken to hospital either early or after all other means of treatment have been attempted. Often the young and poorly nourished child with tuberculous meningitis cannot be cured, but the life of these children is prolonged, and they will accumulate in children's wards with an otherwise high patient turnover.

NATURAL HISTORY OF CHILDHOOD TUBERCULOSIS

The natural history of untreated childhood tuberculosis from experience in the UK has been well described (177), and *Figure 79* demonstrates the relationships in time of the various incidents.

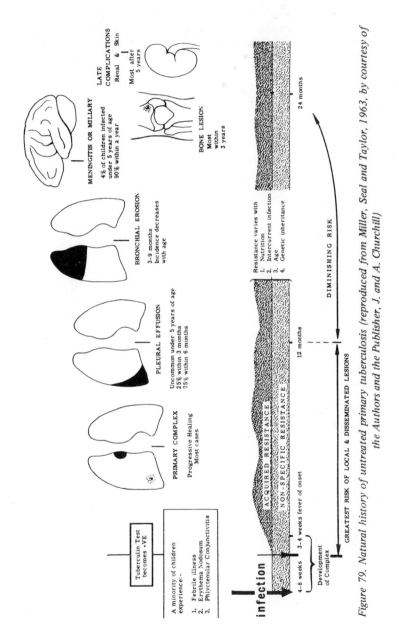

Figure 79. Natural history of untreated primary tuberculosis (reproduced from Miller, Seal and Taylor, 1963, by courtesy of the Authors and the Publisher, J. and A. Churchill)

In developing countries there are some differences from this picture. There is a tendency for infection at an earlier age, the nutrition of the child is poor, and there is a high probability of an intercurrent infection, particularly measles and whooping cough. Low tuberculin sensitivity is frequent and caseation, either in the primary lesion or in the associated lymph glands, is more common.

Fate of the primary focus in the lungs

Certainly the vast majority of primary infections in children over 5 years of age, undergo a benign course with no detectable clinical illness. The complications described here arise for a number of reasons: the more important — nutrition, intercurrent infection and the age of the child — have already been mentioned.

The complications found in a primary focus are set out in *Figure 80.*

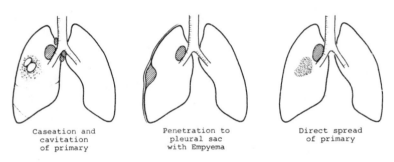

Caseation and   Penetration to   Direct spread
cavitation   pleural sac   of primary
of primary   with Empyema

Figure 80. Complications arising from the primary focus in the lung

If the primary focus forms a caseous mass, this may ulcerate into a bronchus and thus produce a tension cavity. Alternatively it may spread towards the pleura. Due to a low sensitivity a serous effusion is uncommon, but an empyema is a more likely complication in developing countries.

Lastly the primary lesion is more likely to show local extension within the lung parenchyma.

Complication of the glands

The disease may also spread as a complication of the glands *(Figure 81).*

As the glands caseate, they may rupture into the bronchus with aspiration into the lung which is aerated by that bronchus. There may be a segmental sensitivity reaction with little multiplication of bacilli

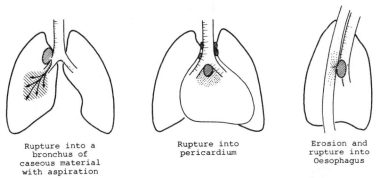

| Rupture into a bronchus of caseous material with aspiration | Rupture into pericardium | Erosion and rupture into Oesophagus |

Figure 81. Complications arising from caseous lymphatic nodes

(epituberculosis), or there may be a tuberculous bronchopneumonia, making the child very ill. The glands may rupture into the pericardium, where it will usually lead to a blood-stained pericardial effusion in a child who is not as ill as the circumstances would suggest. Discharge into the oesophagus lays the child open to a dangerous mediastinitis.

Haematogenous spread

As haematogenous spread is more common in a child who is young or ill-nourished, it is far more common in developing countries *(Figure 82)*.

The finding of a large spleen and liver in a child brought with fever and malaise may by suggestive of haematogenous and miliary spread, a diagnosis that may be confirmed at once by a doctor who has mastered the difficult but valuable skill of examining a child's optic fundus. Such an examination will also exclude papilloedema, a necessary step before undertaking a spinal tap to identify those children in whom the generalized spread has included meningitis. Tuberculosis in the brain substance may lead to a tuberculoma or a more diffuse tuberculous encephalitis.

In some the haematogenous spread will not involve a full miliary spread, but foci develop in bone or kidney *(Figure 82)*. Lesions of the bone are common in young and poorly nourished children in developing countries.

263

Sample case histories

Only too often in such countries the doctor will see one of the clinical syndromes described above. However, as children come more generally under comprehensive care made available through auxiliaries, he will either prevent them through BCG or be able to spot them through early symptoms, particularly an unexplained failure to gain weight, a persistent cough, or as a contact of an adult who is sputum positive. The following case histories, taken from the Imesi study made by the author and his colleagues, are examples of how these both arose in young and relatively poorly nourished children.

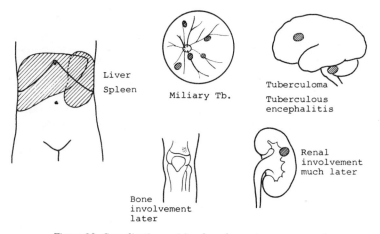

Liver
Spleen

Miliary Tb.

Tuberculoma

Tuberculous
encephalitis

Bone
involvement
later

Renal
involvement
much later

Figure 82. Complications arising from haematogenous spread

Rasaki was an only son: his mother's previous child had died of whooping cough at 5 months of age. Rasaki gained well in the first 6 months of life *(Figure 83)* but then, as so often happens, his gain in weight became less satisfactory. Early in his second year he was away from the village and apparently received a more satisfactory diet and started to gain weight.

From February in his second year of life he lost weight. Examination of his records at this time shows that he had intermittent episodes of fever, cough and diarrhoea. After a period of poor gain in weight for 5 months, a Heaf test was strongly positive and he was found to have minimal oedema of the ankles. He was admitted to hospital for a week. X-ray showed miliary disease.

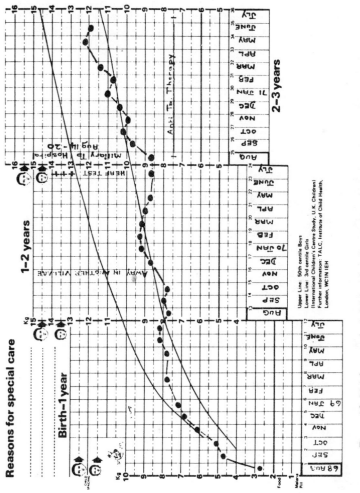

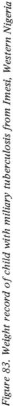

Figure 83. Weight record of child with miliary tuberculosis from Imesi, Western Nigeria

On treatment with isoniazid (INH) and streptomycin daily for a month and then a year's INH he made satisfactory recovery. Experience of children such as this led the author and his colleagues to introduce routine tuberculin testing, using the Heaf technique, for all children showing loss of weight or poor weight gain for 3 months. The brief period of streptomycin used would be criticized by many, but the mother found that bringing her child regularly was difficult, and maintaining her co-operation in giving the full course of INH was considered more important.

The source of this child's infection was not discovered, although he had recently stayed with his grandmother, who died of diarrhoea. In the enquiries as to a possible source of infection in a rural society, as well as enquiring for living relatives with coughs it is also most necessary to enquire specifically about recent deaths. In societies with more adequate medical resources the majority of deaths from tuberculosis occur in hospital. This is not so in rural (and most urban) societies of developing countries, and during the final weeks of the illness the sputum will be particularly heavily infected and the adult confined to the house, so that any children who live there or who visit are likely to become infected.

Taiwo and Kehinde were identical twins. At 15 months Kehinde had 2 weeks' cough and was found to be tuberculin positive. Taiwo was positive and an x-ray of their mother showed a cavity at the left apex. Her sputum was positive for acid-fast bacilli (AFB). The twins were started on INH and their mother on full adult therapy. She was encouraged to continue breast-feeding. She gained weight rapidly and her lesion healed. The weight gain of the twins remained satisfactory, their coughs cleared, and a chest x-ray was considered unnecessary.

DIAGNOSIS OF TUBERCULOSIS IN THE YOUNG CHILD

Tuberculosis in many children is difficult to diagnose; this is true in Europe, where the disease is now rare. Even in developing countries, where this possibility is in the forefront of the mind of every children's doctor, it is easily overlooked.

In reaching a decision, reliance will be placed on a careful and detailed history. Fever and cough will be noted, but considerable reliance will be placed on a decline in activity and the development of unhappiness in the child. Time spent in taking this history from more than one member of the family may be rewarding. Physical signs, except in advanced disease, are rarely dependable. X-rays may be helpful, but may also be misleading. A weight chart can be most useful *(Figure 83)*.

Tuberculin test

It is perhaps fortunate that this reaction was first studied in countries of Northern Europe, where non-specific reactions are less common and its meaning can be more simply defined. Common ways of undertaking this test are the Mantoux intradermal test, or alternatively the percutaneous Heaf or Tine tests.

Mantoux test

This test is the most accurate and most widely used, and is the only test satisfactory for epidemiological studies. Into the superficial layers of the skin 0.1 ml of a standard dilution of old tuberculin (OT) or purified protein derivative (PPD) is injected. The solution must have been made up recently or contain Tween 80, and care is necessary to ensure that the injection is intradermal and not subcutaneous. Special syringes are kept for this purpose only. In clinical work 10 TU (0.1 ml of 1:1,000 OT or 0.0001 mg PPD) are usually used. In surveys only half this strength is universally used. In reporting the test a reading is made in millimetres of the indurated area after 72 hours. Induration in excess of 6 mm is usually considered significant. In developing countries with widespread non-specific sensitivity reactions the figure may need to be reconsidered,

Heaf test

In this test a small amount of undiluted OT or special undiluted PPD is spread on the skin and the needles of the Heaf apparatus *(Figure 84)*

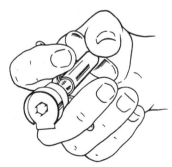

Figure 84. The Heaf apparatus – only the magnetic model is recommended

carry this through the skin. The advantage of this test is its simplicity. The magnetic type of apparatus is tough and not always damaged by a fall on a floor (the 'concrete' test to which much apparatus in developing countries may be subjected)! In this model a small plate carrying six small needle-like blades is held on by a magnet. A number of these plates should be available and they are sterlized between sessions. The blades on the plate do not easily become blunt.

In the author's experience this magnetic variety is useful, but the alternative, carrying needles, should be avoided. The latter is easily damaged, or the needles become blunt or bent. This makes the test both useless and misleading with false negatives. In the Heaf test either old tuberculin or PPD may be used. Undiluted old tuberculin (containing an antiseptic) will keep indefinitely at room temperature and is preferable for health centre use, and also because it is more economical.

The Tine test is similar to the Heaf test, but the disposable apparatus is too expensive for general use in developing countries.

The results of the Heaf test are classified in terms of induration *(Figure 85)*. This should be felt for and a test of both 0 and 1 considered as a negative reaction.

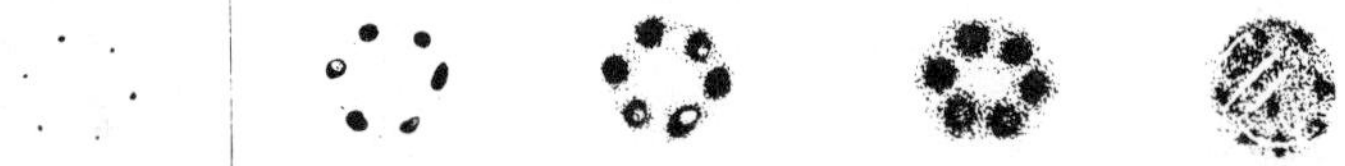

Negative	Increasing degrees of positiveness ⟶			
0	1	2	3	4
−	+	++	+++	++++
Faint marks No induration	4 or more discrete palpable papules	Papules have coalesced, normal skin inside circle	Normal skin obliterated	Blistering present

Figure 85. Results of the Heaf test, classified in terms of induration which are felt as well as seen

Non-specific reactions

If a population of schoolchildren in a country such as Denmark had received a Mantoux test (10 TU) some 30 years ago, and the diameter of induration had been measured 72 hours later, the distribution of the reaction is likely to have been that seen in *Figure 86*. These children consist of two groups, one the non-reactor component on the left, and the second the reactor component, with a tuberculin reaction varying from 8 mm up to 28 mm in diameter.

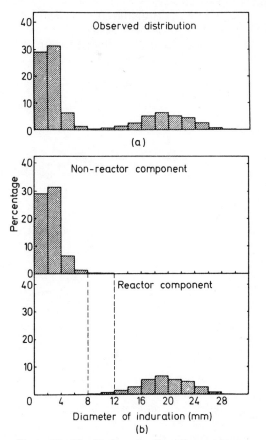

Figure 86. Distribution of tuberculin reaction to Mantoux test in an area where non-reactors and reactors are easily separated. (a) Observed distribution. (b) Non-reactor component and reactor component. A minimum of reactors in the zone between non-reactors and reactors makes the test more satisfactory (reproduced from Nyboe, 1960, by courtesy of the Editor, Bulletin of the World Health Organization)

In such a population, it is safe to consider that the majority of children in the non-reactor component have had no experience of tuberculosis, and that those in the reactor component for the most part are undergoing or have undergone their primary infection. In such populations, the tuberculin reaction can give valuable information at all ages. Unfortunately, such a distribution is frequently not found in schoolchildren in tropical countries. *Figure 87* shows the response found in several developing countries, and the wide range of reaction that may be found due to a non-specific reaction (208).

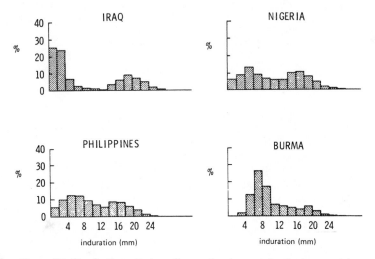

Figure 87. Distribution of tuberculin reaction in some developing countries

In the examples given here, Iraq shows a distribution not unlike that of Europe. In Nigeria and the Philippines the differentiation between reactors and non-reactors is not clear-cut, because of a biphasic distribution with a mode between 4 and 10 mm as well as between 14 and 18 mm. In Burma the most common size reaction is between 4 and 10 mm.

This intermediate grade of tuberculin sensitivity is believed to be due to infection with non-pathogenic or non-specific mycobacteria and possibly antigens from other sources.

In such countries the tuberculin test in schoolchildren and adults is of limited value, because positive reactions, especially in this intermediate range, do not necessarily indicate contact with the tubercle bacillus. Strongly positive reactions, however, are most likely to be due to contact with miliary tuberculosis. In infants and pre-school children reactions of 6 mm or more probably indicate tuberculous infection, while at any age a reaction of 20 mm is indicative of active and serious infection.

Isolation of tubercle bacilli

In the past, methods of diagnosing the disease by culture have been relatively less used in children, because of the difficulty of obtaining suitable material and undertaking culture in developing countries. In children with tuberculosis, a swab taken from the laryngeal area will frequently be positive, and at those centres where such a technique is possible this method has a great deal to commend it (156).

Adult sputum examination followed by identifying contacts

The priority in the diagnosis of tuberculosis in a community is the person who has tubercle bacilli demonstrable on a direct sputum smear. In India 92 per cent of those with positive sputa are aware of symptoms, and 52 per cent have made some contact with health services. Examination of such a film by laboratory auxiliaries should cost only 2 cents ($0.02) a smear and ought to be a routine and much-used investigation at health centres. Cultural methods would only demonstrate 18 per cent more cases, and these are less infective. Once this test is available, childhood contacts may be discovered and treated.

MANAGEMENT OF TUBERCULOSIS ON A NATIONAL SCALE

Tuberculosis is a disease of national importance, and number of developing countries have examined how it may be tackled in a manner suited to their resources. One of the simple and effective plans in a country with limited resources is that which has been undertaken by India (199). In that country, the situation may be simplified and set out as in *Figure 88*.

This diagram is not to scale, nor was the sputum examined or chest x-rayed of children under 5 years of age. The inset values represent what happens without treatment. The influence of these rates on decisions to be made in developing countries where resources are so limited may be different from those in industrial areas. For example, 6 per cent breakdown of suspect cases may have a different significance if resources are too stretched to care adequately for sputum positive cases. The priorities in tackling the disease — BCG and out-patient chemotherapy — are indicated by the two thick arrows (272).

Around 60 per cent of the population will not have experienced any infection with tuberculosis. Among this section of the population BCG will provide effective protection, and an appropriate proportion of the national effort against tuberculosis should be spent in this way.

The other group to need special attention is those who have a positive sputum on smear examination. These are the source of further spread of the disease. For them the need is a low-cost, simple but effective out-patient treatment, now available in India, through tablets containing thiacetazone and isoniazide. For the supervision of this group a simple but efficient record system has been evolved. Those who fail to attend first receive a postcard reminder, and later their nearest health post is informed.

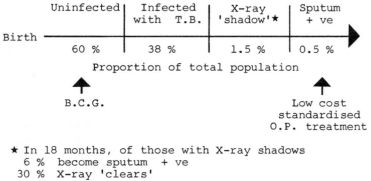

★ In 18 months, of those with X-ray shadows
  6 % become sputum + ve
 30 % X-ray 'clears'

Figure 88. Action to control tuberculosis in the Indian population of 550 million

The remaining 40 per cent of the population include those who have undergone a primary infection and built up their resistance. There will be a proportion (1.5 per cent) with x-ray shadows. However, seeking them out with mass radiography is not widely practical and should not be undertaken until more 'cost-effective' procedures such as BCG vaccination, sputum examination and thorough out-patient treatment of those with positive sputa have been achieved on a national scale.

Unfortunately these results are unacceptable to many doctors who depend for their livelihood on traditional methods of management of the disease. They persist in wishing to spend 80 per cent of their nation's budget for tuberculosis on confining patients with tuberculosis to hospital (160). It has been estimated that the cost of treating one tuberculosus child in hospital will provide BCG vaccination for 7,000 children and give them 80 per cent* protection for 10 years, and possibly some protection against leprosy (143).

*The arguments for the use of BCG have been taken for granted in this chapter The 80 per cent protection quoted here comes from the Medical Research Council trials (1964) (175). It should be noted that in these trials, protection against severe tuberculosis was complete, and in the 20 per cent in which there was evidence of infection, it was of a very mild nature

Use of BCG

In taking BCG to the thousands of villages in one country in Asia, the tuberculosis workers have been through three phases, which are set out in *Figures 89, 90* and *91*.

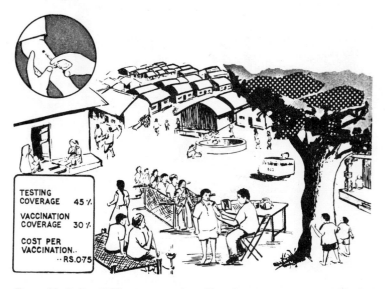

TESTING
COVERAGE   45 %

VACCINATION
COVERAGE   30 %

COST PER
VACCINATION..
         ··RS.0·75

Figure 89. Indian BCG mass campaign: Phase I, an attempt to assemble the community

It will be seen in *Figure 89* that attempts were made to inform and advise the villagers that tuberculin testing and the giving of BCG was going on, and they were brought together in the middle of the village to have this undertaken. As shown in the diagram, a central space in the village was used, and publicity had been carried out first. The inset drawing (top left) is included to show that preliminary tuberculin testing was undertaken. The results were disappointing, in that only 45 per cent attended at the centre and 30 per cent returned for BCG on the third day.

Subsequently, as these results were considered unsatisfactory, Phase II was instituted. BCG vaccination was undertaken by visiting each house in the village to contact the people *(Figure 90)*. The BCG team visited the houses twice, on the first occasion to undertake the tuberculin testing, and on a return visit to read the test and to give BCG to

273

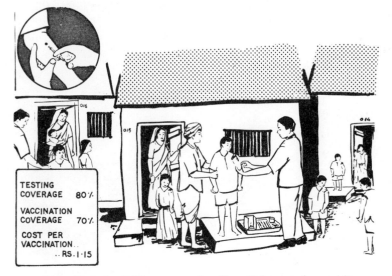

Figure 90. Indian BCG mass campaign: Phase II, house-to-house visits

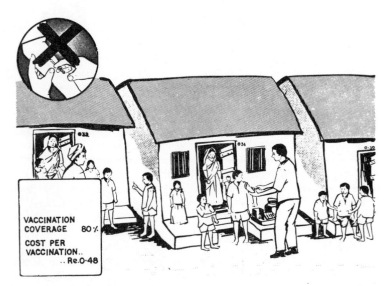

Figure 91. Indian BCG mass campaign: Phase III, house-to-house visits, direct vaccination

those with a tuberculin reaction below 100 mm. While this method was far more effective — 80 per cent were tested and 70 per cent vaccinated — it again proved unsatisfactory, due to the high cost of giving the BCG, on account of two visits being made to each house and fewer vaccinations achieved.

Over the last 10 years it has become apparent in many countries that the use of a preliminary test with tuberculin is unnecessary, and as a result in most mass campaigns BCG is given direct, that is, without prior tuberculin testing *(Figure 91)*. BCG given to tuberculin positive children is harmless. During Phase III only one visit was paid by the BCG team and those between the ages of 0–19 years who were considered eligible for vaccination were vaccinated without a tuberculin test. In this way an 80 per cent coverage was still achieved, as no follow-up visit was necessary, and at the same time the cost was reduced to $0.06 for every BCG inoculation given. The number of vaccinations achieved by the team was doubled.

Further developments since these three phases include combined smallpox and BCG vaccination, given at first separately but perhaps in the future as one vaccine, a step which will further reduce costs.

TREATMENT OF ADULT TUBERCULOSIS

The MRC Madras studies on the management of adult tuberculosis have emphasized the overriding importance of the antituberculous drugs in the control of this disease. They have shown that the homeless patient who continues to live 'in the street' on a most indifferent diet, earning his living by at times strenuous work, does no worse that a well-fed patient confined to rest in hospital designed to manage tuberculosis (85). Home treatment is more acceptable to the community, as it does not lead to family disruption. Nor did the failure to segregate the sputum-positive case during the early months of treatment cause further spread within the community, because within a few weeks of starting drugs, the number of virulent tubercle bacilli being coughed up is so diminished as to make further infection in the community not a serious matter. Unfortunately, these findings are still not acceptable to many doctors.

TREATMENT OF CHILDHOOD TUBERCULOSIS

In childhood tuberculosis, these findings are relevant, although here it is likely that improving nutrition, as in every other childhood disease, does play some part in restoring the child to a state of normal growth.

Coincidence of poor nutrition and intercurrent infection does make tuberculosis in children a greater danger in developing countries. A well-documented example of this is the record of a Durban hospital, where an epidemic of measles was responsible for a 30 per cent mortality amongst children with severe lesions, in spite of anti-tuberculosis and other therapy (304).

Of the drugs available in the management of tuberculosis in childhood, isoniazide (INH) is outstanding. The child can take this drug in the large dose of between 10 and 20 mg/kg taken as a single daily dose, a dose which would have toxic effects in the adult. In the adult on isoniazide it is now well recognized that with this drug alone, after 6 months, between one-third and two-thirds of patients will show drug-resistant bacilli in their sputum. There are two reasons why this argument against the use of isoniazide alone may not apply so well in the child.

(1) In the child, most primary lesions contain relatively few bacilli and it may be necessary to hunt through a primary lesion for a long time before a single bacillus can be found.

(2) In the child, the lesion is usually vascular, and there is not the fibrous tissue found in the adult. The drug, if taken adequately, should be in contact in a high concentration with any bacilli that are present.

The same is not true for the adult, in whom the usual lesion involves a cavity containing many billion bacilli, with a relatively poor blood supply. If it is accepted that there is a good correlation between the number of bacilli in a lesion and the chance of resistant organisms developing, in the child the chances of resistant organisms developing are small.

For this reason, and because a primary lesion in a child is normally a self-terminating lesion, there are good arguments in a 'two dollar a year health service' for using isoniazide alone in the straightforward primary over a period of 1 year or 18 months, particularly in all asymptomatic conversion under 5 years. This was the author's practice, and it has been confirmed by one study (205).

The drug most useful in combination with INH is thiacetazone. Although useful, this drug is rather more toxic than isoniazide, and this toxicity apparently has racial differences. The expense of this drug is also small, and combined tablets with isoniazide are possible. However, considerable care must be taken in the dosage, and the relative dosages of thiacetazone and INH used in the adult are quite unsuitable for the child. Relatively much more INH is required in the child's tablet if treatment is to be successful. In the seriously ill child, and particularly the child with tuberculous meningitis, the use of streptomycin and PAS with INH is essential for an initial period of at least 6 months.

In developing countries with limited finances, management of childhood tuberculosis on a large scale calls for thought, ingenuity and skill in planning. In practice, the cost of the drug therapy is small compared with all the other costs, such as those of personnel. One costly procedure, the necessity for which needs to be particularly examined, is the use of x-rays in childhood. In a child with satisfactory clinical evidence of a primary tuberculous lesion, who has a known contact, several weeks' cough, an unsatisfactory weight gain, but is not severely ill, the additional information that may be obtained from an x-ray is marginal. Even if no lesion can be seen on the x-ray, this does not exclude a primary lesion, as this may be either somewhere else than in the chest, or possibly hidden behind the heart shadow. As the cost of taking and reporting on even one x-ray film is greater than that of treating two or three children for a year with INH, or INH combined with thiacetazone, it was the author's practice not to x-ray children unless the child was particularly sick, or the history suggested that caseation and perhaps cavitation had developed with the 'adult' type of lesion. In the average child with primary tuberculosis, more reliance in assessing recovery should be placed on the weight chart than a series of x-rays.

Therapeutic trials

Difficulty in the diagnosis of childhood tuberculosis in developing countries may be so great that the use of therapeutic trials in its management is highly justified, particularly when drugs of low cost and low toxicity, such as INH, are available. In the future, it may well be that it will be the doctor's responsibility to decide whether and when a child can come off antituberculous drugs, rather than solely to decide when they should be started. Any ill child who fails to respond in a few days to antibiotics and after all available tests have proved unhelpful should be treated with INH. Doctors who accept such a policy would be widely criticized by many of their colleagues. Auxiliaries, particularly those working away from doctors, should be encouraged to start children on isoniazide whenever they have adequate suspicion of tuberculosis, or a child with what appears to be an acute pyogenic condition of the cervical glands is not responding to treatment with the antibiotics that the auxiliary has available. Such children, when they improve, require to be assessed by a doctor, who with his additional skill and experience can then make the difficult decision as to whether recovery was related to the use of antituberculous drugs and whether it is necessary to continue these for the year which is the minimum satisfactory period of treatment.

TUBERCULOSIS IN PUBLIC HEALTH TEACHING

The pitfall of teaching people about infected sputum and inferring that they are 'witches' in one community has already been mentioned (see Chapter 3). The great need in public health education is to build up the understanding in the population at large that this is a disease for which we can offer satisfactory treatment, but that to be effective the treatment must bu continued for a year or more. This teaching is more important than efforts to stop people spitting in public, which though necessary is unlikely to be effective. As in other diseases, the most effective educator will be the treated patient. His knowledge and, if successfully motivated, his concern for others with the disease, may make him the best advocate to persuade others to come for help.

In developing countries the patient with tuberculosis or leprosy will be a feared 'outcast', as people with alcoholism and drug addiction consider themselves to be in Western communities. At the start of a meeting of Alcoholics Anonymous, the speaker will get up and say 'I, John, am an alcoholic'. In this way he has identified himself as one who has been a sufferer in the past and still could be. Similarly the patient with tuberculosis or leprosy who is well motivated can use a similar phrase and become the most effective communicator to fellow sufferers. He can tell them how he came to accept and then, with help from doctors, himself overcame the disease − and how he learnt that those near and dear to him could be protected. This chapter has laid great emphasis on the value of drug therapy. Releasing the patient and society from fears of the disease is also essential.

CHAPTER 16

Common Skin Diseases

In communities with a high child mortality, facilities tend to be concentrated on prevention of deaths, and little time is set aside for treating the common and everyday skin conditions which affect a high proportion of children. Skin disorders in childhood can be a cause of considerable discomfort and morbidity, and, indirectly they may cause more mortality than is generally considered. This description is limited to the infections common in children.

Possibly more than in other disorders, the experience of common skin conditions in the large teaching hospital is a poor guide to their incidence in the community. The management of skin diseases may be different in the community from that in the hospital. With a limited budget, simple but effective treatments have to be supplied at a low cost, and there must be alternatives to expensive preparations in elegant tubes and jars commonly found in the cities.

SKIN INFECTIONS

Infection with bacteria, fungi and infestations is the most common cause of skin disease in children. *Figure 92* represents the frequency of these in a village survey undertaken by a dermatologist compared with findings in his hospital out-patient clinic (250).

In the two studies the overall proportion of the population with infections was not dissimilar but the type of infection such as leprosy, large tropical ulcers and severe pyoderma, would reach the hospital skin clinic. In the hospital widespread tinea corporis was the most common fungal disease seen, while the most common infestation was a chronic onchocerciasis. Conditions seen in the village were usually mild pyoderma, and the most common fungal infections were tinea capitis and pityriasis versicolor, diseases rarely brought in to the hospital skin clinic.

COMMON SKIN DISEASES

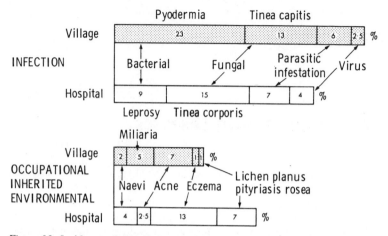

Figure 92. Incidence of skin disease caused by bacteria, fungi and infestations in a village survey compared with a hospital out-patient clinic (250)

Bacterial infections

Bacterial infections of the skin are common and at certain ages in many rural areas almost every child will be affected. These infections are frequently secondary to minor injuries. In the case of young infants carried around by their mothers, many of the lesions may be on the scalp; this is the site most accessible to the mosquito and much of the infection follows the bites and the rubbing caused by the irritation produced. Amongst older children, infections of the leg are ten times as common as those of the arm. Skin lesions are more common in boys who take up farming early, where they use sharp implements without receiving sufficient instruction, and are at risk from abrasions from thorns and bushes. Their sisters engaged with their mothers in household duties are more fortunate because they are less likely to receive injuries which could later become infected. Wearing shoes may reduce the number of skin lesions by as much as 20 per cent. Encouraging the use of simple footwear and so avoiding minor injuries leading to infection is an important preventive measure

Tropical ulcers have been found to be more common in malnourished and debilitated children. Vincent's organisms *(Borrelia vincenti* and *Fusiformis fusiformis)* are responsible. The ulcer is usually surrounded by much oedema, is very painful, and keeps the child awake at night. Treatment with penicillin or other antibiotics will remove much of the pain. Other than this a dressing which is non-adherent and not occlusive is required and, if possible, the leg should be raised and rested for much of the day.

The most frequent bacteria producing skin infections, however, are haemolytic streptococci and pyogenic staphylococci. These streptococcal infections are an important 'missed' tropical disease. They have been particularly studied in Trinidad (213), and these studies have shown that 15–20 per cent of children in some rural schools had streptococcal lesions at any one time, and that the rate of new streptococcal infections was approximately one for every six weeks for each child throughout the year. The infections were successive and mixed, and were so frequent that when a child was admitted to hospital with acute glomerular nephritis, there was a one in three chance that a different streptococcus would be isolated from the current lesions. The route of infection was from skin to skin, and respiratory colonization was mainly secondary to the skin infection.

This early and frequent skin infection may be the reason why acute streptococcal infection in school children and young adults is so much less frequent in these rural communities, as the children have already developed immunity to the majority of the streptococcal antigens. In India it was noted that in some areas severe scabies was followed by nephritis, whereas in other areas this complication did not exist. On investigation glomerulonephritis was common in those areas where streptococci were superimposed on the scabies, while this complication was not seen elsewhere because staphylococci were present. In Trinidad there have been six waves of acute glomerular nephritis over the last 25 years. The streptococci responsible for these epidemics of acute glomerular nephritis were M-type 55, 49 and 57. These are quite distinct from the type 12, which is associated with nephritis following respiratory infection in the more economically developed countries (327).

In some tropical areas acute rheumatism is uncommon, this may be due to immunity to streptococcal antigens being developed through skin sepsis; this skin streptococcal infection does not lead to acute rheumatism. As hygiene improves and skin sepsis is less common, acute rheumatism may be serious as in Singapore. Finally, as standards of nutrition improve, acute rheumatism again becomes uncommon.

Skin infection with diphtheritic corynebacteria is also common, which may be the reason for the low incidence of severe diphtheria in rural societies of tropical countries. Immunity is acquired through the skin, or through sub-clinical mitis infections of the throat.

The prevention of skin sepsis depends on adequate washing facilities which will only be possible when water is piped to each individual house. Spread can take place through the communal use of towels and clothes, or through small abrasions, and the education is necessary to encourage protective measures.

Topical chemotherapeutic agents are the most successful in treatment, and these should be available, perhaps as some locally prepared low-cost ointment base, in every village dispensary or sub-centre. Polymyxin B or neomycin which are effective against a wide range of Gram-negative organisms may be combined with bacitracin or tyrothricin which are effective against Gram-positive organisms. A more widely used but less effective method is 1:1,000 aqueous gentian violet solution.

Neonatal infections

Special care must be given to pyoderma in the neonatal period, first because this infection may at this period of life easily spread and become a septicaemia, with the development of an osteitis or other internal staphylococcal lesion; secondly, at this period of life many of the infections will arise from umbilical sepsis which, if the mother has been delivered in a hospital or health centre, will almost certainly be resistant to penicillin and probably a number of other antibiotics.

Fungal infections

Tinea capitis may be frequent and more than 10 per cent of the children in a school may be infected. The prevention of this condition depends first of all on the maintenance of barbers' combs and clippers in a clean state, and secondly on treatment of cases as they occur. This may be achieved with griseofulvin, and it has been shown that a single large dose of 3 g will cure about 80 per cent of cases. Tinea capitis may provoke a severe inflammatory response, which can mimic a boil; this is called a kerion which heals leaving a bald scar, and will also be relieved by the use of griseofulvin. Untreated tinea capitis usually resolves spontaneously in one to two years.

The finding that tinea capitis usually occurs only in children is probably because the majority of children have acquired an immunity before puberty.

The frequency of animal species of ringworm will depend on the presence of domestic animals living with the population. Cats, dogs and cattle are the most frequent source of these infections. There are now a number of suitable preparations which may be applied locally in the treatment of these conditions.

Tinea corporis can usually be treated with topical therapy unless it is very extensive, when griseofulvin will also be required.

Parasitic infections

The frequency of parasitic infections will depend on environmental factors. It has been suggested that body lice occur only in the tropics, where the temperature is sufficiently low to require heavy clothing, and where this is worn close to the body. Pediculosis capitis infection will also depend on many factors and, for example, is uncommon in West Africa, partly due to the frequency of shaving the hair, and also the fact that the women may weave their hair into intricate patterns, which leads to any extraneous matter being combed out.

Scabies may be endemic, but is often an epidemic disease. In common with other infectious diseases in tropical areas, it appears to develop more frequently at an early age; scabies in small babies is not unusual and may present different features to those seen in older children. Particularly it may be seen on the cheek which presses against the mother's breast, and on the hands and the soles of the feet. The characteristic distribution of the rash in scabies — between the fingers and toes, on the ulnar side of the wrist, the buttocks, and other warm, moist sites — is important in diagnosis, particularly where, as so often happens, a heavy bacterial infection is superimposed. Treatment of this condition with sulphur ointment is almost useless. Application of benzyl benzoate emulsion is not satisfactory, as frequent treatment is required, and when applied to the more tender skin of the body may cause some pain. An alternative and more suitable method was found to be adding a scabicidal substance such as Tetmosol to the local rubbing oil. The use of Tetmosol soap instead of ordinary soap for all washing purposes may control an epidemic. A case can be made for exploring the use of rubbing oils and other local substances as possible vehicles for treating the common and widespread skin infections found in the children of rural societies in developing countries.

RESPONSIBILITY OF THE DOCTOR AND DERMATOLOGIST

In rural areas, and also in peri-urban slums, skin diseases are so frequent as to make their management difficult, and the majority should be cared for by auxiliary personnel. Given guidance and supervision, these workers have an excellent opportunity to manage and reduce these conditions that can cause so much discomfort and misery, particularly to young children.

CHAPTER 17

Common Anaemias

Anaemia is among the top ten causes of death in childhood. At least half of the children dying from other causes will also be anaemic. This is not an easy subject to write about, for the following reasons.

(1)   There is no satisfactory way of measuring anaemia that is suitable for the small hospital or health centre. Although one or two techniques exist, e.g. the Spencer, Lovibond and the low-cost haematocrit methods, none of these have gained general acceptance, and some of the methods of measuring anaemia that are still widely used, e.g. those of Sahli and Tallqvist, or counting red cells, are so inaccurate as to be of little value in measuring response to therapy.

(2)   The incidence and prevalence of anaemia have rarely been documented, and records of the natural history of the common anaemias found in developing countries are lacking.

(3)   In the last few years, the suggested symptomatology of adult anaemia (tiredness, dyspnoea and palpitations) have been shown to be unrelated to haemoglobin levels. In children the symptoms of anaemia are similarly vague. Nor have the long-term effects of chronic anaemia on growth and intellectual development been assessed. Mild or moderate anaemia in adults is not associated with a detectable increase in morbidity or with easily measurable impairment of body function (77). The same may be true of children, but during their period of growth they are particularly susceptible to such changes.

After a brief description of normal haemopoiesis, this chapter will be confined to the recognition and suggested management of the common anaemias of early childhood.

NORMAL HAEMOPOIESIS

The level of haemoglobin at birth is extremely variable, particularly if the cord is cut late and the baby receives a 'transfusion' from the placenta. Even when the cord is clamped at once, levels between 12 and 22 g per cent must all be considered normal. From later childhood onwards there is a mechanism that sets the haemoglobin level for that individual. The range of these 'normal' values will overlap in any community in which anaemia is common with the range found in patients who can be shown to have a haematological disorder (292).

The haemoglobin level is unrelated to maturity at birth. By the age of two months the haemoglobin in all babies should reach a similar figure of about 11 g per cent. This is the lowest level reached, and from this age there is a slow rise in the mean level, which is reached around puberty. Throughout childhood, the haemoglobin levels are lower than in adults, and the normal range is usually considered to lie between 11 and 13.5 g per cent. Capillary blood from a finger prick, which is usually used in young children, will produce a wider range of values than venous blood.

For a long time excessive haemolysis was considered responsible for the fall in haemoglobin in the weeks after birth. It is now realized that the amount of erythropoietic activity of the marrow rapidly declines with increased availability of oxygen, and it is this which is responsible for the fall. The level of this activity is governed by the need to maintain the oxygen content of the blood at a constant level of around 11 g of haemoglobin per cent.

In low birth-weight babies, the fall in haemoglobin is increased, so that although they may start with similar cord blood, their haemo-globin levels fall more than that in the full-term baby by the end of the second month. This is due to a slow response of the marrow to the stimulus of anaemia, and is increased by the rapid growth of the low-weight baby and the need for a greater blood volume. If iron is given to full-term or premature babies, the normal fall in haemoglobin is not reduced, but in low birth-weight infants it is. Even the most premature infant has an iron store sufficient for at least the first month of life, provided that there is no haemorrhage or haemolysis, and it is therefore satisfactory to delay iron supplementation until after the first month. The need for iron is two or three times as great in the first year as at any later period in life. Even in the best nourished infant the iron reserves at one year are likely to be nil (310).

CLASSIFICATION OF ANAEMIA

Table 45 classifies childhood anaemia which falls into three groups: (1) depletion of haematopoietic factors; (2) blood loss; and (3) excessive breakdown (131). Those conditions that are likely to be found perhaps ten times more often in a developing than in an industrialized country are in italics. Because the prevalence of any type of anaemia varies from one area to another, the first priority of any haematological unit which is concerned to serve a community will be to define the frequency of the different kinds of anaemia in different age-groups and to suggest methods for their management. It should be difficult to gain support for research on conditions such as leukaemia in developing countries,

TABLE 45
Classification of Childhood Anaemia

Depletion of haematopoietic factors
Iron, protein, folic acid, vitamin B$_{12}$, vitamin C, thyroid.

Ineffective haemopoietic tissue
- (a)   Primary. Marrow aplasia or hypoplasia.
- (b)   Secondary.
  - (i)   Exogenous poisoning – *lead,* sulphonamide, *chloramphenicol* and other drugs. Also by irradiation.
  - (ii)   Endogenous – *infections.* Chronic illness such as nephritis. Interference with marrow function, leukaemia, neoplastic deposits.

Blood loss

(a)	Acute.	Blood loss (foetal) from the placenta, *umbilical cord,* trauma, epistaxis, *circumcision.*
(b)	Chronic.	Particularly bleeding into the gastro-intestinal tract – *hookworm infection, chronic dysentery,* oesophagitis and oesophageal varices, peptic ulcer, Meckel's diverticulum.
(c)	Blood diseases.	Haemorrhagic diseases of the newborn, scurvy, haemophilia, purpura, leukaemia.

Excessive breakdown
Malaria
Infection
Glucose-6-phosphate dehydrogenase deficiency leading to sensitivity to certain drugs such as *vitamin K analogues, aniline derivatives (sulphonamides, phenacetin, sulphones) primaquine, pamaquin and fava beans.*
Sickle cell diseases
Thalassaemia
Hereditary spherocytosis

After Jolly, 1971

when much higher priorities exist. Studies on the prevalence of anaemia have been undertaken in Europe (76) (90) but in the developing countries few are available. Some good surveys limited to hospital patients have shown marked differences in anaemia between tropical areas of West and East Africa (104), and emphasize the need for local studies, using careful sampling methods (291).

Iron deficiency anaemia

The most common anaemia is the microcytic hypochromic anaemia due to iron deficiency. It is particularly prevalent in infants and young children of low socio-economic status (292). Of the many causes, the most important factor is insufficient iron intake. Deficiency of iron in the diet occurs with breast-feeding when other foods are not taken. In India many mothers give no other food till the child is a year old. Because low birth-weight is also a factor, iron deficiency in developing countries is almost universal in early childhood. Maternal anaemia is not apparently a direct cause of anaemia in the newborn child, but in the presence of anaemia the small but well-absorbed iron content of human milk is reduced, and for this reason a child fed exclusively from the breast of an anaemic mother is particularly liable to become anaemic. Children in developing countries suffer from infection of one kind or another for a third or even half of the first two years of life. Infections also play a part in causing anaemia by interfering with digestion and absorption, by reducing appetite, by increased use of folate, by hyper-splenism, and also by depressing the bone marrow. In the presence of infection iron is diverted from the marrow and immobilized in the tissues.

Recently the importance of various foods as sources of iron has been reinvestigated. Iron from vegetable sources is poorly absorbed and even in the iron-deficient individual the ranges are as low as 1 per cent for the iron rice and spinach and up to 5 per cent for that in wheat. The only vegetable source of iron that is well absorbed is soya bean (10 per cent). The absorption of iron from animal foods is 10–20 per cent, or 20–30 per cent in those with latent iron deficiency (148). Calculations suggest that an adult male in Thailand would have to consume 2–5 kg of dried rice per day and an Indian of Central America 2 kg of corn to absorb their iron requirements. Food of animal origin is thus important in nutrition for its iron content and also because in a mixed diet it increases the iron intake from vegetable sources. A long period of combined cereal and breast-feeding may thus be important in maintaining a child's iron stores during periods of rapid growth and high requirement.

Iron deficiency anaemia is stated to cause irritibility, anorexia for solid foods, and is also claimed to be a cause of pica. These are, however, uncontrolled clinical impressions.

Prevention of iron deficiency anaemia will arise with improved socio-economic conditions and medical care, particularly as the weight of babies increases in developing countries.

Protein lack

As protein is necessary for the formation of globin, the world-wide shortage of protein for children in developing countries can be expected to play some part in the widespread anaemia. However, the formation of haemoglobin probably takes priority over that of plasma protein, and protein must be deficient for a long time before its lack plays much part in anaemia. Where protein lack is sufficient to cause anaemia, the increased severity of infections may result in the anaemia of infection being a more important contribution to the anaemia than protein lack.

Many children with kwashiorkor have a moderate anaemia on admission to hospital, which becomes more severe as they are treated, probably in part due to haemodilution. Fortunately transfusion is rarely necessary, as cardiac failure is particularly liable to follow in these patients.

Folic acid deficiency

Following iron deficiency, folic acid deficiency is probably the most common cause of deficiency anaemia in areas where malaria is endemic. Folic acid is deficient in a diet which lacks green vegetables, liver, meat and milk, foods which are rarely taken by a large proportion of the world's population of children. Folic acid deficiency may also play some part in the anaemia of scurvy, and is also seen frequently in kwashiorkor. Folic acid deficiency anaemia may arise where there is an increased requirement for folic acid, as in sickle cell disease, due to the rapid destruction and formation of red cells. This rapid turnover of cells is also seen in thalassaemia and chronic malaria.

Folate stores in the body are quickly depleted by malaria and other infections and are low in children with sickle cell anaemia. For these reasons folate should be given to children with malaria, malnutrition and any chronic infections. Children with sickle cell anaemia require some folate throughout their lives. Fortunately folate dificiency, unlike iron deficiency, can be quickly made good by mouth.

Vitamin B_{12} deficiency anaemia

This is uncommon in most parts of the world, except in areas where populations live on a very strict vegetarian diet. In India a syndrome of Vitamin B_{12} deficiency is recognized in which the child is admitted with severe megaloblastic anaemia, hyperpigmentation of the knuckles and neurological changes. This is a serious condition, as it has lasting effects on the intellect.

Vitamin C deficiency anaemia

The anaemia of scurvy is due partly to bleeding, and partly to a specific effect of vitamin C on the marrow. The anaemia may be megaloblastic, and frequently requires treatment with both vitamin C and folic acid

Anaemia from exogenous poisoning

Lead poisoning is common in some developing countries and is often overlooked. Lead poisoning may arise from many factors, and outbreaks due to the use of car batteries for fuel, in the primitive methods of extracting gold and from lead paints have been described. A great danger to the child is the use of black lead sulphide as a cosmetic. This is used in West and North Africa, where it is placed on the eyelids of young infants. 'Kajal' is similarly used in Northern India and is safe if prepared at home, but when purchased may contain a high proportion of lead. Legislation on lead content of these substances is urgently needed.

Anaemia due to blood loss

Local knowledge on the prevalence and age incidence of hookworm infestation will suggest whether this is the likely cause. While hookworm anaemia is most common in children of 6–10 years old, it has been reported even in the first few months of life where a child has been born directly onto heavily infected earth. Blood loss after circumcision can cause profound anaemia and a child may be brought for care after the bleeding has stopped and the foreskin healed. Danger from haemorrhage from the umbilical cord was mentioned in Chapter 5.

Treatment to stop further blood loss is an important first step, although in hookworm infestation the giving of tetrachloroethylene (TCE) is usually delayed till a child is no longer in heart failure.

Anaemia due to infection

Malaria

In malarious areas most childhood anaemia is likely to be due to malaria. The anaemia arises from both parasites breaking down red cells, a haemolytic anaemia in which the non-parasitized cells are destroyed, and also a pooling of the blood in the spleen. The malarial infection leads to a folic acid deficiency and there may also be some iron deficiency as well. In holo-endemic areas, the anaemia fluctuates during childhood, starting at or before 6 months and persisting into the fourth year, when immunity may be established. As described in Chapter 14, antimalarials are needed by all children in such areas.

Other infections

A child born in a developing country is likely to suffer from measles, whooping cough, repeated respiratory infection and diarrhoea concentrated in the first three years of his life. The interaction of protein-energy malnutrition and these infections has been intensively studied and is continually referred to in preceding chapters. The interaction of anaemia and infection may be of similar importance in some societies. Anaemia may make the infection worse and the majority of infections that persist more than a few days may reduce the circulating haemoglobin, and this makes the anaemia worse.

Infections that produce rapid anaemia include all those in which pus is formed, particularly empyema, osteomyelitis, and any subcutaneous collection of pus. But anaemia also regularly develops in tuberculosis, and many infants with typhoid present with anaemia (197). Children with acute onset of anaemia, either with or without jaundice from haemolysis, should be treated as infected, unless there is overwhelming evidence to suggest some other cause. The younger the infected infant the more rapid is the onset of anaemia and the greater its severity. If a blood film can be examined a polymorph leucocytosis is likely if pus is present. Most other infections, including those due to malaria and viruses, will show a mononuclear response, which in the case of whooping cough will be distinctive.

Treatment will first depend on overcoming the infection. Only then will correction of any underlying deficiency of iron, folate, or protein be effective. The child on a well-balanced diet can make good his deficiency from his food, unless his anaemia is severe, but the child on an inadequate diet needs supplements of iron and folate and supervision until his haemoglobin has returned to 10 g or his packed cell volume to 30 or 33 per cent.

Sickle cell anaemia

Haemoglobin electrophoresis should be done at district hospital level; indication for this will be on (1) clinical grounds, and (2) where the packed cell volume is below 30 per cent, particularly if response to treatment is unsatisfactory in an area where the sickling trait is frequent.

TREATMENT

Treatment of iron deficiency anaemia will be a major responsibility of all health workers. Iron can be supplied in many forms, but as it is absorbed in the ferrous states, ferrous salts are preferable. The dosage should be calculated in terms of elemental iron, and 6 mg/kg/day is required, divided into three doses. Various iron salts differ in their content of elemental iron. Ferrous sulphate contains 20 per cent, whereas salts such as ferrous gluconate contains only 10 per cent. Probably the most suitable salt is ferrous sulphate, a dose of 30 mg/kg/day. However, in solution this is not stable, and has to be freshly prepared. Ferric ammonium citrate is more stable, but is expensive. To overcome iron deficiency may require 3–6 months' treatment with an effective oral preparation. The changes in colour of the stool over a long period with oral iron therapy may not be easily accepted in some cultures. Prolonged oral iron therapy is difficult and perhaps impossible in some countries, and for this reason other routes may need to be used. Parenteral iron replenishes the iron stores much more rapidly than oral iron, and except for its expense has considerable advantages given as an intramuscular injection as long as the instructions are carefully followed. The dangers associated with this injection are now considered to have been overstated. They include a small chance of immediate collapse, but virtually no chance of cancer. In one study (311) five daily injections of 50 mg as iron dextran (Imferon) were given to infants, starting on the second day of life. With care, 6,000 injections were given in this study without complications. In the follow-up period the treated children had a significantly higher haemoglobin level from the age of 4–26 months *(Figure 93)*. The control group had significantly more hospital admissions, particularly from respiratory infections and diarrhoea. The giving of iron should produce a reticulocyte response and a rise of between 1 and 2 g per cent per week, being rather more rapid in severe anaemia. The giving of iron should continue until two to three months after the haemoglobin has returned to normal, in order to replenish the iron stores in the body. In areas where thalassaemia is common there is some danger of iron overload.

Transfusions of blood in iron deficiency anaemia are required only if the symptoms are very severe, and haemoglobins as low as 4 g per cent, or even as low as 2 g per cent are safely treated with oral iron in the UK. Should a transfusion be necessary, it must be given extremely

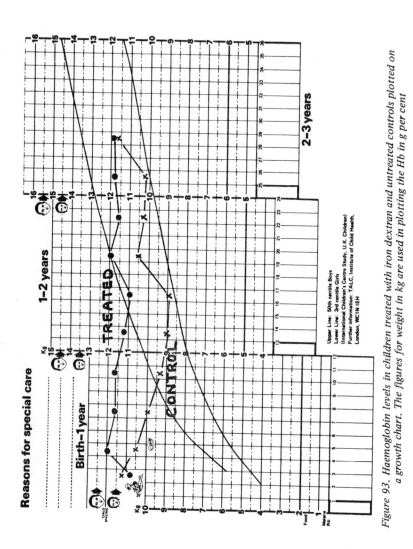

Figure 93. *Haemoglobin levels in children treated with iron dextran and untreated controls plotted on a growth chart. The figures for weight in kg are used in plotting the Hb in g per cent*

slowly if the anaemia is chronic, as there is a very real danger of cardiac failure being precipitated. The dangers of heart failure have been much reduced and the need for exchange transfusions largely eliminated by the intravenous use of quick-acting diuretics such as Lasix (frusemide 1 mg/kg) with slow blood transfusions. As far as possible, avoid cutdowns, and if other methods are not possible the intraperitoneal may be safely used.

THE FOLLOW-UP OF THE CHILD WITH ANAEMIA

The widely practised 'cafeteria' approach to child care has been repeatedly criticized throughout this book. Such an approach, in which the doctor is content with making a diagnosis and supplying treatment 'on a plate' with little attempt at follow-up, is deplorable, but particularly so in the management of anaemia. The Under-Fives' Clinic

TABLE 46

Relationship between Haemoglobin Levels and Haematocrit for Use in Recording Changes in Haematocrit Level in the Weight Chart

Kilo (or Hb) level	4	5	6	7	8	9	10	11	12	13	14	15
Equivalent Haematocrit		12	15	18	21	24	27	30	33	36	39	42	45

(Chapter 19) is an attempt to offer comprehensive and continuing care. Anaemia is not particularly emphasized in the description of Under-Fives' Clinics, as in the areas where they were first developed most anaemia was due to malaria and this was overcome by suppression of malaria. By giving routine antimalarials it is possible to reduce dramatically the prevalence of anaemia. The difficulty is to maintain this routine use of antimalarials over 5 years (Chapter 14). In those children who did not respond, investigations for other causes of anaemia were made. The haemoglobin or packed cell volume, like the child's weight, may need to be regularly measured and, also like the weight, plotted on a weight chart with the following small alteration.

The 10 kg line on these charts is reinforced in red ink to make a level below which haemoglobin levels will be considered abnormal *(Figure 94)*. The haemoglobin is plotted in red against the relevant months in the same way as the weight. If the packed cell volume is used, the same chart can be used, but the relevant packed cell volumes (3 times the haemoglobin) are first written down the right-hand side of the chart against the relevant kilogram line (Table 46). In this way the road-to-

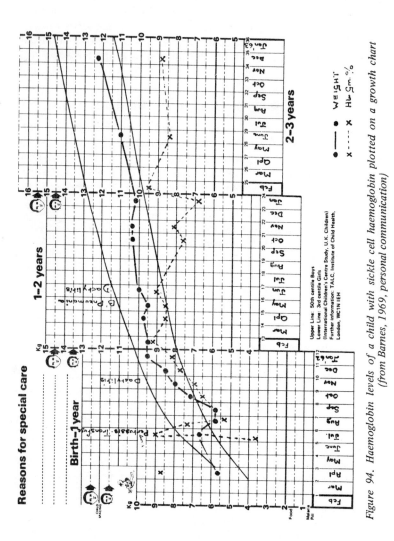

Figure 94. Haemoglobin levels of a child with sickle cell haemoglobin plotted on a growth chart (from Barnes, 1969, personal communication)

health chart will record the changes in haemoglobin level and will show their relation to the child's growth and major diseases which are also recorded on the card. The road-to-health chart is primarily intended for the medical assistant or other health worker in a rural society. For this reason, do not use them to record anaemia until the health workers have thoroughly understood their use in 'achieving adequate growth'.

MANAGEMENT OF ANAEMIA IN THE HEALTH CENTRE

The 'package' principle

The majority of health care for children will be provided through health centres. As already mentioned, most health centres do not yet have the staff or equipment to measure anaemia with sufficient accuracy. To make good this deficiency a new book has been published (312). This has been written on the 'package'* principle in that it describes laboratory tests that have been well tried out using auxiliary laboratory technicians, and it lists the equipment required, which has been selected to minimize both initial and running costs. Also available with this 'package' will be teaching aids to help those training the large numbers of auxiliaries who will be needed if anaemia and other illnesses requiring simple laboratory services are to be managed through health centres in rural societies.

*A 'package' has been defined as an integrated series of components promoting the application of a particular health care technology

CHAPTER 18

Birth Interval and Family Planning

The rapid increase in human population that is now afflicting the world is much discussed today. Estimates such as the doubling of the present world population by the end of the century are put forward. The change in speed of increase is diagrammatically illustrated in *Figure 95.*

THE HISTORY OF POPULATION GROWTH

Estimated rate of population growth
1650 - 2000 A. D.

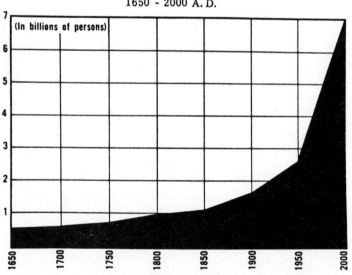

Figure 95. Estimated rate of population growth, 1650–2000 AD

At the present time on this exponential curve a million more people are being added to the planet Earth every five days. The growth rates are compound, that is the rate of population growth increases dramatically as we move from an 0.5 per cent increase per year to a 3 per cent increase. This is well shown in *Figure 96*.

There are those who still do not appreciate the results of exponential growth. To illustrate its effect, we can refer to an old Persian story. A

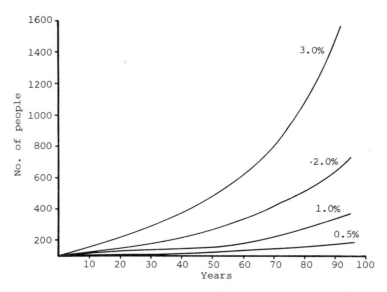

Figure 96. Compound growth rate of population. The 3 per cent level is so much more serious than the 2 per cent

clever courtier presented to the king a beautiful chessboard, with the request that in exchange the king give him one grain of rice for the first square on the board, two grains for the second square, four for the third, and so forth. The king agreed to the request and handed the courtier eight grains for the fourth square, 512 for the tenth and 16,384 grains for the fifteenth. When the twenty-first square was reached, over one million grains of rice had to be handed over by the king. The total rice supply had long since been depleted before the king reached the sixty-fourth square. Had the courtier, in contrast, asked the king to return him one grain for the first square, two for the second and three for the third – a linear progression – on the sixty-fourth square the king would have owed only 64 grains.

From this we can see that in exponential growth numbers increase extraordinarily fast. Population growth can no longer be viewed in time-honoured perspective.

POPULATION GROWTH IN THE UNITED KINGDOM

As a small country with only 1.5 per cent of the world population and a growth rate of only 0.5 per cent, the problem may not appear serious However, many consider that we are already overpopulated in terms of population per square mile, and the increase in the UK of population per square mile is eight times that of the USA, with a growth rate of 1 per cent per annum. At the present time the population of the UK is 55 million, and at present rates this may increase to 66.5 million by the year 2000 (78). At the time of writing, the Government of the UK appears to be moving towards integrating full family planning services within the National Health Service.

POPULATION GROWTH IN DEVELOPING COUNTRIES

At the present time the majority of developing countries fall either into a group which are generally accepted as being 'over-populated', or into those in which the population is relatively sparse.

The over-populated developing countries

Most of these countries are found in South East Asia. India, Pakistan and Indonesia are examples. Reasonable governmental stability over more than a century, associated with the removal of some of the major endemic diseases, has led to rapid population growth, often well up on the 3 per cent growth line *(Figure 94)*. Family planning is today a part of national policy, but is held back by the low levels of economy and the lack of an 'infra-structure' of relevant health services and education, together with the continuing high child mortality which motivates the subsistence farmer to have a large family. These factors (59) interrelate and *Figure 97* suggests where medical services through Under-Fives' Clinics may interrupt this cycle.

The under-populated developing countries

These include most countries in Africa, and some in South America. In these countries there are large tracts of undeveloped land, and the beginnings of industrialization. For national prestige, there is a desire to have a larger population, and even amongst educated people little understanding exists of the difficulty or impossibility of raising standards of education, health and social welfare, while the population is increasing rapidly, in some cases at 3.0 per cent annually. This attitude is particularly evident in countries of South America, where industrialization is spreading. This industrialization cannot absorb the present increase in population, and with the trend towards industry with fewer operatives in modern high-cost factories (Table 5, page 37), it offers no outlet to a rapidly increasing population. In India, at one time, population growth was exceeding economic growth, and improved standards of living for most people became unattainable.

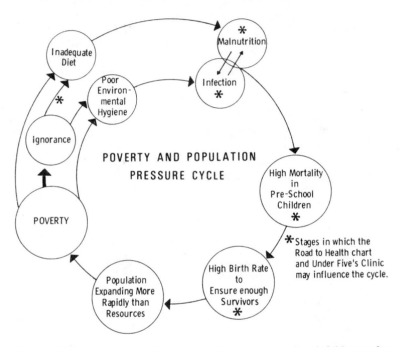

Figure 97. Poverty and population cycle. Comprehensive care of children under five and birth spacing may influence this cycle at a number of points

The rate of population growth increases as mothers move away from traditional rural societies, where long experience has encouraged breast-feeding to be maintained for 1½–3 years, and where the birth rate is well spaced. The mother moves into a situation where bottle-feeding is accepted as the norm. Of many factors involved, the insidious encouragement to artificial or formula feeding of her infants should not be underestimated as a contributory factor in the reduction of the birth interval.

EMPHASIS ON BIRTH INTERVAL RATHER THAN FAMILY SIZE

A large family is a *fait accompli*. We can do nothing except try and help the mother with her large family and persuade her not to have any more children. But when we find a mother has had a short birth interval, we may persuade her to space her children and in so doing we shall reduce the size of her family. The mother who has used family planning methods to separate the births of her children is unlikely to have an over-large family. *Medical workers, when caring for a mother and her young child, will come to realize that delaying the next conception and extending the birth interval are quite as important a part of health care as seeing that the latest child is adequately immunized.* Those caring for children are in an ideal position to counsel about 'birth spacing'. They see the mother regularly, and they speak from the context of concern for the child, and are therefore less likely to be misunderstood as interfering. Most important of all, the mother is coming for help for her child, adn family planning is an answer to a 'felt' need. This chapter is mainly concerned with the birth interval, the disadvantages of a short birth interval to the children, and practical steps the child health worker can take to meet this problem. The birth interval is seen as a fundamental concern; the dangerous level of population growth at 3 per cent previously mentioned is only found in countries where children are born at short intervals in a family. However, as relatively little information is available on the subject of short birth interval or its effect, a brief look will first be taken at the results of a large family. Most of these figures are taken from an excellent review (297).

The large family

There are many correlations between family size and morbidity. As an example, a study of family size and diarrhoea in Ohio (64) showed that in families consisting of three people, each individual could expect just under one attack of diarrhoea a year, but in families of eight it was over two attacks per year. Probably it is in the field of nutrition that we have the best information on the effect of family size. In Africa (192) it was shown that after the seventh parity, there was a marked increase in the chances of malnutrition. In Bangkok, a similar study (297) showed a higher incidence of malnutrition in the larger family. In India, children admitted to hospital with malnutrition came from predominantly large families (98). An interesting study (5) related the sum of money available per head for food, the number of children, and the proportion of malnourished children. These findings are shown in *Figure 98* which suggests that as a subsistence farmer grows older he may have less to spend on food per head and have more malnourished children.

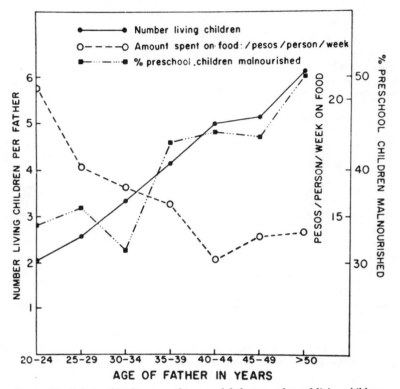

Figure 98. Relationship between the age of father, number of living children, expenditure on food and proportion of malnourished children (reproduced from Bryant, 1969, by courtesy of Cambridge University Press)

As a man's age increases, the number of living children increases, but the amount spent per person on food declines, and the proportion of malnourished pre-school children increases. It is likely that similar figures could be produced for most developing countries where the man's productivity, in a subsistence economy, if there are limitations on the land available, does not increase over the years; and as families grow, the food available has to be divided between a greater number of mouths.

Mortality in infancy and the second year of life is related to position in the family. This was clearly shown in a study of 11 Punjab villages (299) (Table 47).

TABLE 47
Mortality of 1,473 Children Born in Eleven Punjab Villages by Parity of Mothers, India, 1955–1958

Parity of mother	1	2	3	4	5	6	7–12	Totals
Number of births	230	209	210	197	165	136	326	1,473
Infant mortality (deaths/1,000 infants up to 1 year)	172	117	145	124	172	164	206	161*
Second-year mortality (deaths/1,000 pop.)	76	16	24	92	96	77	95	68*

*Average mortality for all parities
After Wyon and Gordon, 1971

This table shows that in each age group mortality rates increased with parities over one. This increase is particularly marked in the second-year mortality figures, which increase four- to fivefold amongst children born after the third. There is a particularly marked difference between second and seventh parities. This increase in mortality after the second or third birth is also present in industrialized countries, as shown in *Figure 99* (195). This diagram shows that in the more fortunate socio-economic groups, including the professional and managerial classes, there is apparently little increase in mortality up to the third child, but considerable increase in deaths from infection thereafter. In the other groups there is a steady increase with parity. Closer examination of the variables in more developed countries shows that in the young mother aged less than 25 belonging to the professional group, the mortality increases more dramatically than in the working class group. Perhaps the young working-class mother has the advantage of support from a more closely-knit joint family system.

Physical growth may also be related to family size. In Britain this association is seen in all but the 'upper' and 'lower' middle classes. In the 'upper' and 'lower' working class the difference between the first child and the third or later child is around 10.2 cm (4 inches) at five years (70). It has been found that the smaller size of children in larger families is common to all of them, and that the first-born does not achieve the height and weight of first-borns who remain 'only' children. These findings suggest that the advent of each additional child to a family acts as a check on the growth of all preceding children. Menarche has also been found to be later in the larger family (264).

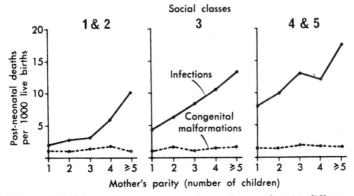

Figure 99. Relationship between parity and mortality in different socio-economic groups

Good evidence is available that family size is related to intelligence. A number of studies, both American and British, show that whereas the average intelligence of the single child in a family will give an IQ score of 105, from approximately the sixth child onwards it will be around or below 90.

Many workers have seen evidence (129) of what has been called 'the maternal depletion syndrome' in women who have had a large number of pregnancies. This may well contribute to the lower birth-weight of later children and a poor performance in lactation (192). Similarly in developed countries large families may correlate with poorer health in the parents.

The effect of birth interval

Far less information is available on the effects of birth interval than on size of family, but there is still excellent evidence for the serious effect on the health of the children when the birth interval is short. The effect of short birth interval and mortality on the preceding child is shown for two areas in *Figure 100*.

From this chart it is clear that the mortality after a short birth interval is far higher in a developing area of the world than in a more economically fortunate region. This is perhaps not surprising, as the good health of the small child in the Punjab depends heavily on a sustained period of breast-feeding, which is not possible with a short birth interval. The largest study to be undertaken in this field was one in the USA (300a). This drew attention to the fact that when the birth interval is below a year, conception for a full-term infant would have to

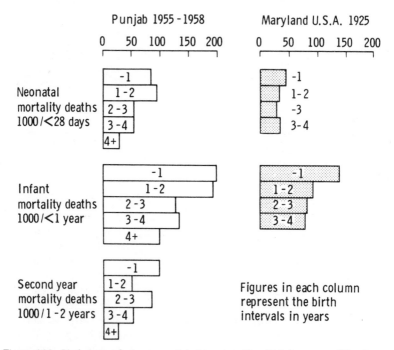

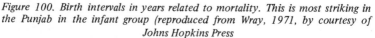

Figure 100. Birth intervals in years related to mortality. This is most striking in the Punjab in the infant group (reproduced from Wray, 1971, by courtesy of Johns Hopkins Press

take place within three months of delivery. However, babies born premature could be conceived within four months of delivery and still be born within the year. For this reason, the mortality under a year is likely to be artificially inflated by this large number of small premature babies. In the calculations for this study (300a), the intervals between birth and the next conception were related to mortality, as shown in *Figure 101*. This study was able to show a striking difference in mortality both in the first year and up to the age of five in children born after a short interval. As intervals increase, so do chances of survival increase.

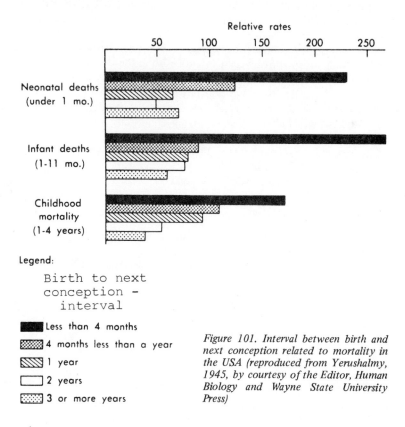

Legend:

Birth to next conception - interval

■ Less than 4 months

▨ 4 months less than a year

▧ 1 year

☐ 2 years

▦ 3 or more years

Figure 101. Interval between birth and next conception related to mortality in the USA (reproduced from Yerushalmy, 1945, by courtesy of the Editor, Human Biology and Wayne State University Press)

The effect of birth interval on morbidity has been little studied. In the field of malnutrition it is well known that kwashiorkor is particularly likely to develop at the time or shortly after a new baby is born. The word 'kwashiorkor' in the Ga tribal language is usually interpreted as 'the disease of the deposed baby when the next one is born' (283). One small study has been undertaken on this question in Columbia (296) where it was shown that when the birth interval exceeded three years there was a fairly marked decline in the incidence of malnutrion.

In the UK, social class difference in the risk of prematurity was found to be relatively unimportant. Risks were, however, greatest in two well-defined groups of working-class women, namely the primiparae aged 20 or less and the multiparae with closely spaced pregnancies. Approximately half of working-class mothers in the UK spaced their pregnancies either so closely or so far apart that they ran an abnormally high risk of giving birth to a low-weight infant. If they could all have been persuaded to allow for intervals of 3–6 years between births, the proportion of low birth-weight infants born in the UK could have been reduced by a fifth.

Just as large families were associated with lower intellectual scores, the same is true of birth interval. One study (70) investigated the effect in middle-class families in which living conditions would deteriorate relatively little even when births were closely spaced. This study showed that in middle-class families of different size the vocabulary scores of the children were relatively high when births were widely spaced and relatively low when they were close together.

BIRTH INTERVAL AND MOTHER CARE

In developing countries, a wide range of birth intervals occurs. The author has had the opportunity of gathering experience from rural societies in a country in Africa and one in South America. In Africa the

TABLE 48

Distribution of Birth Interval in a Country in Africa and South America

Country	No. of births	Months between births								Mean	Median
		9—	12—	18—	24—	30—	36—	42—	48+		
Africa	248	–	1	9	24	127	52	20	15	35.5	34.7
South America	170	9	82	31	18	10	9	2	13	23.3	17.25

The South American data from Perry and Frey, 1971–72, supplied when involved as Peace Corps workers

sample represented all mothers giving birth in a village during a two-year period. In South America the figures came from a survey of all families on two sugar estates (307). The figures are not presented as being representative of either continent, but are given as examples. The results are given in Table 48.

In both countries there is a fairly wide variation in the length of birth interval. The median in Africa, where abstinence for cultural reasons was strong, amounted to 34.7 months, while in South America it was only 17.25 months. A further breakdown showed that the median birth interval for one-third of the families in the South American group was only 14.8 months.

Observations, in developing countries suggest that 'mother care' is largely concentrated on the youngest baby. In Africa the mother is likely to carry the baby around with her for most of the day, and throughout the night he will sleep close beside her and suckle at intervals. At a very rough estimate, the mother gives approximately a sixth of her 'mothering time' to each of her children under five, and the rest of this to the youngest baby.

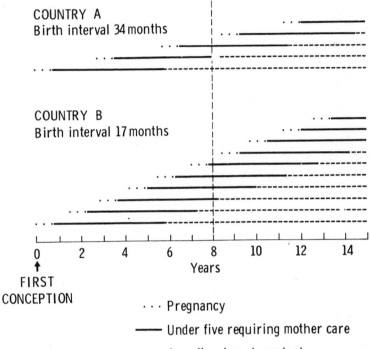

Figure 102. Build up of families in countries with a long and short birth interval. In country B the mother will either have 4 children under five years of age, or if she has 3 she is likely to be pregnant again. In country A she will only have 1 child under five years of age when she is pregnant. Each child in country B is likely to get much less mothering than in country A

Assuming that, as suggested, the mother concentrates her care on children under five, then *Figure 102* represents the way her care will be divided differently in these two communities. *Figure 102* shows that in the African village there is a birth interval of 34 months, so that there will never be more than two children under five for the mother to care for. In the South American estate, however, if all the children survive, the mother may have up to four children under the age of five on her hands, and when she has only three she is likely to be well on in the next pregnancy. With the longer interval the youngest infant will have a high proportion of his mother's 'mothering time' for nearly three years. With the shorter interval he will get a share of his mother's time for under 18 months. The child may get only half as much 'mothering time' for half as long as when there is a longer interval — there may be an approximately fourfold difference.

Effects of a short birth interval

In countries where there is a short birth interval, breast-feeding is usually brief, and may last only three to six months. In these circumstances, malnutrition occurs early, and is not uncommon in the first six months of life. In societies with a long birth interval, malnutrition is more common at the age of 18 months to three years. The malnutrition occurring in the first year of life is likely to be more serious than occurring at a later age, because of its adverse effects on physical growth and full intellectual development of the infant. Failure of growth due to malnutrition in the second or third year may be made up later, when nutrition improves. This 'catch-up' phenomenon is believed to be less in evidence after malnutrition in the first year of life, and children who have been severely malnourished during the first six months or year of life may grow up physically stunted (269). Observations in areas with a short birth interval show that many adults who have grown up in rural areas where malnutrition is common are shorter than those who have grown up in the better environment of the city (302). In these countries short and stunted adults are more common in the rural societies than in those countries with long birth intervals.

Possible effects on the intellect are more serious than those on stature. Not only is the child growing quickly in weight and length during the first months of life, but at birth the brain is growing rapidly, and poor nutrition in the early months of life may lead to smaller brain with fewer cells and the likelihood of poor intellectual development (54, 67, 328).

HOW CAN WE APPLY THIS KNOWLEDGE?

The knowledge of birth interval and its concern are essential for the health of the children in industrialized countries, but even more so in the developing countries. Birth intervals vary from area to area, and the first step is to study the local situation, and from local data calculate percentiles. The data given in Table 48 has been calculated in this way in Table 49.

TABLE 49
Duration in Months of Birth Interval Expressed as Percentiles

Source and number in sample	5%	10%	25%	50%	75%	90%	95%
West African mothers (588)	27	29	31	34	38	45	50
S. American mothers (247)	12	12	13	16	23	36	51

From Table 49 it will be seen that in the West African mothers 5 per cent had a birth interval of 27 months, and family planning needs to be instituted at $27 - 9 = 18$ months after the birth of a child. In the group of South American mothers, contraception needs to be available before the child is three months old.

In *Figure 103* the relationship of the timing of the birth of an infant born in November 1972 is related to the likely time of birth of a succeeding infant in the West African community where the median birth intervals are as given in Table 49. The fifth centile, that is when we could expect 5 per cent of the siblings to be born, is 27 months. Therefore in the case of this child January 1975 would be the month in which there is a 5 per cent chance of a sibling being born.

If a mother wishes to maintain a satisfactory birth interval between her children, she may start some method of contraception soon after the birth of her infant, but in many societies with a long birth interval cohabitation immediately after birth is the subject of a strong taboo. In these circumstances, the mother may see no need for, and be unwilling to accept, methods of contraception at the time of delivery. In order to postpone the next conception, we must discuss the matter with the mother, and through her with the father. In our example this dialogue should reach its peak in the month of March 1974, immediately before the time when 5 per cent of the next infants are likely to be conceived, as shown in *Figure 103*. This is a time when the parents may wish to resume sexual intercourse, and may welcome a supply of condoms for the husband, or an intrauterine device or an injection of a long-acting contraceptive agent for the wife.

The practical application of this concept is shown in *Figure 104*, developed in India (59). Here we see the weight record of a child through the first three years of life. At the same time, along the top of

309

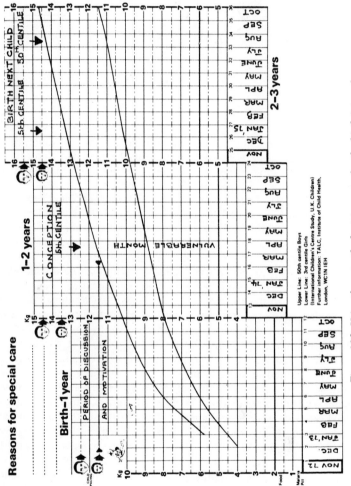

Figure 103. Using the growth chart to supervise the birth interval

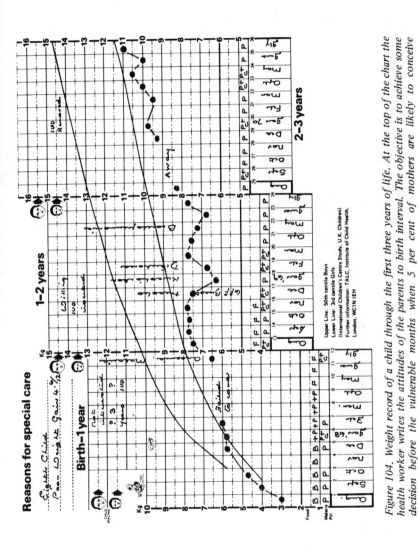

Figure 104. Weight record of a child through the first three years of life. At the top of the chart the health worker writes the attitudes of the parents to birth interval. The objective is to achieve some decision before the vulnerable months when 5 per cent of mothers are likely to conceive

the chart the nurse seeing the child keeps a regular record of the attitudes of the father and mother to birth interval. When the child was only a few months old, the father was uninterested in the interval between births, and the mother was hoping for a period of three years. This dialogue continued, and in the second year the mother was prepared to have an intrauterine device inserted to prevent conception. This was removed in the third year, so that she could conceive her next baby with a birth interval of just over three years. Although still based on surmise rather than scientific studies, the consensus of opinion suggests that a birth interval of three years, as practised in many rural societies, is about optimal both for the mother and her children.

By relating the use of contraceptives to the road-to-health chart, we are introducing, so to speak, the time element into increasing the birth interval, and anyone supervising the clinic will, by looking at the child's road-to-health chart, be able to see whether the nurse seeing the child is maintaining and is recording a dialogue with the mother on maintaining her birth interval. As the emphasis is placed by the nurse on birth interval rather than family size, this method will be acceptable in most communities. The emphasis in the dialogue with the mother may not be on limiting the size of her family, but rather on the length of birth interval and the expectation that if she wishes to do so, she may have more babies later on. Perhaps it is analogous to an adult managing a child, who will be more successful if he says 'Perhaps later' rather than 'No more'.

In most societies in the future we can hope that those responsible for caring for children will by carrying on a continuing discussion with the mother on family planning at the same time as the child's growth, development and immunization are being discussed. It is so easy for the child health worker to say:

Your child is doing very well now; it would be a pity if you became pregnant again before he can walk and look after himself. These first two years are so important to him. The size and strength he grows to and how well he does in school depends on your caring for him and giving him good food at this time when his brain is growing. Have you considered . . . (Family planning advice given if requested.)

Or:

Your child is not doing quite as well as he should; it would be most unfortunate for him if you became pregnant again before he was really strong. These first two years are so important to him. The size and strength he grows to and how well he does in school depends on your caring for him and giving him good food at this time when his brain is growing. Have you considered . . . (Family planning advice given if requested.)

Involvement of the father

Population pressures are so serious that every discipline must examine how their expertise and personnel can be involved. The presence of the weight chart in the home may allow the agricultural extension officer, the teacher, pastor, or other male worker who has been trained and motivated, to start a discussion on birth spacing with the husband on a 'one-to-one' basis. In this he would discuss the weight and growth of the child, and draw attention to the advantages of a satisfactory birth interval, and suggest to the husband how this may be achieved. In doing this the information in the road-to-health chart he finds in the home will be a useful starting point for a discussion.

Reducing the desired family size through Under-Fives' Clinics

Elsewhere in this book, in describing the road-to-health chart (Chapter 7) and comprehensive care through the Under-Fives' Clinic (Chapter 19), a description was given of the work undertaken in the

TABLE 50

Surviving Children and Median Number of Additional Births Desired by Imesi-Ile and Oke-Imesi Mothers (1967) (253 responses)

	Median additional births desired	
Surviving children	Imesi-Ile (where Under-Fives' Clinics were first developed)	Oke-Imesi (Control Village, see page 145)
1	5.9	10.2
2	6.3	8.5
3	4.6	6.8
4	3.6	3.6

Reproduced from Cunningham, 1971

village of Imesi-Ile. In this village, where over the years there has been a relatively high standard of child care — higher than in most other parts of West Africa — a study was made of the desire of mothers for additional children (57). In an analysis of 253 responses given in 1967, highly significant difference was found between this village and the neighbouring one (Table 50). As has been found in so many other communities, once the mothers realize that their children are likely to survive, their desire for a large family diminishes.

BIRTH INTERVAL AND FAMILY PLANNING

The Under-Fives' Clinic through the road-to-health chart promises to be an efficient channel for the delivery of health care through which the 'reproductive community' can be effectively kept under supervision.

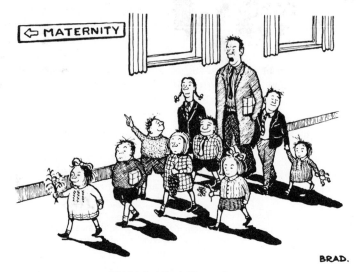

'Alright stupid!—dad knows the way.'

Figure 105.

NATIONAL ATTITUDES TO FAMILY PLANNING

An outstanding statesman, President Nyerere of Tanzania, a sparsely populated African country, has this to say in guiding his people towards limiting the speed at which they increase their country's population:

'It is very good to increase our population, because our country is large and there is plenty of unused land. But it is necessary to remember that these 350,000 extra people every year will be babies in arms, not workers. They will have to be fed, clothed, given medical attention, schooling, and many other services for very many years before they will be able to contribute to the economy of the country through their work. This is right and proper and is in accordance with the teachings of the Arusha Declaration. But it is obvious that just as the number of our children is increasing, so the burden on the adults – the workers – is also increasing. Giving birth is something in which mankind and animals are equal, but rearing the young, and specially educating them for many years, is something

314

which is a unique gift and responsibility of men. It is for this reason that it is important for human beings to put emphasis on caring for children and the ability to look after them properly, rather than thinking only about the numbers of children and the ability to give birth. For it often happens that men's ability to give birth is greater than their ability to bring up the children in a proper manner' (209).

India commits the largest population of her health budget to family planning, and other countries can learn much from her experience. The Chinese Government has been advocating family planning for 10 years, and claimed in 1972 that the population growth is down to 1 per cent in the cities, but is still 2 per cent in the rural areas (43).

Both the developing and the industrial countries of the world have a long way to go in regulating their population size satisfactorily.

CHAPTER 19

The Under-Fives' Clinic —
Comprehensive Child Care

The cost of medical care given through the clinic or out-patient department is only a fraction of that for in-patient care. Trials in many countries have shown that items of care such as operation for the repair of a hernia, or care of most tuberculosis, including tuberculosis of the bone, can be effectively carried out with equal success in the out-patient clinic as by admission to hospital. This is a field in which further investigation is urgently needed. With perhaps $1 per head to spend on health in developing countries in 1970 and $3 by the year 2000, the proportion of money usefully spent and the emphasis placed by doctors on out-patient care is likely to increase in these 30 years.

The clinic as described here attempts to offer comprehensive care for all children under the age of five. As will become clear, it is different from a traditional out-patient clinic, which it replaces. Adult out-patient clinics in developing countries were designed to separate out the more severe conditions for specific therapy and to offer symptomatic relief for the rest. So often clinics for children have been developed along similar lines. Because the Under-Fives' Clinic attempts to offer curative and preventive services, the mother will receive teaching at a number of stages as she passes through the Clinic. Her child will be weighed and the weight charted, and any immunizations that are due will be given. The child will also receive curative and symptomatic treatment for the symptoms his mother presents, and this treatment is her felt need. She is unlikely in the first few years of attendance to understand the need for prevention. The Under-Fives' Clinic will be a major part of the maternal and child health work undertaken by the hospital, health centre or sub-centre where it is held. If possible, it should be run in conjunction with an antenatal clinic and family planning services, all of which need to be available to the mother at every visit. The antenatal clinics for mothers without young children will usually only take place once or twice a week, but the Under-Fives'

316

Clinic facilities should be available at any time for children, and able to care for pregnant mothers as well as their children.

At Ilesha a family planning clinic is now open at the end of every morning. The mothers know that they are welcome to attend this clinic after attending the Under-Fives' Clinic. For them this has a considerable advantage as they can obtain family planning advice inconspicuously, without making a special visit. In a community where everyone's movements are usually known, this visit need not necessarily become a matter of general gossip.

The Under-Fives' Clinic completely replaces both the welfare clinic and the out-patient clinic for all children under 5 years of age every day of the week. As long as children under 5 years of age are still seen in a separate out-patient service, an Under-Fives' Clinic does not exist.

THE OBJECTIVES OF THE UNDER-FIVES' CLINIC

The Under-Fives' Clinic aims to extend low-cost curative and preventive care to as large a proportion of the population as possible. The basic services it offers will be the same whether it is situated in a remote village or in a hospital complex in a major city. The clinic described was developed over several years to meet the paediatric challenge presented by the young children of the Ilesha area of the Western Region of Nigeria. This challenge is inherent in a birth rate of over 40 per 1,000 that is common to the whole of this region, and a childhood mortality of 30–40 per cent, which means that in the past no less than a quarter to one-third of all the children born there died before they were five. The experience from Imesi is compared with other areas in Table 51 (246).

The Ilesha hospital, where this clinic evolved, serves a town of 100,000 people in Nigeria. This meant that had none of them died, there would have been no less than 20,000 children under five in the town, a figure that death did in practice reduce to the hardly more manageable number of about 17,000 – still a formidable task for one small hospital. Though the main clinic is in Ilesha itself, it was developed from the findings of an intensive study of child health carried out in the nearby 'research village' of Imesi. The figures for Imesi (Table 51) confirm the importance of diarrhoea, pneumonia and malnutrition. Table 52 shows that the starting of an Under-Fives' Clinic there coincided with the reduction of all deaths in the first five years of life to about one-quarter of their previous number. An independent study (56) showed a striking difference between Imesi and a neighbouring village. Curative services alone can cut such gross under-five mortality by half, among them being sulphadimidine or penicillin for

TABLE 51
Major Causes of Death in the Under Fives (Percentage)

	Imesi Nigeria (1957)	Luapula Zambia	North Sumatra	Pusan South Korea
Diarrhoeal diseases	12	18	25	15
Pneumonia	12	10	11	9
Malnutrition	12	16	26	14
Malaria	8	15	8	3
Whooping cough	8		2	4
Measles	8	13	7	16
Tuberculosis	5		6	8
Smallpox	5			
Anaemia		7	5	
Other, mostly neonatal	30	21	10	24
Total number of children	–	340	1,282	1,036

Note: All the conditions *underlined* can be prevented in an Under-Fives' Clinic. Health education and early diagnosis and treatment can reduce mortality from the others

Reproduced from Shattock, 1971

TABLE 52
Child Mortality, Imesi Village, Western State, Nigeria (Population 1963–1964 = 5,476)

	Prior to 1957	1962–1965	1966	UK 1966
Stillbirths/1,000 total births	41	36.4	21.7	15.3
Neonatal deaths/1,000 live births	78	21.9	22.2	12.9
Infant mortality/1,000 live births	295	72.0	48.1	19.0
1–4 mortality/1,000 alive at that age	69	28.1	18.9	0.84
Population (natural) increase/year %		3.5	2.9	

bronchopneumonia, and chloramphenicol for early whooping cough, but its further reduction to one-quarter will only follow the introduction of preventive paediatrics. This is the whole purpose of an Under-

Fives' Clinic, and the enormous number of lives it saves is the entire justification for what follows.

ESSENTIAL ACTIVITIES AND AIMS

The essential activities of an Under-Fives' Clinic rest on the four corner-stones of Treatment, Immunization, Weighing, and Health Education. Of these, weighing is exceptional to the others, as the weight curve that results acts as an evaluation of the other three activities. The aims of those who run Under-Fives' Clinics may be summarized as follows.

(1)   The supervision of the health of all children up to the age of five.

(2)   The prevention of malnutrition, malaria, measles, pertussis, tuberculosis, smallpox, poliomyelitis, diphtheria and tetanus.

(3)   The provision of simple treatment for diarrhoea, with or without dehydration, pneumonia and the common skin conditions.

'Reproducibility'

At one time it was suggested that these clinics were suited only to the conditions of church-related hospitals, and not for general use, for only there, it is said, is found the combination of staff continuity and high motivation that is required for success. While it is true that the idea and practice of Under-Fives' Clinics has spread quickly to other church-related hospitals in four continents over the last six years, the author has always believed that they were suitable for more general use, and it has been reported that large numbers of these clinics have now been started by many governments, particularly in Malawi, Sarawak, Sierra Leone, Zambia and elsewhere. Here the locally trained nurses and medical assistants have taken up this work with its clearly defined objectives with a new zest and enthusiasm. Given guidance, leadership and supervision, these clinics can be started in any developing country that may benefit from them. Thus, there are signs that they are spreading, and so making it possible for the lives saved over the last 14 years at the original clinic in Ilesha to be saved in other countries too.

THE BUILDING

The staff of an Under-Fives' Clinic will have to spend long and exhausting hours in the building available. The doctor in charge must be concerned with the details of the building if his staff are to function efficiently. While these remarks are true of the whole health centre, they are particularly important in the wing of the building used for the Under-Fives' Clinic, as this is likely to be the most crowded area. As around 60 per cent of those attending the health centre will be children under five, an area needs to be set aside for this group for use every day. In this description of Under-Fives' Clinics, no mention is made of facilities such as a laboratory or room for dressings, as these facilities will be shared with the rest of the health centre.

An architect defined the purpose of a building as a structure to protect those who live or work in it from the weather. In most tropical countries this implies protection from the heat of the sun. Some of the important ways by which a room may be kept cool and dry and 'friendly' are so often ignored that doctors need to be familiar with them.

(1) Light means heat, therefore windows should be small, and wooden louvres may be preferable to glass. The roof should be over-hung with large projecting eaves. Where possible the length of the building should be across the direction of the prevailing winds. A knowledge of the direction of storms may suggest modifications which will keep out the worst of the wind and rain.

(2) When the sun hits the roof the air under the roof is warmed, thus there should be ample allowance along the sides of the building for circulation of air between the ceiling and the roof, with vents at the gable end. A layer of silver paper on the upper surface of the ceiling *(Figure 143)* will reflect back infra-red rays.

(3) The out-patient clinic will contain many people generating heat. This must be allowed to escape upwards and clearly the height of the room is important. There is also need for vents (at least one foot square) in the walls near the ceiling to allow the hot air to escape. In some hot countries a 'Dutch barn' type of structure, with few if any walls and only screens, has been successfully used.

(4) If there is any choice of building material, the heavier material such as mud or mud brick is a better insulator than the concrete block.

(5) The health centre or out-patient building will be the first and most frequent contact that the local people have with medical services. They are more likely to feel at home if it is constructed along the same pattern as their own houses. This will vary from area to area, but the mud-wattle-dieldren-and-whitewash building recommended for some areas of East Africa (139) is a good example. This can be a highly durable structure, and yet it can be extended or altered by local labour who are expert in such building methods. Out-patient waiting space is often inadequate. A simple construction is suggested and has been designed so that the use of the rooms may easily be altered *(Figure 106)*.

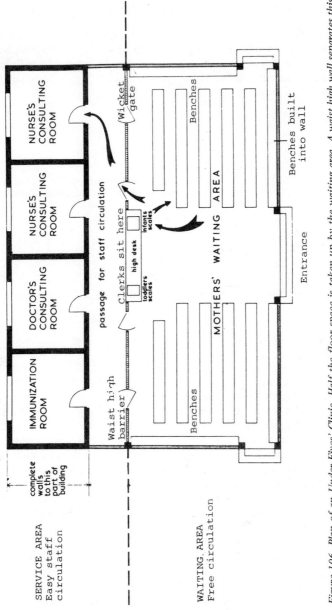

SERVICE AREA
Easy staff
circulation

complete
walls
to this
part of
building

IMMUNIZATION
ROOM

DOCTOR'S
CONSULTING
ROOM

NURSE'S
CONSULTING
ROOM

NURSE'S
CONSULTING
ROOM

Waist high
barrier

passage for staff circulation

Clerks sit here

Wicket
gate

toddlers
scales

high desk

infants
scales

WAITING AREA
Free circulation

Benches

MOTHERS' WAITING AREA

Benches

Entrance

Benches built
into wall

Benches

Figure 106. Plan of an Under-Fives' Clinic. Half the floor space is taken up by the waiting area. A waist high wall separates this from the service area

COMFORT OF THE MOTHERS AND STAFF

In the waiting space and in the rooms where the mothers are being seen, the seats should not be higher than 14 inches (35 cm). The mother with a child on her lap is uncomfortable on a chair of standard height; she tends to sit with her heels off the ground and her legs become painful *(Figure 107)*.

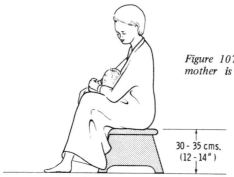

Figure 107. A low seat is needed if a mother is to be comfortable with a child on her lap

30 - 35 cms.
(12 - 14")

An easily visible and accessible tap, so that she may get a drink for herself or her possibly feverish child, is essential. Not only is adequate and clean latrine accommodation essential, but a modified unit may be necessary which can be used without fear by the children.

One feature that is particularly valuable is a low wall separating the area of staff activities and circulation from the waiting space. In this are placed small gates. The waiting mother should not feel too far from the place where she will be seen, but the staff will not be surrounded by a crowd as they work. The registration desk will be in this low wall. The clerk carrying out the registration is seated on a high stool behind the registration desk, which is 40–50 inches (100–120 cm) high, so that his eye level is the same as that of the mother *(Figure 108)*. This level is important. The mother who will be standing to register with a clerk sitting at a table at a normal height may not see more than the top of his head, unless he looks up. The clerk sitting on a high stool has his eyes on the same level as the mother, and as she comes forward he smiles and greets her in the manner traditional to their society. Such a first reception at the clinic is invaluable. The mother who may be so anxious about her child finds with relief that she is welcomed, and the staff want to help her.

COMFORT OF THE MOTHERS AND STAFF

The weighing station may also be set in the low wall. Either a beam balance scale with weights moving along an arm or a modern spring suspension scale* on which the child can be suspended in special trousers or in a bowl is the best. If trousers are used, several pairs will be required, so that mothers can put their children into them while another child is being weighed. If the space for the scale is situated in a 'well', the child when perched on the scale is less likely to be frightened, as he is at the same level as the working surface on either side. For older children an adult scale with a toddler bar is required. This latter scale may also be used for antenatal and adult weighing.

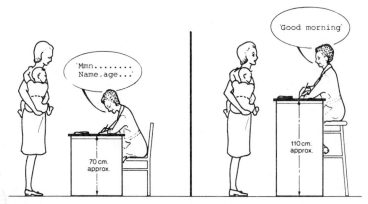

Figure 108. Registration, the first and perhaps the most important contact with the health service

The system in which the mothers form a sitting queue on the benches and slowly shuffle their way along is only slightly more satisfactory than a standing queue While waiting they should have an opportunity to attend a discussion with the health teacher or just to socialize. This will be possible if they deposit their green clinic cards in a pile knowing they will be seen in this order. It is better to have a 'queue of cards' than a queue of mothers. The mother may also appreciate high and clearly visible shelves on which to deposit belongings, and if these are visible to themselves and their friends, the risk of thefts is reduced. If possible, the mothers should be called into the consultation room in groups of 10; there, while they wait to be seen, they should 'learn by overhearing'.

*Salter Scale No. 235, 25 kg x 100 g, with special (King) dial face, including four pairs of strong plastic trousers, cost approximately £9, and is available from CMS Weighing Equipment Ltd., 18 Camden High Street, London NW1 0JH

In more than one rural area doctors have reported that the level of attendance was improved when specific days in the week or month were set aside for different villages or areas, and on those days as complete attendance as possible was attempted. This is similar to the system now used in some European schools where children from one village work together to increase a sense of community.

RECORDS

There are few hospitals in developing countries that keep adequate record filing systems for their out-patients. Maintaining a file of more than five thousand records, where the identification of people by name is not clear-cut, can be difficult and expensive both in personnel and waiting time for the children. Experience from many countries emphasizes that the mother will care for her child's own records once she has learned of their importance. These records must not resemble a 'bus ticket', designed to take the child through one disease incident only, but should record his growth (on a weight chart), his major illnesses, his immunization state and any 'reasons for special care'. Each record card should be supplied in a strong polythene envelope 10 cm longer than the card together with a clinic card on which the staff can write details of minor illnesses and their management. Such records (Chapter 7) are becoming more widely used in many rural areas where there is a planned service and these records are likely to replace other types of hospital out-patient records in many areas in the next decade. A staff of clerks is essential, although they will not be needed for filing records. They will complete the record cards, weigh the children and call groups of mothers to the nurses. Cards neatly made out with clear weight curves will be their responsibility. In all developing countries there are many unemployed young men with primary education. As clerks in the Under-Fives' Clinic they may be brought into the health service and from experience gained there go on to training in other fields. Successful recruiting NOW and training of intelligent and well-motivated young men is essential if medical services are to expand in rural areas. In some societies girls or married women clerks may be used. The latter have the advantage that as married women they are more acceptable for discussions with the mothers on controlling the birth interval (Chapter 18).

The road-to-health chart is an integral part of the Under-Fives' Clinic. As described in Chapter 7, the objective in using these cards is to promote adequate growth rather than to prevent malnutrition. The author is familiar with the 'family record' folder, and all the advantages proposed for such a system, but in his experience, the logistics of the service prevent such records being adopted outside certain demonstration or teaching areas. In no country has their use spread widely to the majority of centres.

Records other than the road-to-health chart should be kept to a minimum. Unfortunately, many governments still demand detailed returns which serve no useful purpose, and are often difficult to maintain with the limited facilities available; they also absorb staff time that could be more effectively used. In many countries the phrase 'medical records' brings to mind 'visions of inky-fingered clerks covering, in an infinitely laboured hand, page after page of a dogeared ledger; of out-patient forms so grubby, porous and ephemeral that they almost melt in the hand' (139). Two types of record exist; the patient's own record, such as the road-to-health chart, with its accompanying clinic card, which is 'home-based', and the files and ledgers which record the work of the clinic or hospital, both for its own use and for the State. These 'hospital-based' records also need to be simplified.

Hospital-based records

The hospital records system needs to record the patients, old and new, seen each day. This can be done by a simple tally system *(Figure 109)* as developed in Zambia (246). If for legal purposes a record of the patient's attendance is needed, then only the patient's number will be recorded. If a numbering system encoding the date of birth of the child is used (139) the records of attendance may be used to identify the distribution within age groups of the children attending.

As well as recording the old and the new patients in the Under-Fives' Clinic, the children attending Zambian clinics whose weight falls on or above the lower line on the road-to-health chart are also recorded. These, when expressed as a percentage of all attendances, make an excellent monitor of the changing nutritional status of the children between seasons of the year and from year to year in each area of the country. This is an example of vital information needed in planning health services, which is sadly lacking in many developing countries.

The immunizations undertaken are also recorded by a tally system. A further useful record now being included in the Zambian system is a notification of each child completing their immunization programme. Such a child is called the 'protected child'. If this latter figure is expressed as a percentage of new attendances, the success of the service in maintaining contact with the children providing a full immunization can be gauged.

The majority of infectious diseases of children brought in contact

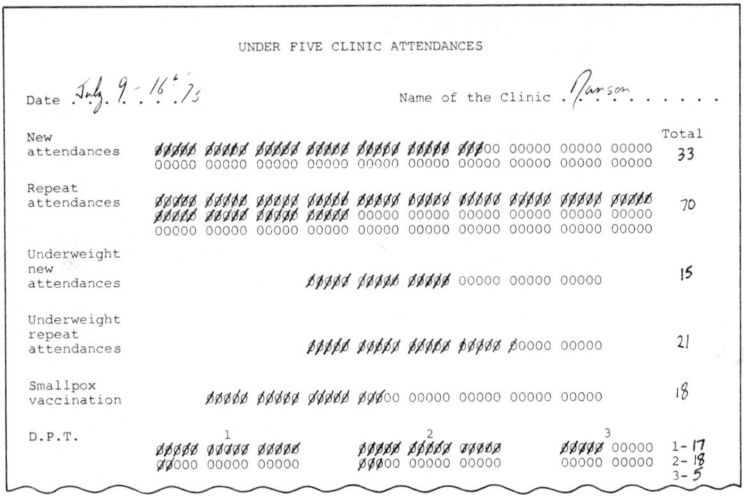

UNDER FIVE CLINIC ATTENDANCES

Date July 9 - 16th 73 Name of the Clinic Narson

	Total
New attendances	33
Repeat attendances	70
Underweight new attendances	15
Underweight repeat attendances	21
Smallpox vaccination	18
D.P.T.	1- 17 2- 18 3- 5

Figure 109. Part of Under-Fives' Clinic attendance form; a tally system is used (after Shattock, 1971)

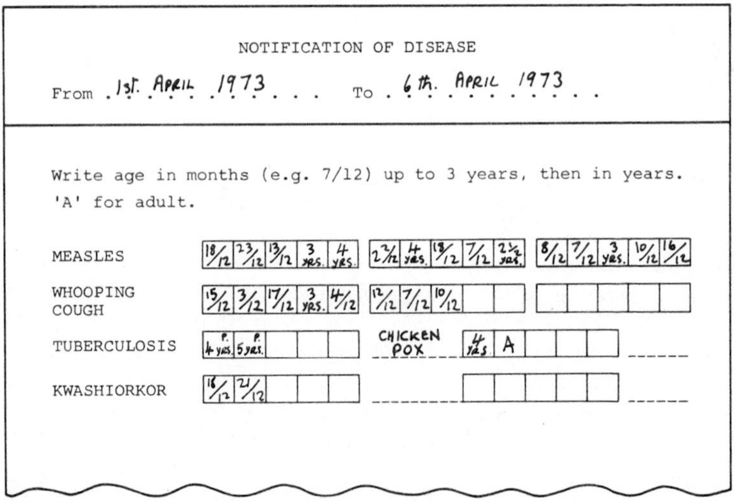

NOTIFICATION OF DISEASE

From 1st. APRIL 1973 To 6th. APRIL 1973

Write age in months (e.g. 7/12) up to 3 years, then in years. 'A' for adult.

MEASLES	18/12, 23/12, 13/12, 3 YRS., 4 YRS., 2 2/12, 4 YRS., 13/12, 7/12, 2½ YRS., 8/12, 7/12, 3 YRS., 10/12, 16/12
WHOOPING COUGH	15/12, 3/12, 17/12, 3 YRS., 4/12, 12/12, 7/12, 10/12
TUBERCULOSIS	P. 4 YRS., P. 5 YRS.
CHICKEN POX	4 YRS., A
KWASHIORKOR	16/12, 21/12

Figure 110. A notification of disease form giving the age incidence of the children. A fresh form is started each week

with the medical services will be seen at the Under-Fives' Clinic, and a simple record of these is needed. Records of the individual child's name and address will not be required (exceptions are perhaps only smallpox and rabies), and any system of individual notification as used in some industrialized countries is unnecessary and wastes the valuable time of the clinic staff. A tally system may also be used for these records, although a slightly more involved system, such as that shown in *Figure 110,* will give the age incidence of the children. From this information a breakdown of the age incidence of infectious and other diseases in each area by week can be made. This is necessary information if the planning of immunization programmes is to be efficient and effective.

Whatever system of records is used the time involved in their preparation needs careful study. One study (65) of a medical assistant's working time gave the following breakdown for each working minute *(Figure 111).* Of all his time that spent in listening and talking to the patient is likely to be the most valuable.

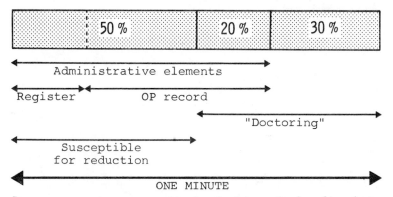

Figure 111. Medical assistant's working time; breakdown of each working minute. Can his time be better used? (reproduced from Dissevelt and Vogel, (1970) by courtesy of the Director East African Literature Bureau, Nairobi, Kenya)

USE OF PERSONNEL FOR CONSULTATION

A doctor involved in clinical work will spend more time in consultations than in anything else. Ways must be found to reduce this by delegating the diagnosis and standardized treatment of common conditions to less skilled personnel. The step described below is the most urgent and important change in the method of delivery of health care if our objective is to serve the whole community and not just those who come to hospitals asking for help.

The traditional European out-patient clinic is a referral clinical and not the primary medical contact. In most developing countries the hospital out-patient clinic is the first contact with the medical services for the majority of patients. The doctor must devise a system by which his time can be kept for the following necessities.

(1)   Giving detailed care to 10–20 per cent of the children attending. This will include the more complex conditions and the more seriously ill children.

(2)   Spending time in training and encouragement as a doctor ('doctor' = 'teacher') to the nurses or medical assistants and to all levels of staff with different qualifications and degrees of training who will care for the majority (in practice 90 per cent) of those attending the Under-Fives' Clinic.

This pattern of care is brought out in *Figure 112;* the quotations are taken from Spence's writing (253).

CONSULTATIONS

".. all else in the practice of medicine derives from it "

A. Traditional Pattern

Mother & child ⟷ 100% Doctor

B. Alternative Pattern

Mother & child ⟷ 90% 'Nurse'

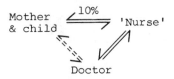

Mother & child ⟷ 10% 'Nurse'

Doctor

"The purpose of a consultation...
shall give explanation and advice...
not the diagnosis or the technical treatment."

Figure 112. Consultation. The role of the nurse or medical assistant and the doctor

Nine out of ten consultations are between the mother and the 'nurses' or medical assistants. These are 5–10 locally trained women who ideally will themselves be mothers. They should have five minutes available to spend on each child. They personally accompany all ill children to the doctor.

During the consultations in which the doctor is involved, together with the nurse or medical assistant, he is making double use of his time by teaching and raising the standard of care offered by the nurse. If he sees that the nurse supervises the treatment he prescribes, he will increase the respect given by the mother to the nurse. The nurses are not acting just as a filter allowing certain patients through. The doctor is working with and through the 'nurses' and guiding them in the continuing care of the children who will visit them regularly. This daily contact between the doctor and the auxiliary worker will lead to a high standard of work. The doctor is here fulfilling his role as manager (Chapter 21) and effectively delegating to those with less training.

A doctor who has additional training in paediatrics is likely to have the responsibility for children from a population of 100,000 in which there will be 17,000 children under five. He cannot attempt to know individually all the children and their mothers. This will be essential with only two groups; those needing hospital admission, and the children of the hospital staff. The latter must receive special attention, as their robust health will be such a valuable example in educating the local people. In a town in West Africa it was known by the people that no child belonging to the staff of the hospital had died over a period of five years. The doctor may ask his staff to look out for another group such as the children of the indigenous practitioners. Caring for the children of these indigenous practitioners who can be so powerful in the community may be the step through which he can gain a rapport and friendship with these traditional health workers whose co-operation can be so helpful.

Mother–nurse relationship

To the mothers of sick children the locally trained nurses from their own locality inevitably become the most important people they meet at the hospital. The great importance of the nurse is the critical factor in the whole psychology of the clinic and is something that the doctor does all he can to promote. Spence held that consultation *(Figure 112)* is the quintessence of the medical art, and in the Under-Fives' Clinic this is certainly true, except that here it is consultation not between mother and doctor, but between mother and nurse. Spence maintained that the true purpose of consultation is to give explanation and advice, and that diagnosis is usually but a means to achieve this and must never become an end in itself. Such explanation and advice leads to the right action by the mother in matters concerning the health of her child; this action is much more likely to follow careful and sympathetic explanation than an ill-understood and peremptory command. Because she comes from the same culture as the patient, a well-instructed and supervised nurse is the best person to explain and offer sympathetic advice to the mother. Her cultural proximity to the mother will make discussion of birth interval (Chapter 18) particularly meaningful if the nurse is well trained and herself has a family.

The mother–nurse relationship is so crucial that it must be strengthened wherever possible. Thus, every time a mother comes to the clinic it should be to see the same nurse, and each time she consults a doctor this nurse *must be present,* the doctor ensuring that in all he does or says he always supports her in the eyes of her patient. This is difficult for the doctor who has not been trained in the team approach and sees himself as the clinician in a 'one-to-one doctor–patient' relationship, and not as a teacher, manager and leader, working with a team of auxiliaries. The flow of communication in the triangle *(Figure 112)* needs careful consideration. Where possible, the doctor must gain much of his information from the nurse, and use her to verify that the mother has understood his instructions. The success of the Under-Fives' Clinic depends heavily on a high level of 'one-to-one nurse–patient' relationships. Unfortunately, this delegation is a recognized or unrecognized 'threat' to the doctor (Chapter 21) and the success of the clinic may largely depend on his coming to terms with his own attitudes.

From experience, the most likely cause of failure in these clinics is because the doctor does not have the nurse present and does not fulfil his obligation to teach and support her. If the child has to come into hospital, he should return to this same nurse on his follow-up visits. This vital continuity is maintained in practice if the child's card bears upon it the number of the table where sits the nurse assigned to that family, or if these tables are distinguished by some special colour. Such a system allows the nurse time to offer preventive care through discussion of the child's diet with the mother, and she can at the same time ensure that the required immunizations are undertaken and discuss the birth interval. The doctor will supervise this work by personally checking that inoculations have been given, discussion on birth interval has been undertaken and by enquiring from some of the mothers brought to him how they feed their children.

The greatest economy can be achieved in employing staff to the utmost of their skill and ability. It is clearly wasteful to employ a nurse for weighing children when in a week or two a clerk can be trained to do this just as well, or a doctor to see the common conditions when these may be more adequately taken care of by a nurse specifically trained in their diagnosis and management, who is also trained to undertake preventive care.

Those responsible for the organization of the Under-Fives' Clinic need to work out a consultation plan to be carefully followed by the auxiliary nurse as she sees the child. A possible step-by-step method is set out here and is designed to be as simple as possible. *(Figure 113)*. The nurse must be encouraged to spend as much time as possible in discussing and, particularly, listening to the mother.

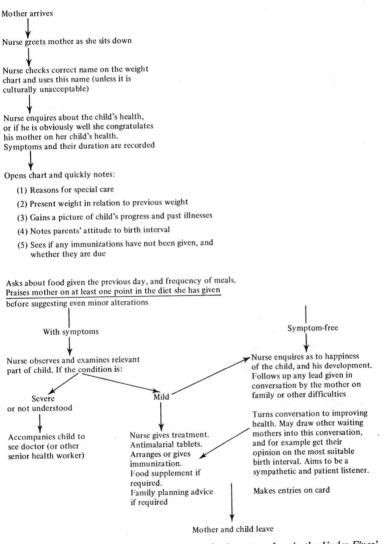

Figure 113. A suggested sequence for consultation procedure in the Under-Fives' Clinic

331

This plan of the consultation, when agreed upon, will be set out in the nurses' manual and will be a central core of the training programme. For example, as part of their training, a child's symptoms and signs and his road-to-health chart are given to a group of student nurses, so that they may discuss what action they would take, and bring their decision to the tutor for further discussion.

Lines of flow

The happiness and good temper of those who work in the clinic, and of the mothers, will depend on the thought and careful observation given to the lines of flow. A mother with a sick child should not have to

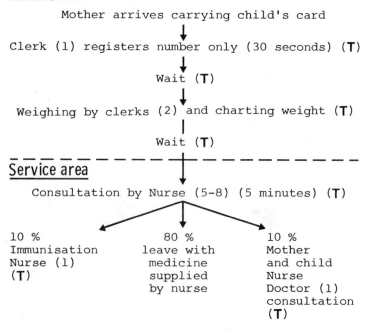

Waiting area

Mother arrives carrying child's card

↓

Clerk (1) registers number only (30 seconds) (**T**)

↓

Wait (**T**)

↓

Weighing by clerks (2) and charting weight (**T**)

|

Wait (**T**)

– –

Service area

Consultation by Nurse (5–8) (5 minutes) (**T**)

10 %	80 %	10 %
Immunisation	leave with	Mother
Nurse (1)	medicine	and child
(**T**)	supplied	Nurse
	by nurse	Doctor (1)
		consultation
		(**T**)

(**T**) Teaching introduced whenever the opportunity arises

Figure 114. Lines of flow in an Under-Fives' Clinic averaging 300–500 visits per day. The figures in brackets relate to the number of personnel undertaking each function

force her way through a crowded door; passageways used for staff circulation must be left clear. *Figure 114* should be examined in relation to the suggested waiting and service area in the clinic lay-out shown in *Figure 106*.

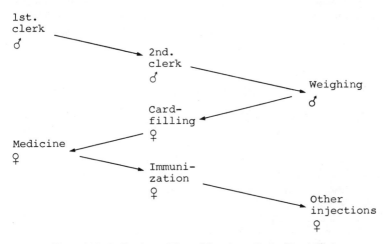

Figure 115. Badly planned line of flow in an Under-Fives' Clinic

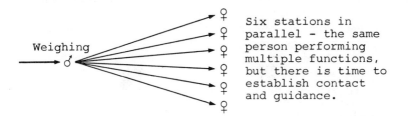

Figure 116. The same Under-Fives' Clinic as shown in Figure 115 with a reorganized line of flow

An example of what may happen if thought is not given to planning is shown by the line of flow that existed over several years in one clinic *(Figure 115)*. Here the mother was making brief contact with seven people and the average consultation time was 50 seconds; no wonder such a contact with scientific medicine bewildered her. The same clinic was differently organized *(Figure 116)* and subsequently a good rapport was achieved.

The large Under-Fives' Clinic is run with the activity sequence shown in *Figure 114,* with a daily attendance growing from 400 to 500 per day over ten years. In this the immediate contact with a clerk on arrival is brief, but the mother knows her presence has been recorded. Her child is then weighed by one of two clerks and has a consultation with one of six nurses, who will always attend her on subsequent visits. From there she may go for immunization, leave with her medicines, or accompany her nurse with other referred mothers to see the doctor.

HEALTH TEACHING IN THE UNDER-FIVES' CLINIC

Health teaching is an important function of all members of staff and must permeate all activities of the clinic. Specific talks with cooking demonstrations are best carried out informally in the waiting space. The mothers should be involved in the food preparation and feed their children with any food prepared at the demonstration. Teaching may be effective during the consultation; here not only the mother but also eight or ten other mothers waiting to be seen are involved. These mothers are 'learning by overhearing'. The teaching is built on the mother's existing knowledge. A discussion with several mothers in which they unfold the course or natural history of the common diseases of childhood will be popular. The role of the nurse will be to guide this discussion and particularly to offer advice on the management of the condition at home, and to emphasize those symptoms that suggest the need for a visit to the Under-Fives' Clinic.

Immunization is often a neglected opportunity for teaching. Here as elsewhere the mother must be involved, and the nurse will build on her present knowledge of the disease being discussed. A blown-up picture of a child with smallpox, or a nurse, who with practice can give a good imitation of a child with whooping cough, may start what should be a 'discussion' rather than a 'lecture'.

Of the 300 children with malnutrition in the population of 100,000 already mentioned, a few will require hospital treatment. The majority are better and more economically treated in nutrition rehabilitation centres, and in some areas these centres are becoming integrated with the Under-Fives' Clinics (255). They may be day care, or residential, depending on the distance from the mother's home. In the nutrition rehabilitation centre emphasis is placed on the mother rather than the child. The mother is involved in the production and preparation of suitable foods. The 'stethoscope and syringe' are not in evidence. The teaching is largely undertaken by mothers whose children have recovered from malnutrition, who are guided by staff with a knowledge of nutrition and teaching methods. If possible, mothers who are leaders in the community are encouraged to stay and join in the activities of the centre.

The formal teaching period

Although special emphasis has been placed on the informal teaching by all the staff of the clinic, a more formal period in which teaching and group discussion take place is still needed. The rota of instruction in an Under-Fives' Clinic in South India (58) is given as an example (Table 53).

TABLE 53
Under-Fives' Clinic – Teaching Rota (South India)

Monday	Child health and weight cards. The importance and use of the cards.			By staff nurse
Tuesday	a) Immunization b) Scabies and skin sepsis		Alternate weeks	By Public Health nurse
Wednesday	a) Diarrhoea b) Sore eyes	Prevention and home management	According to season	By staff nurse
Thursday	Feeding infants and children			By nutritionist
Friday	a) Family planning and child health b) Intestinal parasites and hygiene		Alternate weeks	By Public Health tutor
Saturday	Prevention of protein-energy malnutrition			By nutritionist

When teaching remember the following points.
(1) Be Brief – 5 to 10 minutes is enough in a busy clinic.
(2) Be Simple – make one or two points clearly, do not confuse with too much information.
(3) Be Seen – use visual aids and actual foods when possible.
(4) Be Heard – speak really loud and capture their interest and attention.
(5) Be Remembered – where possible emphasize your teaching with one of the well-known proverbs we have chosen.
(6) Call the doctor just before you begin; he is interested to hear and support your teaching.

Reproduced from Cutting, 1971

The weekly staff discussion

A weekly meeting of all members of staff involved in running the out-patient department may do much to achieve efficiency and economy. The value of such discussion groups, both in improving morale and in implementing new ideas in an ever-changing situation, is now well recognized in the UK (46). At this meeting discussion should take place on the following points.

(1)   Reducing the waiting time for mothers. A line of flow diagram is valuable in seeing how mothers pass through the out-patient department and in discovering how the mother's contact with different members of the staff can be made more effective, even if it has to be brief.

(2)   Ensuring that urgent treatment is given to the seriously ill child. All staff, including the cleaners or sweepers, are encouraged to identify such children, and when they bring a child to the doctor and urgent treatment is instituted they are congratulated on playing an important part in saving the child's life.

(3)   Uncovering points of friction between members of the staff and bringing these out for discussion.

(4)   Educating all members of the staff on matters such as nutrition and the natural history of common diseases, and discovering ways in which every activity can have an educational content. When off duty and away from the hospital all members of the staff, from the cleaner or sweeper upwards, will be asked for advice on medical problems, and for this reason even the most junior should receive this type of education.

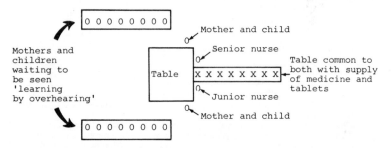

Figure 117. Arrangement of furniture which allows teaching and supervision of staff in training

Training personnel in the Under-Fives' Clinic

Make this a major concern of the doctor and be prepared to give up time to plan it. Some of the teaching will be by discussion, as in the weekly staff meetings, some by reading and short courses, and rather more when he is seeing referred cases brought by the nurse.

The more experienced nurses or medical assistants will also take a part in this training of new staff. The following arrangement of the furniture, developed in Sierra Leone (50), was found to make this teaching and supervision possible *(Figure 117)*. The senior nurse shares her medicines and tablets with the junior nurse, and can keep an eye on the children she is seeing and tactfully intervene if necessary.

REDEPLOYING MONEY SPENT ON PHARMACEUTICAL PREPARATIONS

As the clinic becomes more 'preventive' in its outlook, a greater proportion of the money spent on drugs will need to be spent on vaccines, and less on injections and tablets. In the majority of cultures, including that of the UK, the bottle of coloured and strongly smelling medicine has greater appeal than the tablet. While the injection may be impressive at the time, it cannot be carried home and passed round to be examined by the relatives, as can the bottle of medicine. By offering such medicines to the mothers of the children we care for, we are not 'teaching them to rely on the bottle of medicine'. In their own culture they will almost certainly regularly use herbal and root teas, just as we may use unnecessary vitamins, and we should be substituting something that we know to be at least harmless for something which is unlikely to be beneficial and may be harmful (as has been shown in the case of the Jamaican herb teas which led to hepatic cirrhosis). We may be able to persuade the mother that her child is healthy and her concern over some minor symptoms was unnecessary but she may have difficulty in passing this message on to her relatives. If she arrives home bearing a bottle of 'tonic', her time at the hospital will be justified among her relatives, who may have had to undertake some of her household chores for her, and perhaps have supplied the cash to make her visit to the hospital possible. The child may come with some trivial symptom, and if he is due for an inoculation he will receive this. The inoculation may well prove life-saving in the next epidemic, but to the mother the bottle of red-coloured peppermint water costing 3 ¢ a gallon to make in the pharmacy may be a more significant medication.

Of the liquid medicines given, the 'saline mixture' for diarrhoea may be the most valuable. This consists of a concentrated solution of sodium and potassium chloride and a colouring agent, and is diluted by the mother to make up a drink for the child if he has diarrhoea.

Tablets are best pre-packed, as this reduces the problems of checking their distribution. Directions for their use may be stamped on the pack with a rubber stamp, or small duplicated slips included if they are packed in polyvinyl (139).

To the cost of the injection must be added the cost of employing the staff to give it, and the sterilization of the syringe. Clearly the number of injections given must be cut to a minimum and the senior staff should lay down criteria for their use.

A most important economy is for the common and simple medicines to be given out by the nurse herself. This saves particularly the mother's time, as she does not have to queue at a dispensary to receive her medicines. In this as in other activities, the senior staff will continually observe and discuss with other personnel what innovations or changes may lead to greater efficiency. For example, in dispensing liquid medicines a wide-mouthed container into which a scoop will pass allows the nurse to measure out and dispense, through a funnel, into the mother's own bottle a known quantity of medicine *(Figure 118)*. When instructing the mother in the quantity to give the child, locally available demonstration spoons are required. Holes are drilled in the handles of the different sized spoons; three spoons attached together with a key-ring are less likely to disappear than one unattached spoon! The road-to-health chart described in Chapter 7 is supplied with a polythene envelope and is also shown in this diagram.

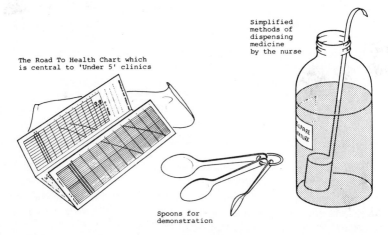

The Road To Health Chart which is central to 'Under 5' clinics

Simplified methods of dispensing medicine by the nurse

Spoons for demonstration

Figure 118. Simplified method of dispensing liquid medicine by the nurse. Spoons for demonstration. The road-to-health chart and its polythene envelope

THE ECONOMICS OF THE UNDER-FIVES' CLINIC

The cost of a visit to the clinic is approximately the same as that calculated for a health centre attendance and amounts to about $0.21. In arriving at this figure, salaries were costed at the local Nigerian rate, and the annual budget of about £6,000 ($17,000) was divided between the 80,000 patients attending the clinic at the research village of Imesi during the year. These figures include many adults, who take longer to see than children, and make no allowance for the research activities of the clinic staff. The true cost of a visit to an Under-Fives' Clinic may well be less than 5p ($0.14). So far few others have been successful in reducing it further. In India (58), with a higher proportion of ill patients, clinics were costed at $0.20 per visit. In Malawi they have recorded a cost of $0.11 for each visit (47).

TABLE 54

Examples of Recent Cost in Nigeria in ¢ of Some of the Material Used in the Under-Fives' Clinic

	¢		¢
Triple vaccine, one injection	9	Road-to-health chart in polythene envelope	5
BCG	20	Old tuberculin for Heaf test	2
Pyrimethamine, one year	7		
Chloroquine treatment for malaria	3	INH for one month, 200 mg/day	11
Sulphadimidine, 12 tablets in packet	6	Tetmosol to add to rubbing oil to treat scabies	12
Saline mixture or other medicine, 100 ml	1		

As already mentioned, most developing countries at present have around $1 (40p) to spend on health for each citizen, and are unlikely to have more than $4 by the year 2,000. Both these figures are in the region of 1 per cent of what is spent on medical budgets for health in Europe and North America.

The present expenditure on Under-Fives' Clinics is probably better spent in terms of cost benefit than most other expenditures in the health field. However, it is still too high. Probably the greatest economy will be through training village mothers to run Under-Fives' Clinics in their own village. Their satisfaction may be through the responsibility and prestige they receive by helping their community with only a small financial incentive.

In the Under-Fives' Clinic the majority of conditions could be prevented or treated at low cost. Table 54 contains figures that were first published in 1963 (184), but the prices have been brought up to date. The items may all be purchased through normal channels.

DESIRABILITY OF COMBINING A CURATIVE AND PREVENTIVE APPROACH IN ONE CLINIC

Some experienced workers are still concerned with the possible danger of bringing all children together under one roof. Undoubtedly there is a slightly increased risk of infection. However, the author believes it is justified on the following grounds.

(1)   Measles, whooping cough and many other infections are more infectious in the prodromal stage, when the child is not 'ill', and he is just as likely to be brought by his mother to the well-baby clinic. It is the mother who makes the decision where he should be taken.

(2)   In most traditional communities, unless preventive services are integrated with curative, the majority will not receive the preventive services.

(3)   Personnel and facilities are so limited that more effective care can be given to most children through a comprehensive service.

(4)   The separation into preventive and curative clinics arose historically because doctors in Europe failed to show interest in providing preventive services, particularly advice on feeding methods, and this function was taken over by the child welfare movement. This movement, which was run by voluntary agencies and town councils, developed a network of welfare clinics in the first half of this century. The doctors were adamant that the child welfare clinics should not offer any curative care. This separation of curative and preventive services did not arise out of any idea of removing the danger of infection to the well baby. At first only a minority of doctors were involved. Strict rules were enforced to prevent the two services being combined (284).

CHAPTER 20

Nursing

If as doctors we claim to be the leaders of the health team, all its
shortcomings are ultimately our responsibility. This includes nursing,
and if this is bad, as it is in so many developing countries, then the
development and welfare of the nursing profession is no less important
to the care of the sick than the development of the medical profession.
It is also the justification for this chapter being written by a doctor.
Doctors designed the present health services and the relatively back-
ward state of nursing and the poor facilities for training nursing
students, compared to those for medical students, is *their* concern. If
nurse training is to be quickly improved, doctors must be involved,
although once a strong corps of senior nurses is available the doctor's
responsibility will be reduced to that of encouragement and assistance
when this is required.

WHO IS A NURSE? WHAT IS NURSING?

A sick child needs much looking after. He needs to be examined,
investigated and diagnosed. He may require a variety of medications
and treatments and he has also to be watched over and comforted as
well as fed and cleaned. Provided it is to the ultimate good of the child
community as a whole, there is no *a priori* reason why any part of these
tasks should necessarily be done by any particular cadre of health
worker. Here we would include mothers, as well as the various kinds of
doctor and nurse as being perhaps the most important health workers
of all in the care of the sick child. Just who does what in this team will
depend upon how many of each kind of workers there are compared
with the total number of children to be cared for. When, as in the
developing countries, there are so many children and so few trained
staff, doctors have to delegate more tasks to nurses, which on many
occasions include routine diagnosis and treatment. Nurses in their turn
have to delegate much routine hospital nursing to mothers. For the
mother, the nurse is a person who works either in the hospital or clinic,

341

or may occasionally visit the home. The nurse will usually be distinguished by some form of uniform, and the majority will be women. If all the people involved in this wide concept are included, we are dealing with a profession or discipline that is already playing a major part in improving the health of the children, and one that has the greatest potential to expand further and raise the standard of health.

The local people in a rural society see the nurse in two situations — working in the hospital ward, or in a clinic either away from or attached to the hospital. From this clinic she may under certain circumstances also visit the people in their homes. The great difference in her work in these two roles lies in emphasis on the skills that the nurse possesses. In the hospital setting, she will need more of the traditional specific nursing skills. In the clinic situation, she will frequently require to have many of the diagnostic skills for which she has usually been less well trained. Here she may ultimately carry different, and at times greater, responsibility than those held by her colleague in the wards of the hospital.

Midwives

The separation of the midwives from the main body of the rest of the nursing profession has arisen largely for historical reasons. In the rural societies of developing countries such a division must be deplored. Modern drugs and vaccines and understanding of nutrition are so effective that a student, while training as a midwife, can at the same time learn enough about child care to enable her subsequently to reduce child mortality to a greater extent than she can maternal mortality. For this reason, in training programmes designed for the future, it is likely that the child health element ought to be at least equal to that given for midwifery training.

THE HOSPITAL

The hospital today is responsible for moulding the attitudes and expectations of society to illness and health, aging and death. Nursing is the pivot on which the whole practice of good hospital care depends, provided that the doctors offer the nursing staff the opportunities and respect it deserves. As the nurse is so central to the hospital, the following paragraphs examine its function.

The hospital has been described as a place that has served on various occasions down the centuries as a hostel, a prison, a religious retreat, an asylum, a poor house, a social assistance agency, a school, waiting room for death and therapeutic community (285). Looking more closely at the tasks of the hospital there are three among many which may be considered of primary importance for an institution. These have been set out in *Figure 119*. Thus in an accident hospital, a surgical ward, or a tuberculosis unit, the primary task is cure; in a geriatric ward or hospice for the dying, it is care; in a teaching hospital, the educational role is primary. In general, all three tasks are usually interwoven, but in the developing countries it is the first and third that predominate. In the future we may hope that the concept of every hospital as a teaching centre will continue.

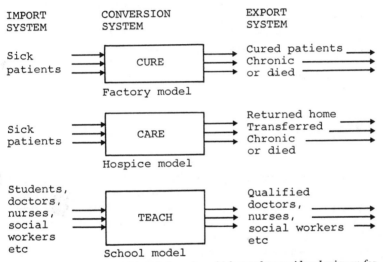

Figure 119. *Three types of hospital service which may be considered primary for an institution (after Wilson, 1971)*

THE HOSPITAL IS A LIVING LEARNING ARENA

When a nurse gives an injection she may be curing; at the same time her gentleness is an act of care, in addition she may also be teaching a student nurse how to give injections, and teaching the patient the effect of the injection in helping his body to recover. It is now suggested that there is a fourth way of looking at the task of the hospital as an institution. Because the inputs and outputs are human beings, we (and our families) respond to events, experience them, and learn from them. The staff are also involved in this learning process which is represented in *Figure 120*.

This description of the hospital as a living learning arena is even more important in developing countries. In Europe and America, the people have a certain understanding of the causation of disease and the approach of scientific Western medicine. They can compare their experience in a hospital situation with their previous contacts with medical care, and can assess their experience in the light of this previously established attitude and experience.

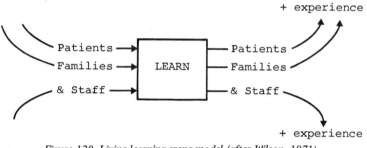

Figure 120. Living learning arena model (after Wilson, 1971)

In the developing country, the mother who brings her infant to a children's ward may never have undergone a previous experience of medical care, and her whole attitude to scientific medicine will be moulded by the way she is first greeted on arrival, and her experience thereafter. During her stay with a dehydrated child, we can hope that a sympathetic nurse has sat down with her and patiently helped her to spoon-feed her child with a saline solution, and at the same time explained dehydration in a way that she can understand. This mother, when she returns to her own community, will take with her some comprehension of modern medicine and the attitude in which it may be offered. She may also have become convinced of this way of looking after her own and other children during periods of dehydration. Her stay in hospital will have *strengthened her confidence in herself* and she will have learnt how she may care for both her own and her neighbours' children if they become dehydrated. This ability to increase and strengthen a mother's confidence in herself and her own ability to cope is greatly lacking in much of European paediatrics. In the developing countries it is an area in which research is badly needed if the existing health facilities are to achieve their potential to enlighten rural societies.

THE HOSPITAL IN SOCIETY

This psychosocial approach and its implications for the structure of the hospital has been described as 'medicine's contemporary growing point'. The frame of reference is no longer the individual patient; it is the patient in society, it is the society which is learning, not just the patient. This is particularly true in developing countries where traditionally the individual's concern is primarily for his family, and secondarily for his village or other community. The wider concept of care and concern for individuals from other areas, frequently with a different religion and language, is not easily accepted. If such a brotherhood between races can be practised in the hospital environment, the example will spread to the community outside.

SOME HUMAN FACTORS IN NURSING

'We can cure our patients these days without even knowing their names'. This remark applies to a small proportion of human illness, where a single action such as an injection, or an operation, may seem appropriate, but such a complete disregard of human factors is more appropriate to the conveyer-belt of a factory than in a hospital ward. However, the attitude of the person giving the injection or administering the anaesthetic will influence readiness with which the patient, his family and friends will consult that form of health care in the future. This is only too well appreciated by those who purchase medical care through private hospitals. The frequent disregard for human factors in public hospitals, as opposed to private health resources, is one reason for government services being so often held in low esteem by the general public, and also for governments being less ready to vote money for health care.

A nurse requires much factual knowledge and skill in numerous techniques, but her training must also equip her to manage her personal relationships with patients and colleagues. Classroom instruction cannot teach her to do this. She learns it as she forms her ideas about health, illness, aging and death from her personal experience in ward and clinic, usually accepting but occasionally rejecting what she is told by senior nurses and doctors.

THE NURSE AS A HUMANIZING AGENT IN THE HOSPITAL

The hospital has been described as an important socializing agency, within which a whole range of attitudes to health, sickness and medical technology are unconsciously learnt (305). This is even more so in a rural society, where the person has few alternative areas of learning. Lambourne writes:

> The hospital is one of the most significant of those institutions which are powerful humanising instruments through their persuasive influence on "faith and morals". I use "faith and morals" in the wide sense of the generally accepted idea about "what's done and not done", and "what life is like". The hospital shares with other institutions such as schools, universities, churches, press, television and theatre this power of socialisation. But because of the dramatic nature of hospital work, and because of its special combination of personal commitment and modern technology, the influence of the hospital, disseminated progressively through journals, novels, press and all the other mass media, may be deeper and more far-reaching in this twentieth century than we appreciate. Nurses can be more important in this humanising process than the doctors because they spend more time with patients, there are more of them and they should have a better opportunity to build up an effective relationship with the patient.

For developing countries there is surely an argument here for the simple 'homely' hospital where man—medical care confrontation can take place. The multi-storey concrete and glass block, accessible only by lifts, is unpopular with the majority of patients. The large hospital has also accentuated the problem between members of the health team.

IMBALANCE BETWEEN NURSES, DOCTORS AND ADMINISTRATORS

Nurses, even more than doctors, have perhaps been caught unprepared for the immense changes which have taken place in medicine over the past two or three decades. In most countries, the turnover of patients has greatly increased. As the demand and cost of services have rapidly risen, the hospital has become restricted to the acute and seriously ill patient who requires much nursing. Senior nursing administrators emphasize the escalation in fatigue, frustration, disappointment, disillusionment and despair of the nursing profession. This has arisen partly due to the enormously increased demands made on it, and also to a deterioration in communication within the hospital.

In Birmingham, the ratio of doctors to nurses has increased within a year from one doctor to 9.2 nurses to one doctor to 8.8 (223). If this problem is serious in Britain, where there is such a large number of nurses to each doctor, it is many times more serious in those countries where the number of nurses being trained is less than the number of doctors. One step that is being taken in the Western world to ease the burden on the nurses is the increase in number of supporting staff. From 9 a.m. to 5 p.m. on a weekday in a hospital in the UK these may exceed the number of nurses on duty, but for the rest of their 24-hour service for 365 days in the year, nurses have to work without their help. For this reason, such supporting staff can be only a partial answer to the increased work load of the nurses, unless they too are employed on a 24-hour basis. Such situations require to be more widely understood throughout the health team.

DETERIORATION IN RELATIONSHIPS WITHIN THE HOSPITAL

There is a deterioration in the relationship between nurses on the one hand and doctors and administrators on the other (223). There has been a serious imbalance produced in the triangle that represents the care of the patient in hospital *(Figure 121)*.

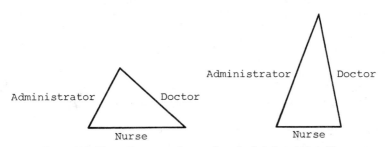

Figure 121. The unfortunate change of emphasis in hospital staffing

Over the last few years, the sides of the triangle that represent doctors and administrators have grown in strength and expertise far beyond that representing the nurses. In this the doctor as the leader of the health team is in part to blame. There can be only one solution. He must *create dialogues in which not only can he express his problems but in which he can also listen to those of the nursing staff.* Just as doctors resent being made to feel that they are under the hospital secretary and his administration, the sisters similarly resent this attitude when they meet it, as they often do, in the course of their duties. To avoid this situation regular discussions between the administrative staff and the senior nurses are essential. The world-wide demand for higher pay by nurses reflects a much deeper need, which is for true recognition as professional colleagues, and for participation in management of the

347

patients and their environment. To achieve this recognition from society she must first receive it from her medical colleagues.

DEVELOPING THE NURSING SERVICES

Health planners, most of whom are doctors, have not allowed the nursing profession the same opportunities to expand as those offered to their own profession. In most regions nursing, both in numbers and standards of training, has tragically lagged behind medicine. Nor has nursing as a profession reached the esteem in which it is held by the people of Europe and America. There are many reasons for this, but one of the more important in some countries is the character of doctors, whose attitude to nurses resembles their approach to a servant rather than a colleague. One reason for this is in the class structure of societies. Doctors come largely from the urban elite, who have failed to provide a corresponding number of nurses due to the popular misconception that their job is menial. Until the doctor changes his attitude, the medical care of the children cannot reach the high standards that are possible, nor can specialized services such as those for intensive care or neonatal surgery, be successfully developed. Not until the doctor treats the nurse as a colleague and thus increases the public's respect for her, as well as the respect of the nurse for her own work, will the standard of child care in hospitals improve. In the process both the government and the public will upgrade the nursing profession.

There are many reasons for the unequal development of the nursing services in different parts of the world; some of them are historical, others cultural. In the nineteenth century, when nursing began to develop as an organized profession in the Western world, it was fortunate in having leaders from socially prominent families. At that time, when the potent drugs of today were not available, nursing care was clearly a major component in the recovery of patients. This has led to nursing being a profession that was both socially acceptable and respected. Because cultural patterns link the duties of a nurse with a menial class in society, governments demand only low educational qualifications, but this is self-defeating, as ease of entry deters the brighter girls from taking up nursing. Those nurses who could by background, education, ability and experience lead nursing to a position of greater acceptance are handicapped by the traditional attitude of non-acceptance of a professional status for nursing.

The doctor's role in recognizing what good nursing can provide, in offering support to the nursing staff and creating a better attitude in the public mind regarding this aspect of health care, cannot be overestimated. As the doctor works each day in the wards and departments of a hospital, the eyes of the patients, and through them of the public, are on him. From the tone of his voice, the expression on his face, and every communication with his nursing colleagues, the public will derive their attitude and respect (or lack of it) for nurses.

In colonial days an attitude was engendered by the expatriate nurses, who did not consider or treat their local counterparts as equals until they were forced to do so. Unfortunately this attitude is being perpetuated by the quite impossible standard being unrealistically required by some countries as a basis for the traditional nurse. This fails to acknowledge the worth of other contributing members of the health team such as the midwife and those at the assistant nurse levels. While in Europe there has been a rapid increase in the use of enrolled nurses and other grades, in some developing countries their training and employment has been stopped. In one of the countries of which the author knows, the district councils cannot afford to pay the salaries of the better qualified nurses and midwives now being trained even if they were willing to work in the villages. As a result, since the training of other cadres has ceased, the villages of that country are rapidly being depleted of their trained midwives.

NURSING CARE OF CHILDREN

The nurse has an essential part to play in the care of every child in the hospital. But she can play this part only if the doctor lets her take her essential place in the health team. Nursing entails the physical care required for comfort, and teaching the patient's mother how to give this care. The nurse will build up the mother's confidence in her own ability to observe the changes in her child. She gives her the emotional support necessary to foster recovery, maintains her confidence in the treatment, giving the treatments prescribed by the doctor, and observes the response of the patient.

The quality of the nursing care that can be provided will be determined not only by the ability of the nursing personnel and the attitude, but also by their number. The world shortage of nursing tutors trained in effective teaching and communication methods is a serious limitation in every developing country. In determining a nurse's functions in particular circumstances a critical minimum level of nursing is what matters, recognizing that with increased staff increased service can be offered.

The major difference between nursing in Europe and America and that in developing countries is the amount of teaching to be done. This is not so much in formal teaching but through the nurses in all their actions assisting the mothers from a rural society who have little understanding and appreciation of scientific medicine and technology. The interpretation of *all* that goes on in the treatment of the child must be the concern of the nurse. The special difficulties of communicating with an illiterate mother are considered in Chapter 22.

To ensure that the experience of the mother and her child in hospital is as beneficial as possible, the nurse must undertake the following responsibilities.

(1) Observing the child, and recording what is found.

(2) Making the hospital a temporary but acceptable home environment. Feeding must be supervised. Cleanliness of the children and their mothers with safe disposal of excreta must be organized.

(3) Giving medicines. (This usually takes up too much of her time; the experienced doctor will know how to reduce medication to essentials.)

(4) Assisting with and/or performing other treatments.

In all these the nurse is concerned to be *communicating, teaching, explaining* and as it is only through this that the experience of hospitalization can achieve its maximum benefit for the child, his mother, the family and the society.

If nursing care is to be effective it must be well administered. To achieve a high standard, routines and procedures must be established, and therefore adequate minimal facilities must be provided. It is part of a doctor's job to ensure that the minimal facilities are available and to encourage and assist the nurses as they establish this routine. For example, the provision of proper nursing care is often handicapped from the moment of admission by the way children are allotted to vacant beds. It is common practice to assign patients to beds allotted to particular doctors. Thus children with infections may be next to children with non-infectious conditions, infants may be next to adolescents, the acutely ill next to the chronically ill. In order to facilitate good nursing care nurses should have a voice in determining who goes into which cot. A policy taking into account the available facilities and the nursing needs of children should be worked out by the ward sister and the doctor in charge.

Control of admissions and discharges

When every cot is full in an acute children's ward the nurses are usually fully employed. The admission of further children in extra cots, 'doubling up', or as 'floor patients' will lead to a rapid decline in standards of care. The staff become frustrated when excess patients and their relatives block free movement on the ward. The knowledge that for every sick or dying child there may be another two or even ten in the community may help in refusing children when the ward is already full. In Cuba this situation was met at ministry level. They found that one reason for an increase in the infant mortality rate was overcrowding in children's wards. Legally, additional children cannot now be admitted, and if necessary they are admitted to medical or surgical beds.

The 'emergency room' or 'round the clock' intensive care service that has now been introduced in many hospitals should play some part in preventing overcrowding. Children can be brought to this service with a minimum of formality, and it is particularly suited for rehydrating acutely sick children. An experienced paediatrician usually goes around once or twice a day to decide which of the children will benefit most from admission to any cots that have become vacant. In some of these services there is a set limit of 24 or 48 hours for which a child may stay, after which he has to be admitted to the ward or sent home. These units are particularly useful in training medical students and medical assistants and nurses to come to diagnosis using side-room laboratory facilities that are available, they can also learn to institute emergency treatment which in their future career they will need to use without expert guidance being available. A disadvantage of these units is their requirement for staff and they are only feasible in larger hospitals. They should include one room which can be used for temporary isolation.

The decision to discharge children in a ward with a high turnover is difficult, and it was the author's practice never to discharge a child without discussion with the ward sister or nurse in charge. So often the good nurse who is working close to the mother and child knows of circumstances which make a further day or two in hospital necessary. Similarly she will recognize the mother who can cope and follow instructions, allowing some children to return home early.

The doctor who has frequent discussions with his ward sister on the number and level of training of the nurses available should, in consultation with her, be able to maintain a busy ward with always sufficient in reserve to allow for the unexpected emergency admissions.

Assignment of nursing duties

Another practice which radically affects the care of patients is the method of assigning nursing duties. While there are various methods of doing this, such as functional, total patient care, or team nursing, the functional system will predominate for many years in the developing countries. This is unfortunate, as it is both inefficient and uneconomic. Team nursing is much more effective, particularly in countries with few graduate nurses. Functional nursing has become the traditional method of assignment in most countries because it was introduced by a 'westernized' group. It is generally not practical to attempt to introduce advanced methods of nursing. However, it is equally unsatisfactory to adopt a *laissez-faire* attitude, using the limited number of nurses as an excuse for no efforts to improve. It is worth considering the possibility of continuing to use the functional system, but in addition assigning each nurse specific patients for whom to take general responsibility. That is, functional nursing will persist and there would continue to be 'a medications nurse,' 'a kitchen nurse,' 'a treatment nurse,' etc., but in addition each of these nurses would be assigned a limited number of patients in whom to take a special interest. These patients would continue to have their medicines, treatments and diet given by different nurses, but in addition they would have a particular nurse to take responsibility for all incidental care they might need. If the number of nurses is adequate, every patient should be given such a nurse. If the number is limited, only the seriously ill or those with special problems will be able to have one. Alternatively, accepting the principle of disaster nursing, assignments should be made to mothers anxious to learn, or whose children are admitted with preventable conditions. This will have the most lasting effect in the community. Under no circumstances should the nurse be given so many patients that it is impossible for her to offer any additional care.

A doctor must know which nurses are assigned to each of his patients and make a point of discussing them with each nurse in terms of diagnosis, plan of treatment and its expected outcome. He should also try to gain from her the insight she achieves from daily contact with the mother and child. In this discussion of the plan of treatment the sister or nurse in charge of the ward at the time will be involved. As well as her expertise in the nursing field, she will bring a greater knowledge of the mother and the family, and how the delivery of health care must be moulded to meet their knowledge and living conditions. In this way the patient should receive improved care and the nurse should develop a feeling of self-esteem which will be reflected in the quality of her work. The doctor should receive the benefits derived from knowing that his patients are well cared for and eventually of seeing a widespread improvement in health services. However, such a system will fail unless there is enough time for the nurse to report back regularly to the sister or doctor.

All policies affecting the nursing of patients should be within the field of the doctor's interest. This can be demonstrated by discussing policy with the ward sister and giving his support in whatever nursing practices are instituted.

Each of the points previously listed will be considered in terms of the doctor's role in providing support to the nurse as she attempts to implement satisfactory policies for patient care.

Cleanliness

Place emphasis on cleanliness, it is vital in preventing cross-infection, in preventing recurrence of disease in discharged patients and in maintaining morale. Too often the doctor ignores the facilities available for the washing, bathing and excretion of patients, mothers and the staff. It is within the responsibility of the doctor to know what facilities are available, what difficulties exist in use of these facilities, and what the nurse thinks could be done to improve the situation. He will only become alive to these problems by regularly examining the facilities available with the nurse in charge. If as a visitor the author is shown round a ward, he always asks the sister to see the toilet facilities. The state of these may give a better indication of the level of care being offered than what can be observed in the ward. The doctor should press for the improvement of facilities, but no matter how limited the situation is, the staff should strive to make the best possible use of what is available. This involves planning for such things as the storage of water for periods when the taps are not operating, for frequent cleaning of the latrines, for instruction of patients and families in the use of the available facilities. To keep the latrines and wards clean there must be an adequate number of sweepers or cleaners, who should be known by the doctor and respected by him as essential to the care of the children. They are at least as important as anyone else in the prevention of cross-infection. Together the ward sister and doctor should plan how the staff and patients are trained in the use of the available facilities. It will be the nurse's responsibility to implement planning, and the doctor's responsibility both to encourage her efforts and to see that the behaviour of the medical staff sets an example of hand-washing and general cleanliness which can be followed. In a similar manner there needs to be a plan for the cleaning of the wards, the walls, furniture, equipment, kitchen and treatment rooms, and maintaining, repairing or replacing worn items of equipment.

Ward linen

Finally, some consideration must be given to linen. Clean linen is a major factor in nursing care and it too needs to be within the concern of the doctor. Because of inadequancy of supplies, limited laundry facilities and the danger of linen being stolen, maintaining adequate supplies is extremely difficult.

In most hospitals the responsibility for the ward linen stock devolves in the senior nurses and much of their time is taken from their vital nursing duties to check clean or dirty laundry. In some hospitals they must replace any deficiencies out of their salaries. The doctor must know the system used for washing linen as well as of the problems which the ward sisters encounter. Depending on resources, the ward sister should plan how linen will be handled. The responsibility for this should be shifted to non-nursing personnel, with the doctor encouraging any change which would result in nursing staff being freed for more vital nursing duties.

The mother's shelter

Many of the mothers staying with their children will be far from home and need a place to store their belongings, wash themselves and their clothes, and possibly cook their food. A mothers' shelter built to meet these needs is an essential adjunct to most children's wards. Usually lockers are required, to which the mother can bring her own padlock. The day-to-day control of this shelter may be undertaken by a married woman under the supervision of the sister. This woman can also teach the mothers. The functioning of such a shelter will be improved if the doctor pays an occasional visit of encouragement, and discusses their problems with the sister and the staff concerned.

Child feeding

An adequate diet and clean handling of food are essential. Since many children in developing countries are admitted to hospital with nutritional diseases, and most patients will have some degree of deficiency of diet, this matter is of the utmost importance. The doctor should inform himself of what food is provided and study it as to its nutritional adequacy. For example, more frequent and modified meals (or snacks) with milk will be required by a children's ward. One aspect of malnutrition that is frequently overlooked is the infrequency of meals in many societies. Recovery from malnutrition will be accelerated if meals are frequent and food always available for the child who is hungry. Perhaps we can learn from the old English saying, 'Children, like chickens, should always be pecking'.

Cleanliness in handling food is vital. The doctor should aquaint himself with the kitchen facilities and discuss, with a view to their solution, the limitations and problems which the nurse points out to him. He should support her efforts to promote proper handling of food by not conducting activities such as ward rounds during the time when she should be in the kitchen supervising food distribution. Clean handling of food requires instruction of both staff and patients. Although this is the responsibility of the nurse, the doctor should offer encouragement and assistance when necessary.

Medicines and equipment

An important nursing responsibility relates to the dispensing of medications. It is obvious that if the patient does not receive the proper medication at the proper time, his progress may be affected. Although it is within the province of the nurse to work out the routine for this, there may be many problems which she needs to discuss. Limited supplies of medicine glasses, droppers, syringes and needles often handicap her efforts.

When medications are ordered by doctors through nurses, there are often difficulties which need solution. Sometimes medications which are not available are ordered. Once the nurse has notified the doctor of this, he should either see that the medication is provided or that alternative medications are ordered. In some countries certain medications are given only by a doctor; he should be required to note this on the chart himself, or failing this the nurse should note it in his presence.

Nursing treatments present many problems. Equipment is usually scarce and far more delicate than that used for adults. Availability and care of necessary equipment is itself a major factor. In a children's ward examples of this special equipment include the following items.

(1) Fine short lumbar puncture needles, which can be mistaken for ordinary syringe needles.

(2) Fine intravenous needles and canulae, which can also be mistaken for ordinary needles.

(3) Fine scissors and other instruments for cutting down on a vein for transfusion.

(4) Glass syringe and fine aspirating needles for chest work.

(5) Low-reading thermometers.

If problems exist over equipment, the doctor should make himself available to discuss these.

In as far as possible routines should be established for treatments performed by doctors. These routines should be written, beginning with equipment required and continuing with the procedure. The doctor in charge should ensure that those performing treatment do so in a proper manner, so that it serves as an example of good technique to the assisting nurse. All doctors should be encouraged to describe their actions and discuss the purpose of a procedure and the anticipated results with the nurse, as a valuable teaching technique. In as far as possible the treatments performed should coincide first with the needs of the patient and then the convenience of both doctor and nurse. Where possible such practices as taking blood specimens immediately before a child is fed, or when he is deeply asleep, should be avoided. In treatments performed by the nurse, the doctor should be willing to discuss any problems which are brought to him.

Observations made by the nurse

One of the most vital functions of the nurse is her ability to make pertinent observations on the condition of patients. Because she is in contact with the patient, she has a unique opportunity to observe any change in him. All too often her observations are ignored or discounted rather than encouraged and developed. Doctors who observe signs such as the alae nasi working or subcutaneous emphysema in a child have a responsibility to show these and similar signs to the junior members of the nursing team at the bedside and supply a simple explanation of their significance. When the nurse does not volunteer information she should be asked what has been noted and possibly told what to expect. Her education has encouraged her to observe, but frequently her ward experience has discouraged her development of this characteristic, even to the extent of making her oblivious to major manifestations of distress.

If doctors will encourage the development of observation in nurses who need assistance and will seek out and rely on observations of nurses, this could effect a fundamental and widespread improvement in patient care. If it is possible for the nurse to record her observations, then it is imperative that the medical staff pay heed to them, otherwise nurses will not develop this important skill. In the circumstances of a developing country the nurse is frequently in the position of recognizing the signs that distinguish the ill from the well child, and she needs to be encouraged in this skill. Nurses who are astute observers are invaluable in their assistance both in caring for hospitalized patients and in working in the community. This delegation of responsibility for observation is critical in child care. Changes that arise in the child's condition need to be observed by nurse and mother between the doctor's visits.

TEACHING AND COMMUNICATION IN THE CHILDREN'S WARD

Permeating many, if not all, activities of the nurse is the responsibility for teaching. Her role as teacher includes both teaching of the parents and teaching of other members of staff. Most of her effective teaching will be incidental — the word of encouragement to the mother, or praise and thanks given to a student nurse. In both of these types of teaching the support of the medical profession is essential. The nursing profession, by close contact with the mother and child, has an unequalled opportunity to spread a better understanding of disease and its causation and of desirable health practices. Also, because of responsibility for the services of the non-professional staff (practical nurses, cleaners or sweepers, etc.), the nurse has a unique opportunity to instruct.

The mother in the children's ward is vitally interested in her sick child. The opportunity to use every contact with the mother for communicating and encouraging her in better care must not be missed. *Figure 122* suggests how a ward round can be adjusted to improve communication. In *Figure 122a* three professional people are discussing records of the child. In *Figure 122b* the mother and child are together and central to the discussion, and the child sees the doctor on his own level.

The teaching must be at a level which the mother's knowledge and culture will allow her to accept readily. The need for all workers to have a well-founded knowledge of the local beliefs as to the causation and therapy of disease has already been emphasized. In conversation with the mother this information becomes very necessary. The mother knows that her child's condition of dehydration is a manifestation of the 'evil eye', and can hardly be persuaded that the child is undernourished, and that because of this germs which are not dangerous to adults have caused the diarrhoea. However, she may be able to appreciate that his condition is related to loss of water from the diarrhoea and vomiting that she has observed. This understanding will increase as she sees her child recover through her own efforts in spoon-feeding him with a suitable salt solution. If this understanding can be achieved, then she may have learnt the importance of fluid replacement in future episodes, and the need to seek medical help early. Perhaps by the scrupulous care in dealing with the stools taught her by the nursing staff she may gain some understanding of how diarrhoeal infections are spread. In her efforts to become more effective as a teacher, the nurse will do well to remember the saying of Aristotle, 'How can a man learn but from a friend?'.

357

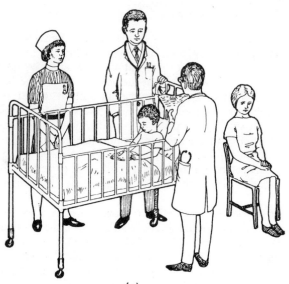

(a)

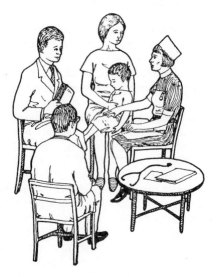

(b)

Figure 122. Better communication on a doctor's round in a children's ward

Effective teaching means involvement

As far as possible the nurse's teaching of the mother should lead to activity by the mother. Teaching the mother the need for a better diet and more frequent meals will be done most effectively by the mother preparing the food herself, as in a nutrition rehabilitation centre, using methods she uses in her own home. However, facilities to make this possible will rarely be available. At least the hospital must provide the same type of food as she will use at home. In every instance, from bathing, to spoon-feeding supplements for an underweight infant, to administering insulin to the diabetic, the emphasis should be on the mother first observing, then doing under supervision, and finally doing independently, those tasks which can be used to foster good health practices. Particular emphasis should be paid to the use of facilities such as the water closet, with which village mothers may have had no previous experience.

If the nurses are to undertake such care, it is imperative that the doctors recognize this as a valid nursing role. Instances of doctors criticizing nurses for 'allowing' mothers to do the 'nurses' work' can seriously hamper improved health practices in the community. Rather, doctors must seek every opportunity to acquaint themselves with the nurse's efforts at this type of teaching and lend support when possible. In the design of children's wards, facilities for this aspect need to be included. For example, the mothers' sluice has worked well in the wards designed at Ilesha *(Figure 123)*. As mothers expect to clear up their children's faeces, facilities need to be available for this. The glass window between the sluices enables any nurse working in her sluice to observe what the mother is doing, and guide her where necessary.

In addition to this incidental teaching, the nurses should be encouraged to undertake some organized teaching of mothers. It is obvious that groups should be as homogenous as possible, that is, mothers should have approximately the same educational and cultural background. If these mothers have children suffering from similar conditions, the teaching would be more effective.

Teaching for all ward personnel

Regarding the ward sister's teaching of other members of the staff, this should be planned not only for student nurses but also for staff nurses and all other categories of ward personnel. The doctor's role falls into two main categories – that of actual participation in a clinical discussion of the care of a patient assigned to a particular nurse, and of

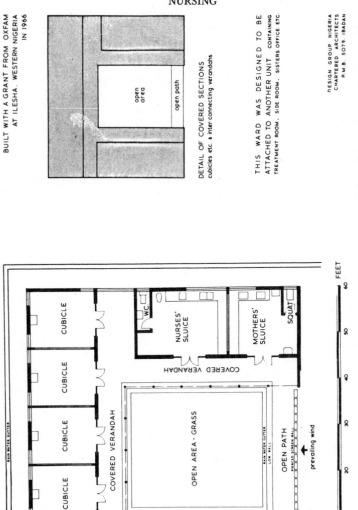

BUILT WITH A GRANT FROM OXFAM
AT ILESHA. WESTERN NIGERIA
IN 1966

DETAIL OF COVERED SECTIONS
cubicles etc. & inter-connecting verandahs

THIS WARD WAS DESIGNED TO BE
ATTACHED TO ANOTHER UNIT CONTAINING
TREATMENT ROOM. SIDE ROOM. SISTERS OFFICE ETC.

DESIGN GROUP NIGERIA
CHARTERED ARCHITECTS
P.M.B. 5079. IBADAN

Figure 123. Experimental cubicle ward for children in a hot climate. Provision has been made for a sluice to be used by the mothers under supervision

general support to the ward sister as she plans the content and arranges the time for in-service programmes, ranging from routine procedures for staff nurses to methods of cleaning the vessels for the kitchen attendant and cleaning the latrines for the sweepers. Finally, if it is possible for the doctor in charge to press hospital administrators to institute instructional classes for all non-professional staff at the time of appointment to their post, the ward sisters would have much more effective control of practices which may be adversely affecting a clean and safe ward environment.

SPECIAL PROBLEMS OF THE NURSE MOVING FROM AN ADULTS' TO A CHILDREN'S WARD

As described above, the nurse coming to the children's ward needs a different attitude, as well as additional knowledge and skills, to those working in a general ward. She will need to accept the high mortality and a quick turnover of sick children, with a speed of illness that particularly requires her observational skills. For example, no longer will she be recording only pyrexia and be on the look out for hyperpyrexia, she must also know the significance of hypothermia.

Among ill children, especially those with malnutrition, cross-infection is particularly liable to arise. In preventing this, the presence of the mother can be a tremendous asset in that she alone will be feeding the child and dealing with its excreta, under the supervision of the nurse. It is in this relationship with the mother that the nurse's greatest difficulty will arise, particularly if she has no children of her own.

Unlike caring for adults, a knowledge of simple nutrition as related to local diet will be needed for the nurse to be effective. She will understand the dangers of bottle-feeding and be patient in teaching the mother to use a cup and spoon.

THE NURSE IN THE CLINIC

Great emphasis has been placed here on the nurse in the ward. At the present time, probably more nurses are to be found within the hospital wards than working outside them. However, as medical care becomes more effective in its planning, it is likely that this situation will be reversed, and a greater number will be working outside in the community, where they can be so effective in raising the overall standard of health care.

In the clinic, the nurse may hold very different positions. She may be no more than a help to the doctor, or on the other hand she may be working as a nurse or midwife in a remote village, with tenuous supervision, and little opportunity for referral. Unfortunately, it is frequently the more skilled and the better equipped nurse who is working in the hospital, while the nurse in the remote village holds the greater responsibility. Just as lack of housing and other amenities deters the doctor, so also the nurse is reluctant to live in a rural society.

The function of the nurse in caring for children in the clinic has been considered in detail in Chapter 19. She undertakes the responsibility of diagnosis and therapeutic skills which have usually been only poorly taught, if taught at all. Just as a plea is made in this book to take much of a doctor's training away from the hospital, so also the nurse needs training in Under-Fives' Clinics and through a period of home visiting in the community she is to serve. This part of her experience must kindle interest in the community early in her nursing career. Unfortunately, many senior members of both the medical and nursing professions regret that she takes on these duties, but in largely rural societies she and the medical assistant must share them, as doctors are not available and would be too expensive to use there.

In some clinics, the medical assistants may care for the small children, but a more natural division will be for the nurse to look after the women, particularly when they are pregnant, and the small children up to school age.

NURSES AS COLLEAGUES OF THE DOCTOR

In conclusion, there must be a further reference to the nurse's role as a colleague of the doctor. It should be obvious from the comments made at the beginning of this chapter that many nurses may not have as privileged a background as members of other professions. It must always be remembered that some nurses will have by background, education and experience much more to offer in the care of their patients. If there is to be an improvement in the quality of nursing care, doctors must give recognition to all that which is so satisfactory in the nursing of today, and press society to invest more resources in nursing. In order to do this, the doctor must realize the handicaps under which discourteous behaviour may place the whole profession. He should learn to identify those nurses who already have much to offer in terms of their professional acumen. He should encourage all nurses to become integral members of the health team, able to discuss their observations of the patient and their problems, both in the care of particular patients and of the ward in general.

Furthering nurses' training

One further way in which doctors can support nurses is by teaching them, and especially by teaching sessions in their training schools where they will be found to be most receptive students. He may be able to assist the sister tutor in many other ways, and she will be grateful for offers of help. Education is one of the chief ways in which the nurse can be prepared for a more responsible role in health care, and the doctor who wishes to improve the care available for children will do all he can to encourage higher studies for his nurses.

If all or any of the suggestions made for the doctor to assist in developing an increased contribution from the nursing profession are to be implemented, then it would be advisable for regular meetings to be held to discuss nursing problems in as far as they are created by or may be alleviated by the medical profession. These meetings should not just become sessions where grumbles can be aired, nor should they be regarded as unimportant and possible of being delegated as the responsibility of a junior doctor. The most senior doctor of the unit should take an active part in these meetings. The subjects for discussion should be prepared by the nurse in charge and should be restricted to those items which can profitably be discussed at any meeting. Any member of her staff should be asked to present a problem and indicate what she considers possible solutions and the support necessary to implement each solution. Following this, discussion should reveal what can and cannot be done. Trial solutions may be implemented and the matter pursued at a later meeting. Over a period of years or decades it will be possible to implement patterns of nursing care which lead to an improved health status of the community.

CHAPTER 21

Management

'Doctors must either manage or be managed'. (Rosenheim, 1971)

In the previous chapters a changed role was suggested for the future paediatrician working in developing countries. He has to be a member and the leader of a health team. Membership in a team gives him more time with each sick child, and thus frees him to use his special diagnostic skills on children who particularly require such expertise. This change to a team approach, which involves the doctor in the study and practice of management, is being adopted increasingly in Europe and North America. The developing countries are in particular need of a team approach, if the few well-qualified staff in rural areas are to make their skills widely available to those who desperately need them.

The idea of management, however, is not universally acceptable. Many of the leaders in medicine resent the need to spend time on management; for them it will be an 'identity crisis' -- 'This is not the way in which a professional person is taught to perceive himself'. And yet good clinical practice has always contained a high content of management skills!

If the doctor is to become an effective leader and manager, he must equip himself with the skills of management. Medical schools must train doctors for this role. Most of the readers of this book will already have been trained, and this chapter can only point the way and suggest a framework within which the paediatrician can develop a manager's approach to medicine. This chapter is written primarily for the doctor working with a team of medical assistants and others who are not medically qualified, as this is likely to be the future pattern in rural areas of developing countries. However, without much alteration, what is said could be applied to units in which the team includes other doctors as a professional unit.

It has been said that 80 per cent of learning the skills of management derive from the experience of being well managed, rather than from lectures or reading. Most of us can remember how horrible it is to be poorly led and to work in a team where there is little understanding of management. Equally we know the excitement and benefit of being well led. If this is so, then those in senior positions who read this chapter and agree with this proposition will realize their responsibility when they next pick up the telephone to speak to a junior, or walk into the hospital and greet the ward sisters. If they can learn to manage well, they will set the pattern of leadership and improved management for the next generation.

Whether we like it or not, the problem of reconciling great medical needs with limited resources exists, and in practice is handled in a variety of ways. Lack of positive action results in misunderstanding, dilution, rationing, and at times exclusion on economic or other grounds. One or usually several of these sanctions can be identified in almost every decision. Some can be identified in every out-patient department or other place in which the medical resources are unlikely ever to meet the need. It is better that decisions involving needs and resources, and the question *who receives what little service there may be,* should be made as deliberately as possible, rather than be left to pressure and prejudice. A manager's role is to make such decisions, to be able to justify them both to those to whom he is responsible and to members of his team who will have to see most of the patients. The wise manager may emulate the traditional African chief, who undertakes discussion sometimes at length, and makes a decision only when he has discovered 'the feeling of the meeting' and has thoroughly involved the people concerned in the decision-making process.

The following process of decision-making through defining problems and the steps in their solution has been suggested (31). *Figure 124* is an extension of *Figure 14* already produced in Chapter 4.

Bryant suggests the need to define problems carefully and then set them out in terms of priorities, considering the following points.

(1)   Community concern: as always we must give priority to the felt needs of the people.

(2)   Their prevalence in the community rather than in the hospital out-patient department. An example of this is measles, which is rarely seen in hospital out-patient (outdoor) clinics in Asia, but is clearly a major problem in the community.

(3)   The seriousness of the problem, in terms of morbidity and mortality.

(4)   Vulnerability to management. Examples of this are neonatal tetanus and whooping cough which can be controlled, unlike sickle cell disease in West Africa and childhood cirrhosis in India. The latter are serious problems, but as at present they cannot be satisfactorily

managed, their control should perhaps receive a low priority in expenditure of limited medical resources.

Continuing Bryant's circle, there is a need to set objectives that can be readily measured, and to do this a target population must be defined. Just as long as medical resources are poured into an unmeasured sea of mankind, real planning and evaluation are difficult

BRYANT'S PROBLEM-SOLVING CYCLE

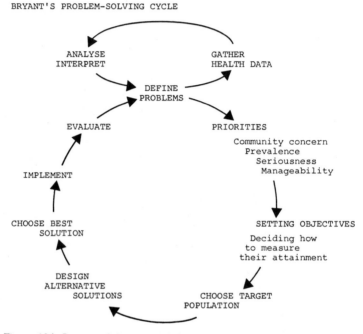

Figure 124. Process of decision-making. More attention needs to be placed on sorting out priorities, setting objectives that can be evaluated and defining the target population

or impossible. For example in the UK, a medical school in an area such as Newcastle-on-Tyne has undertaken important research in a well-defined community from which it draws its paediatric patients – an advantage not held by those working in London, with a number of overlapping medical schools. Several medical schools in developing countries are undertaking the care of a limited and well-defined community. On a smaller scale, a health centre needs a defined area in which it may measure and assess its work. The target population may be, as above, defined geographically, or equally it may be a section of the whole community, such as that under five, which is the target population for this book.

For almost all problems alternative solutions are possible. If neonatal tetanus is taken as an example, the possible solutions in any community may include some, if not all, of the following.

(1) Treatment of cases as they occur.
(2) Training of local midwives where these exist.
(3) Immunization of the mother during pregnancy.
(4) Supplying pregnant women with a sterile cord-cutting and dressing package, with health education.
(5) Making available ½ cc. Anti Tetanus Serum (ATS) to newborns.

The author's experience in West Africa leads him to suggest that more time and energy should be spent on the immunization of mothers than on care and treatment of neonatal tetanus. Where for any reason it was not possible to contact the mother, it was best to give ATS as soon as possible to the newborn. There were no indigenous midwives in this community, so it was not possible to use these.

Having decided on the best solution or solutions and implemented them, a continuous evaluation is necessary as the problem changes. Bryant particularly emphasizes that this is a never-ending circle, as the problems will always be changing and health data needs to be compiled.

DEFINITION OF MANAGEMENT

'The business of management is the efficient allocation of resources'. This definition sounds obvious enough. Another of the many possible definitions, and perhaps the most suitable in the medical field, is that given below (259).

DECIDING WHAT IS TO BE DONE
(after due consultation)
and
GETTING OTHER PEOPLE TO DO IT

If these definitions are expanded a little, we may get the essence of management *(Figure 125)*.

This definition will upset many who quite rightly consider that decisions should be made collectively, and that the best results can be achieved by releasing everybody's creativity, not only the doctor's. The manager has a responsibility to encourage everyone to become practised in decision-making.

367

A community development approach might interpret this as initiating a community process by which felt needs are recognized and aiding the community to obtain satisfaction from these needs being met.

Once the group has become involved in decision-making, difficulties in motivation become less serious. Perhaps the second half of the definition would be more effective if it read GETTING OTHER PEOPLE TO DO IT WITH THE MANAGER.

Such an attitude is still not acceptable in many societies, although many managers will wish to move in this direction, as described later under theory X or Y. In working together with their team, the manager or doctor will always wish to demonstrate his willingness to become involved in any work that is not 'his job'.

In an ever changing situation
{ DECIDING WHAT TO DO
{ GETTING OTHER PEOPLE TO DO IT

(A) To plan and set objectives

(B) To analyse and organise resources to meet the plan

(C) To 'measure' and control the use of resources towards attaining the objectives

(D) To motivate, develop and train staff at all levels to meet changing situations

Figure 125. The essence of a manager's work

These are the different aspects of management in all walks of life. Management has still to go a long way to achieve the status of a science in the industrial field, let alone the medical field. In what follows, an attempt will be made to expand these aspects of management in the fields in which a doctor works.

DECIDING WHAT IS TO BE DONE

TO DEFINE THE PROBLEM AND TO PLAN AND SET OBJECTIVES

Objectives need to be divided into long-term and short-term. Long-term objectives are important, but it may not always be easy to see where they lead. For example, the writer's long-term objective is to improve the standards of health care in the rural societies of developing countries. Short-term objectives are often of greater practical value, such as, for example, to secure the general introduction of the road-to-health card described in Chapter 7. But this may be too distant an objective, as their general acceptance by a population may take several years. A more immediately attainable objective might be to see that all mothers delivered in a particular maternity unit receive and are taught about such a card for their newborn babies before they are discharged.

In deciding both immediate short-term objectives and ultimate goals, the desires and aspirations of the people must be considered. Their felt needs are very real and can be discovered in every community. The real needs often differ, and their definition depends much on the knowledge, experience and culture of the adviser. Real and felt needs can often be linked in the determination of objectives. The felt need held by the mothers may be for there to be a continuing interest and

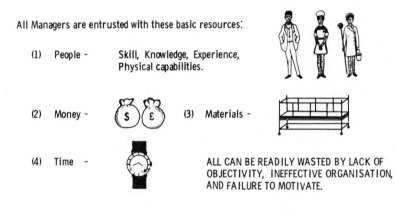

All Managers are entrusted with these basic resources:

(1) People –   Skill, Knowledge, Experience, Physical capabilities.

(2) Money –   (3) Materials –

(4) Time –   ALL CAN BE READILY WASTED BY LACK OF OBJECTIVITY, INEFFECTIVE ORGANISATION, AND FAILURE TO MOTIVATE.

Figuer 126. The basic resources of managers

concern by medical personnel in their newborn babies. When the mothers recognize this road-to-health card as a 'passport' through which the nurses and doctor can better help and care for their babies, they will wish to have them.

A skilful manager will influence and instruct his staff so that they feel that the final decision to introduce the road-to-health card seems to originate from them. In the example already quoted, the paediatrician may have to 'sell' the idea of such a card to his obstetrical colleagues and nursing staff. If he is patient, he may be able to get them to suggest the idea themselves, and the introduction of the cards should be delayed until they are convinced of their value.

TO ANALYSE AND ORGANIZE RESOURCES TO MEET THE PLAN

There are certain basic resources available to *all* organizations, and management is concerned with these just as much in medicine and education as in commerce. They are set out in *Figure 126.*

369

PEOPLE AS A MANAGEMENT RESOURCE

You yourself are one of the greatest resources. Although the short-comings of medical organization are frequently attributed to lack of money and materials, it is the knowledge, skills and attitudes of the staff that matter most. It is you, and how you use your time, and how you can inspire your staff to use their time, that matters. Can you liberate both yourself and them, both from the master—servant relationship and from being so hard-pressed that you can together plan a better service? But before the doctor—manager looks at how the staff use their time, he will need to examine how he uses his own. A doctor's own time is the most important of all, for it is the resource that he can most easily redeploy. When he has analysed how it is spent, he will find that there is a certain fraction, most probably the majority, that is decided for him by the nature of his job, and a smaller part that is largely free for him to dispose of as he wishes. It is on this latter part that he may have to concentrate to improve his efficiency and to attain his objectives.

TIME AS A MANAGEMENT RESOURCE

The analysis of how the manager's time is spent will show where saving by delegation will be achieved and how he can devote more time to longer-term objectives, particularly in the preventive field. This analysis has become common practice in industry, where management studies have shown that a detailed diary is necessary before any true analysis can be made. Some attempts by doctors (321) and other health workers (305) to undertake such studies have been made. A doctor who wishes to become more effective must consider doing the same, although making such an analysis requires more than average determination.

Keeping a diary

For most paediatricians, particularly those in senior posts, the time actually spent in direct care of children, that is in the diagnosis and management of disease, will take up only a part of the day. Those who have set themselves objectives will have included objectives other than those directly concerned with the care of sick children. They will know that if they can reach these objectives, for example the setting up of an immunization programme in a community where it does not exist, this will do more to improve the health of the children than all the time they spend on clinical care. As an example of this, it was estimated that a man with a training limited just to jet injection techniques in a normal working day in West Africa was preventing six deaths from measles – a saving of life that few well-qualified paediatricians could hope to achieve.

If a paediatrician is to spend time on other than clinical care, those responsible for training him will need to know how best he should spend the rest of his time, so that he can be prepared for it. Unfortunately, there are few records of how paediatricians actually do spend their time. It may be, perhaps, through many paediatricians keeping a detailed diary of their activities that we will come to know how they should be prepared better for their many duties. Some of the questions that such a diary may help to answer in as little as a fortnight's observation are given below.

(1) What proportion of time is devoted to the fundamental activities of examining and treating patients in the ward and in the out-patients department (and in private practice, where this is done), in teaching, in large groups or small, in reading, writing, telephoning, and in meetings, travelling, inspecting and interviewing?

(2) To what extent is the pattern of the day governed by prior engagements, and to what extent by emergency or other interruptions?

(3) What interaction is there with other doctors, staff members, students or the general public?

(4) How much time is spent with other people? Are the contacts he makes usually with more than one person?

(5) When not involved in clinical duties, what subjects is he dealing with, and what skills or knowledge does he require? How much time is devoted to these subjects?

(6) Other than in direct clinical care what scope is there for a paediatrician to make decisions, and what is their nature? Where outside permission is required, who has to agree?

(7) Finally, it should be possible to clarify what a paediatrician does, other than his immediate clinical duties. How is the decision reached in the allocation of his time, apart from seeing patients? How much is it from experience, and how much from 'backing hunches'? Does he attempt to analyse his situations and problems in a scientific and logical way?

Before keeping a diary, the future diarist should write down how he *thinks* he uses his time. Experience from the other disciplines suggests that he will be more than a little surprised when he completes the analysis!

How the diary is kept should depend on an initial pilot study of one or two days, and will depend on what information is required. Later on it may be useful to examine one portion of his day more specifically, to

Starting Time	Service Duties (T = teaching also)			Teaching away from children		Read	Write or Dictate	Telephone	Discuss	Travel	Break	Arranged	Remarks
	In O.P.	In Ward	Elsewhere	Groups of less than 10	Groups of more than 10								
7.45 am	✓	✓											Planning & Staff
8.00	✓	✓											Round
9.15	✓												Mainly in U.5.C.
12.30	✓	✓											Treatment in ward & special consultn.
1.30											✓		Lunch and rest
2.30							✓		✓				Correspondence
4.00											✓		Tea
4.15			✓								✓		Consultns. and photographs
5.00			✓							✓			Village Nutrition Follow up.
6.30											✓		Bath and meal
7.45		✓									✓		Night round, whole hospital
9.00													Home
TOTALS	4h	3h	1½h				1½h		¼h	1h			11¼

372

see in greater detail how this is spent. There is little information on how such diaries should be constructed, but *Figure 127* has been adapted from one used by medical administrators when they are attempting to analyse how they spend their time.

Any of these categories can be further broken down, and it may be useful to find the relative time spent in teaching groups of post-graduates, undergraduates, or other staff. Reading can be broken up under such headings as circulars, scientific texts, or original papers. In keeping a diary it is easy to make it too complex at first, so it cannot be maintained. Start by keeping it simple, even simpler than the one suggested. Having achieved the first objective of an overall look at how he spends his time, the doctor can look at parts of it in greater detail. The result of keeping such a diary during a period of one week by a doctor involved in rehabilitation work is given in *Figure 128*.

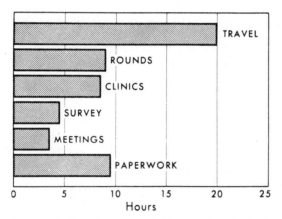

Figure 128. Breakdown of a week's working time of one doctor involved in rehabilitation (321)

It is difficult to keep such a diary. We all believe that we use our time in the best way and seldom waste time. This arises out of our stereotyped idea of what a doctor should do in our particular situation. The very idea that we could use time differently and perhaps more effectively threatens our belief and our ego. Such diaries are clearly for one's own personal use, but if several doctors are prepared to keep diaries, the discussion that comes out of their analysis may be an even more useful exercise.

Analyse the periods spent in different activities and how they contribute to the objectives the doctor has set himself, and the nature and frequency of the interruptions to his work. As most doctors have a given agenda of work, from the responsibilities of which they would not wish to escape, nor could they readily do so, only minor adjustments can be made. Increasing this disposable time can be of the greatest value. The most likely opportunity for increasing disposable time, increasing efficiency and reaching objectives will be through delegation. The diary should therefore be examined for opportunities to delegate time-consuming tasks to those less busy and with less training. It is more important to choose to do what you can do better than anyone else, not necessarily what you can do best.

Few detailed records of how doctors spend their time have ever been made. However, management experience in other fields suggests that almost half will be spent in communicating with other people, hence the reason for the next chapter. We have now to consider management's other resource — materials and money.

MATERIALS AND MONEY AS A MANAGEMENT RESOURCE

European medicine is imbued with the tradition that 'cost is immaterial as long as the doctor is convinced that expensive treatment is for the good of his patient'. In Britain this matter came to serious public notice for the first time with the impossibility of enough kidney machines being supplied by the National Health Service. Statements, such as the following recorded by Professor D. N. S. Kerr, have begun to appear (138).

> Inevitably someone has to select some patients for survival and leave some to die. The job of making these decisions is hard, and it explains why doctors have often been driven against their better judgement to treat all comers on a shoe string rather than face the task of selecting a few to treat properly .

Unwittingly, perhaps, far more serious decisions are made daily in developing countries, and children sicken and only too frequently die from preventable conditions such as whooping cough, measles and tuberculosis, because most of the money that is available is spent on curative services. In Europe, the supply of the most expensive medicine is considered justified, but money for an impoverished family to spend on a special but expensive diet may be impossible to provide. Ineptitudes in deciding how money can be used are met at every turn. Recently, in a South American hospital, it was found that the most expensive antibiotics could be given to a dehydrated child if he was admitted, but it was administratively impossible to provide him with or teach his mother to provide a cheap saline mixture as an out-patient, even though this would have been at a hundredth of the cost.

Doctors are seldom trained in how their patients' and the community's resources can be best deployed. Poor deployment of drugs and equipment is perhaps less serious than the poor deployment of capital, particularly if this is spent without consideration of how it may tie-up recurring expenditure, staff and capital, as described in Chapter 2. As mentioned earlier, the yearly cost of running most medical establishments is equivalent to a quarter of its initial cost, and most developing countries are handicapped by a vast teaching hospital and other establishments which absorb an inordinate proportion of the national health budget.

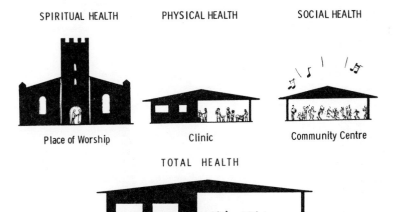

SPIRITUAL HEALTH   PHYSICAL HEALTH   SOCIAL HEALTH

Place of Worship   Clinic   Community Centre

TOTAL HEALTH

One Multi-purpose Building

Figure 129. Can a building be made to serve different needs of a community?

The need for health facilities to be close to the people if they are to use them is now generally accepted. If the rural society is to make the best use of its resources, can buildings, their biggest capital investment, be made to serve many purposes? (See *Figure 129.*)

GETTING OTHER PEOPLE TO DO IT

THE MEASUREMENT AND CONTROL OF RESOURCES IN THE ATTAINMENT OF OBJECTIVES

The staff and their time

A doctor who analyses and manages his own time well, and discusses this with his staff, may well inspire his team to do likewise. For example, he should if possible not keep members of his team waiting unoccupied for his arrival, and should this happen he should be the first to apologize, to impress on them the value of their own time. On his wall he may post the reminder 'Plan Ahead'. In no field is this more important than in that of staff and their continuing training.

Quality of present and future staff

On arriving in a new post and joining a new team, the doctor inherits the skills, knowledge and attitudes that have been implanted in the staff by his predecessors. He has to build on these, but may find that there are severe limitations in the abilities that can be given or imparted to many of the less intelligent members of his team. It will seldom be possible or wise just to dismiss or transfer the less able, but when the

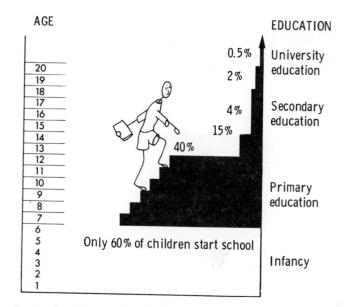

Figure 130. The educational ladder. In each country there is likely to be a 'plateau' above which few from rural societies will rise; this will be the source of most health workers (reproduced from King, 1966, by courtesy of Oxford University Press, Nairobi)

time does come to take on new staff, do it with the greatest possible care. The successful functioning of the unit over the next 30 years will depend on choosing suitable staff, particularly in a situation where there is low staff mobility. Once they have been selected and proved themselves, the manager's responsibility is to train them to make the most of their ability by developing their knowledge and skills. Arranging, supervising and perhaps partaking in this training is the greatest gift and responsibility of the manager to his subordinates.

The ladder of education in rural areas is represented in *Figure 130*. Many start primary education but as *Figure 130* shows, few may complete it. Fewer will go on to secondary school; more of the secondary school places will be available to children from an urban background, and the chances of even a highly intelligent child from rural areas obtaining university entry may be small in some countries. Usually those who go on to secondary education are from families who can afford the expense. For this reason, selection for secondary education or university entry is not entirely by merit, and a number of intelligent and perhaps well-motivated young people with only primary education, who could not afford further study, are available, particularly in the rural areas, if only they can be discovered.

There are several possible methods of obtaining the best workers. In some areas it may be both expedient and politic to ask the local leader or chief for a suitable applicant (who is likely to be a relative of his). If after one or two weeks this person proves unsuitable, it will cause little ill feeling to get a replacement by going back to the local leader. Another possibility is to offer training to literate farmers who are already leaders and have been selected by the community. The training is given in their free time in the season when farm work is light and they receive training in return for limited service. During this simple training those with ability can be identified and offered further training. In this way they may be 'earning while learning'.

The following two steps may also be effective in selecting the best type of staff.

(1) As large as possible a pool of potential candidates are carefully 'aptitude tested'. If possible the help of a vocation assessment service should be obtained. In countries such as Zambia this has been undertaken for trainee medical assistants with excellent results. No completely satisfactory 'do it yourself' set of aptitude tests exists, but the Raven progressive matrices have proved useful to many.*
The small but sophisticated vocational assessment unit in Zambia working along these lines, but using other methods, has done much to raise the standard of medical assistants.

*Further assistance and tests are available from The Californian Test Bureau, Del Monte Research Park, Monterey, California 93940, USA and The Godfrey Thompson Unit for Educational Research, 14 George Square, Edinburgh 8, Scotland

(2) All classes of auxiliary workers should be recruited initially 10 per cent or even 20 per cent over strength, and reduced to size after an initial three months' probationary period. This reduction is quite fair, provided it is made perfectly clear to all concerned. Such a reduction will prevent the employment of misfits who cannot be identified by any selection method.

Staff motivation

A parallel from industry can again be valuable to the doctor as team leader. The results of such a study (113) are given in *Figure 131* and suggest strong positive and negative influences in the motivation of staff. The length of the boxes in this figure relates to the intensity of their effect, while the depth gives some indication of their duration.

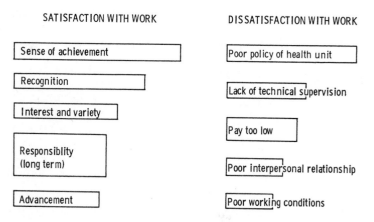

SATISFACTION WITH WORK   DISSATISFACTION WITH WORK

Sense of achievement   Poor policy of health unit

Recognition   Lack of technical supervision

Interest and variety   Pay too low

Responsiblity (long term)   Poor interpersonal relationship

Advancement   Poor working conditions

Figure 131. Comparison of positive and negative influences in the motivation of staff

Positive factors

In the figure some factors, such as achievement, will give considerable immediate satisfaction. Others, such as responsibility, are important; the satisfaction they provide is less intense, but it persists longer. Whatever the post within a clinic or hospital, a worker, whether he is a senior medical assistant or a part-time sweeper, will work better if he feels he is achieving something tangible which is recognized. The doctor's job is to supply this satisfaction if his team is to become more

378

effective. Interest in the work will depend in large measure on each person understanding the objectives of the unit and his part in it, and with imagination some variety can always be introduced. If a worker can feel that he alone is responsible for some part of the work, and that this work is valuable, he is likely to put more effort and interest into seeing that it is well done. The attitude of the doctor to his subordinates can do much to create a better understanding in the unit. This is also promoted if he can provide opportunities both for the team to meet socially and for regular discussion of their work. These regular team meetings are at the same time one of the most neglected and the most important aspects of management in medicine. The regular weekly, bi-monthly or monthly 'inspection' of all larger units, including a discussion and a request for ideas to improve the services, has already been mentioned with reference to the Under-Fives' Clinics. This will be the opportunity to promote satisfaction by praise and recognition, and raise interest and a sense of responsibility. At the same time, the reasons for dissatisfaction can be sought, and where possible eliminated. The team meeting must not be ignored nor used for a show of power by the doctor.

A ladder of possible promotion is an essential stimulus if intelligent workers are to remain happy. There should also be a method by which the worker can up-grade his basic education, so that it does not hold him back. Not everyone can, or wants to, ascend more than one or two rungs on the ladder of promotion, but if this advancement has been gained through personal effort and initiative, the satisfaction of the achievement of moving up one step on the promotion ladder may last a lifetime *(Figure 132)*. This diagram has caused and will cause considerable discussion. It suggests that everyone in the health service should be on some ladder and have the chance of promotion, as the achievement of promotion is a source of job satisfaction. Unfortunately, it perpetuates the idea of 'levels' or 'low grade'. The most important and effective workers in the health service are frequently those at the bottom of the promotion ladder. It is clear that many of the most valuable workers in the health service will never obtain promotion. This diagram also stresses the difficulty and problem of moving from one category over the wall of further education into a higher category of health worker. Doctors only too easily forget that education and the opportunities that arise for those who achieve it come from accident of birth.

The possibility of gaining more skills and achieving promotion is an essentail feature of successful management in Western medical services. However, 'promotion ladders' are largely a Western concept, and the indigenous practitioner finds his satisfaction in the increasing respect and stature given to him in a village society. In the future, as communities are mobilized to become responsible for their health care, they should choose their own village health worker who will be both from the village and remain part of the village. Upward mobility will be less important for him, and he will find much reward and satisfaction from the position awarded to him by his fellow villagers.

The disgruntled staff member can be located in many organizations. His problem may have arisen because he has been promoted above his

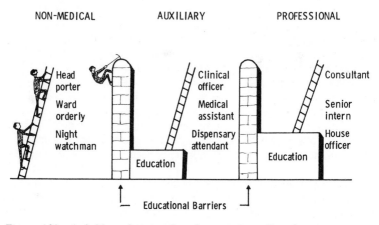

NON-MEDICAL   AUXILIARY   PROFESSIONAL

Figure 132. A ladder of promotion for everyone. Can they surmount educational barriers, or should these be broken down?

ceiling, or for family or interpersonal reasons. As a result, he may appear to go out of his way to be rude, and have difficulty in dealing with his subordinates, peers and superiors, and more important in the long run, with members of the public. In developing countries, the chances of his moving or being moved to another organization where he will be happy are small. The recognition of such an individual is essential to good management. Fortunately some aspect of his work is likely to be good. If only this can be discovered and receive public praise, his general relations and co-operation in the team will improve. In general, if any reproof is required, this should always be given in private. Public remarks should always be limited to approval and praise. Where possible, public confrontation with staff at any level is to be avoided.

Negative factors

The doctor—manager will need to watch out for evidence of dissatisfaction in any of these, and take action if possible to overcome them.

Improving them beyond a point where they no longer cause dissatisfaction will have only a slight effect on motivation. The worker who feels he is out of touch with hospital policy and is not informed of changes, particularly those that will affect his working conditions, will be unhappy. In many cultures, lack of supervision and discord in supervision are a well-recognized and fruitful source of discontent, particularly where nursing sisters are supervising male workers.

The relatively small importance placed on salary in motivation depends on the salary being adequate and on a similar level to others in the same cultural setting. Increasing the salary above the general level is unlikely to yield greater productivity either in industry or in medicine. On the contrary, it may defeat the purpose for which it was intended and give rise to an artificial upper class who will look down on those paid less.

The needs of the worker

The needs of the worker have been summarized (164) into the following hierarchy of need.

Self-fulfilment

By this is meant both a desire for self-fulfilment and an understanding that one's ability is being made use of. It is also the knowledge that one's training has prepared one for the job.

Esteem needs

The worker is encouraged if he has evidence that those both senior and junior to himself believe that he is successful. The understanding of the real need for a job will also lead to an increasing self-respect. The more junior and menial a job, the greater the need for respect from those in authority, and if this is supplied there will be a greater loyalty to the organization and the leader. Equally, those who work close to the top need to remember the isolation of those at the top and that they also need continuing reassurance.

Belongingness and love needs

Few men like to be truly independent. This gregarious tendency needs to be met within working hours and is symbolized by the occasional meeting together of all who work in the unit. If possible, at least on some occasions all the team may have their tea break together.

Insufficient thought in planning health units is given to providing workers with library, canteen and recreational facilities.

Safety needs

The orderliness of the unit is important, and a feeling of security and justice are essential. Just leaders are apt to be forgiven many other shortcomings.

Maintaining a balance

A more difficult function of the manager, particularly for the doctor—manager, is maintaining a balance. In child care one of the fundamental balances to be maintained is between the needs of the children the team is caring for and the needs of the individuals who make up this team.

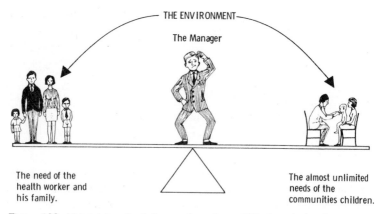

Figure 133. Maintaining the balance of needs, a difficult task for the manager

The suddenness of illness and death in childhood, and the deep emotions of guilt that death may produce in parents and staff, create more difficulties than in the medical care of adults. The urgency of illness in childhood involves more work at night and during weekends, and conscientious staff are unlikely to take time off during working hours to make good the resulting emotional and physical exhaustion. For these reasons, those working in child care may be in particular need for help in maintaining a balance between their personal needs (and those of their families) and the almost unlimited needs of the children in the society they serve *(Figure 133).*

Most doctors with experience in developing countries can remember conditions under which this balance has been upset, to the detriment either of the individuals who made up the team or alternatively of the children for whom a service was being offered. As shown in *Figure 133*, the environment in which the unit works will always be changing and making differing demands on those who work there. The doctor– manager needs to be sensitive to these changes and to the varying needs of the individuals.

However, this is only one of the many balances that have to be maintained. Others will include service responsibility versus teaching and research, the demands of in-patients compared with out-patients, or a balance between capital expenditure on a prestige building and ensuring adequate running expenses.

The dignity of the manager

The manager who wishes to build a strong team will show that he does not consider it below his dignity to undertake any job. If a child vomits, the doctor himself on occasion fetches the mop and bucket and discovers whether the equipment available to the cleaning staff is adequate. For a senior doctor to do this in many countries will be unthinkable (just as it would have been in Victorian England). In the UK or USA it might easily happen, and the doctor would appreciate the strengthening of the bonds between his team, as a result.

Availability of the manager

The manager of an efficient team needs to make himself available at known times to hear complaints and problems. Many of these may be personal and unrelated to the work. Only sometimes will any action be necessary as a result of these complaints, and as long as the worker receives a sympathetic hearing, he will on most occasions be satisfied. Sometimes the experienced manager will learn more from what is not said than from what is said.

To create a system of balance the manager requires monitoring or management systems.

MANAGEMENT SYSTEMS

The simplest system is shown in *Figure 134*. Any procedure or service will depend on various inputs, which must be adjusted if the system is to work efficiently. In this model, if the manager or decision-maker is to make effective use of his resources, then the steps shown by the dotted

MANAGEMENT

line will be needed. A communication system will be created that is both appropriate and swift.

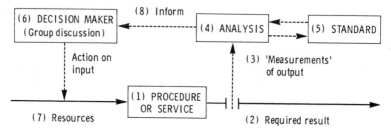

Figure 134. A simple model of a management system

Take for example, the elimination of neonatal tetanus in a community of 50,000 people. Referring to the diagram we can say:

(1) *The procedure or service* is the injection of tetanus toxoid to all mothers by the nurse—midwife in the antenatal period.

(2) *The required result or objective* is the elimination of neonatal tetanus in the community.

(3) *The measurement of output* will be the returns from the clinic of the number of injections given and the number of mothers who have received all three injections.

(4) *The analysis* is made each month of the proportion of ante-natal mothers inoculated, and this will be compared with the standard.

(5) *The standard* will be the number of pregnancies expected from the birth rate in a population of 50,000. However, allowance must be made that reaching the last 5—10 per cent of mothers is likely to be too expensive to be economically feasible.

(6) *The decision-maker* takes this and information on cases of neonatal tetanus still being reported, and uses it to influence the input or resources. One of his more important resources in effective motiva-tion will be through group discussion of those involved, and his action may be modified as a result of this group meeting.

(7) *The resources.* The 'action on input' may involve any of the following considerations.

  (a) The nurse and her skills in encouraging all the mothers to attend to accept the injections.
  (b) Supply of toxoid.
  (c) Supply of syringes, sterilizing equipment, etc.
  (d) The attitudes of the community towards the clinic and their

384

motivation to encourage all their mothers to attend the antenatal clinics.

(e)   Special health education facilities for areas of low acceptance.

In this situation the objectives are to eliminate neonatal tetanus in the community and not only in infants born to mothers who come regularly to the clinic.

With objectives involving the majority of families in the community, a doctor will need to work through the community leaders or council and encourage them to take their part in the programme. Community attitudes to the programme then become a resource in its achievement. *One cannot enter any community by by-passing the leaders because if a leader feels that he has not been given due recognition he can become hostile and unco-operative.*

(8)   *Communication.* For any system of management to be effective, the communication system must be efficient and swift. A manager requires information quickly, rather than with great accuracy. If, for example, a child from his district dies in hospital with neonatal tetanus, he needs to know the name of the village the child comes from, so that he can check their returns, rather than a detailed account of the child's birth.

Efficient management rests on the communication of up-to-date administrative, clinical and therapeutic information. To achieve this, some accurate regular feedback from medical records is essential. Maintaining and improving the standard of care in smaller units can best be achieved by always attempting to improve on past results, and discussing success or failure in this regularly with the staff.

Many of the decisions of Ministers of Health and District Health Departments in developing countries should be based on the experience of people working in smaller hospitals and rural health centres, yet the machinery for such consultation is primitive.

TYPES OF MANAGEMENT

The extreme theories of management have been set out as Theory X and Theory Y *(Figure 135)*. In practice no organization lies at either extreme of these theories; all lie somewhere between. Managers need to consider their own position in the organization and that of the organization itself. How much can they afford to be out of step with their organization in increasing participation and moving towards Theory Y? Institutions and organizations need to be trained, as well as individuals. In some cultures which are accustomed to accepting decisions without question, efforts to increase participation will take time, and involvement of junior staff in discussion over decision-making may at first disturb them. Similarly, in some cultures otherwise brilliant young men when promoted to a position of importance become dictatorial, and perhaps because of a feeling of inadequacy are unable to consult junior staff, with a disastrous effect on the team spirit.

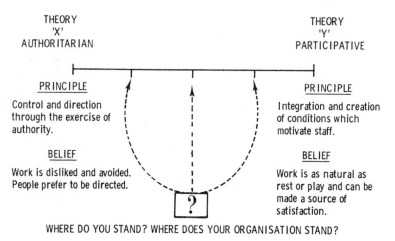

THEORY
'X'
AUTHORITARIAN

THEORY
'Y'
PARTICIPATIVE

PRINCIPLE

Control and direction through the exercise of authority.

PRINCIPLE

Integration and creation of conditions which motivate staff.

BELIEF

Work is disliked and avoided. People prefer to be directed.

BELIEF

Work is as natural as rest or play and can be made a source of satisfaction.

WHERE DO YOU STAND? WHERE DOES YOUR ORGANISATION STAND?

Figure 135. The extreme theories of organizational behaviour (169)

DELEGATION

Delegation is the process of entrusting less skilled 'subordinates' with authority to act in a given field, using their own discretion on behalf of their more skilled 'superiors'. Merely explaining how to do a job and insisting on it being done in a particular way is NOT delegation. In delegation there must always be a content of training and supervision.

The work of a doctor doing an effective job for children in a developing country frequently grows at an alarming rate. Unless he is to be inundated by calls on his time, he will need to keep ahead of this growth by increasing the delegation of his more routine duties to those capable of undertaking them. If delegation is to be successful, three possible difficulties must be borne in mind. In many situations they present as threats, so they have been expressed here as fears. Two are found in the delegating doctor and one can be expected in the person involved in the new duties.

(1) The doctor's fear of having to give up what has become routine

work for him. To step back and not do the job which he has been accustomed to do may be difficult, and requires courage. The most obvious difficulty a doctor meets is when he asks someone else to become 'the first point of medical contact' and to make the first diagnosis. He believes that someone else will miss a sick child, and that only he can cope. Few can appreciate that there are so many children who can never get to any clinic, due to the general failure to organize services. This has been discussed with reference to the Under-Fives' Clinic in Chapter 19, where the one-to-one nurse—patient consultation is considered of more importance than the one-to-one doctor—patient consultation.

(2)   Fear that the person undertaking the new responsibility may become more expert than the doctor himself, who feels his position threatened. A simple example may be the setting up of a scalp vein drip. The person who does this regularly, given average intelligence and manipulative skills, should within a few months become more expert than the doctor who trained him. But the doctor does not lose the respect of visitors if he says 'Go to my nurse if you want to learn about scalp vein transfusions'; rather he gains respect.

(3)   Fear by persons taking on the new responsibility, so that they do not exercise their decision-making within the limits clearly set out by the doctor. Every doctor makes mistakes, and some mistakes must be expected when his work is delegated. Search for the reasons for them. The most likely cause is a failure of communication, or the delegation of too much responsibility after too little training. Whatever the cause, the responsibility must be shared by the doctor, who will need to examine with the person involved how the mistake occurred. The doctor who implies that when a mistake is made it is always the fault of the workers will not gain their respect and will not help them in future decision-making. He must be particularly sensitive to subordinates 'losing face' by being reproved in public.

To remove these three fears an unconscious bond of trust must be developed between the doctor and the staff to whom he delegates responsibility. The worker will be encouraged by suitable remarks of praise to develop his discretion on behalf of the doctor. He must act within the limits set by the doctor, which need to be clearly set out, although the doctor has the right and responsibility to vary them as required.

Delegation should lead to those with less training developing their own ability and skills, as well as greater job satisfaction and a bond of common interest and purpose between the doctor and his team. In this process the doctor will be suffering from an 'identity crisis'. During his training he is likely to have developed a fairly restricted image of himself, fashioned from his teachers. During the process of delegation this image may be upset. The whole process of management is disturbing as the doctor finds himself in a new role.

For effective delegation a doctor requires the following characteristics.

(1) The capacity to communicate the necessary information as well as what decisions can be made without reference first to the doctor. In most circumstances detailed instructions need to be written down, either in a manual or as duplicated notes.

(2) The ability to set out for the worker the order in which he should take the necessary action and decision.

(3) An awareness of what cultural and other difficulties will arise, and the workers' response to them.

(4) The ability to carry out appropriate checks.

(5) The willingness to trust subordinates, to praise their successes and to discuss their problems.

(6) The willingness to take his full share of responsibility for all mistakes made by his subordinates.

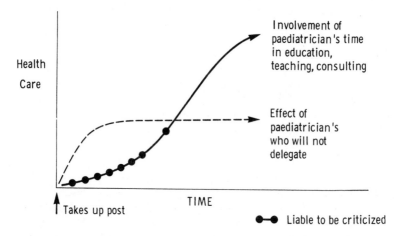

Figure 136. Results of delegation on the amount of health care provided

The effects of delegation will not be immediate *(Figure 136)*, and the doctor who delegates will realize that he must stop 'giving his all' the whole time to his patients. In the early days of educating, teaching and consulting his team, the doctor may come under criticism because he is not spending all his time with the patients. It is a difficult decision to give less of himself to his patients so that he can work through his staff, but once effective delegation can be achieved, the amount of

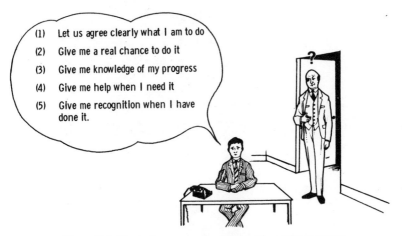

Figure 137. The junior manager's appeal to the senior manager

health care that becomes available to the community will rapidly increase. Effective delegation depends on training before undertaking the job, training whilst on the job, and by supervision with refresher courses.

Effective delegation is only possible with good communication, and the doctor needs to be continually answering the questions set out in *Figure 137*. They may be unspoken and perhaps unformulated, but they exist in the mind of the person to whom responsibility is delegated.

THE SKILL PYRAMID

A hospital or health centre can be considered as a skill pyramid, with those who have had much training and learnt many skills at the apex. This pyramid is arranged in the hierarchal manner with which we are all familiar *(Figure 138a)*. In discussion with Dr. King, who first created this well-known diagram, it emerged that he now believes that it is better reversed, as in *Figure 138b*.

The doctors are then at the bottom and the pyramid is a wedge, and those with lesser skills, but on whom the effective health service in developing countries really depends, are at the top. The arrows have

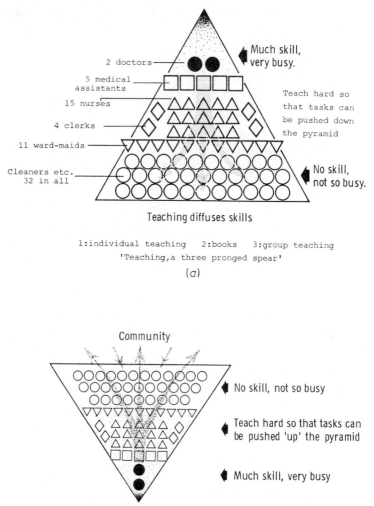

been extended showing how teaching diffuses skills, and that knowledge and the skills from the hospital diffuse out into the community. At the same time, there is information passing back from the community to the hospital, and back from the workers there to the doctors. The hospital now becomes a 'living learning arena' (see Chapter 20). The skills of rehydrating children, the knowledge of better feeding habits and the attitude of a scientific understanding of disease no longer 'leak' but now 'pour out' into the community. Much but not all of this contact can be made by the less skilled hospital workers.

This pyramid is constructed on the rule 'Delegate every task to the humblest and least expensive member of the team capable of doing it satisfactorily'. Often there is no one who can do the job effectively, and the delegation involves teaching or passing skills up (or down) the pyramid.

The skill pyramid can be seen on a smaller scale in the health centre and the small hospital, or in a department within a larger hospital, and every doctor working in a developing country needs to consider how he works in relation to a skill pyramid. Is he desperately busy, while there are others with fewer skills who are comparatively idle? For him there must be a constant striving to push down the pyramid, first through staff training and then through effective delegation, with the necessary supervision that is so essential a part of delegation.

The skill pyramid suggests not only training, but also a re-training programme. At all levels of personnel, a regular re-training is required. In the 'two dollars a year' health care country, the once or twice yearly training seminar can do more to raise standards of health care in an area than any other step. The doctor who fails to bring his staff who are working in more peripheral centres together for this training, however busy he is, may well be considered guilty of professional negligence.

Only too often the doctor will find that in practice the skill pyramid in the service in which he works is in a disordered state, and one of his managerial tasks may well be to build in the missing parts of the pyramid.

Disorders of the skill pyramid

The idea of the skill pyramid has been taken further with diagrammatic suggestions of how it may be at fault (140).

The idealized pyramid (Figure 139a)

This shows staff of each grade of skill in the correct proportion. For simplicity, the different grades of workers have been reduced to three,

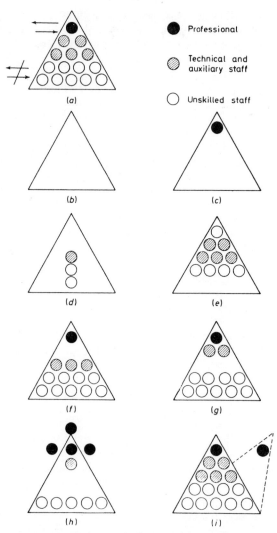

Figure 139. Disorders of the skill pyramid. (a) Idealized pyramid: correct proportion of staff. (b) The empty pyramid: planning gone wrong. (c) 'The lone wolf'; isolated doctor, no teaching, no delegating. (d) 'No officers': auxiliary unsupervised; no teaching. (e) 'No privates'; no cleaners, messengers or clerks. (f) 'No sergeants'; no paramedicals. (g) 'No corporals': no auxiliaries. (h) 'Too many generals': doctors without supporting staff. (i) Divided loyalty (reproduced from King, 1970, by courtesy of the Editor, Journal of Tropical Medicine and Hygiene)

the paramedical and the auxiliary being grouped together. This idealized pyramid may be upset by frequent posting of senior staff, as suggested by the arrows. Administrators seldom appreciate that a doctor cannot develop any improvement in a service in less than two years, and a period of five to ten years is probably optimal for a senior post. To guard against the chaos resulting from the almost inevitable posting of key personnel, the experienced manager will see that someone parallel or one rung down in the pyramid is receiving training as a possible replacement. Just as mobility at the apex of the pyramid is liable to be too great, job mobility at the base may be inadequate. However, if a training programme is available, and some ladder of promotion can be created, the chances of mobility and job satisfaction are increased.

The empty pyramid (Figure 139b)

Only too frequently found, this situation has arisen through construction of buildings for a health service programme which has been planned without adequate estimates for trained staff that will be available. It is commonplace for the politician to promise such buildings without consideration as to the suitability of the site or the availability of staff.

The 'lone wolf' (Figure 139c)

This represents the doctor, usually in private practice, who teaches no one and delegates to no one. He is not using to the best advantage the knowledge and skills he took so long to learn and which were usually gained at considerable cost to his country. Because he is not teaching, his own standard of practice declines.

'No officers' (Figure 139d)

The auxiliary in charge of a health centre, working perhaps with unskilled staff, frequently attempting to do a good job but lacking the stimulus of further training that is a part of good supervision.

'No privates' (Figure 139e)

The trainee nurse doing cleaning and messenger tasks that cleaners might do. Or in the clinic, the use of nurses for weighing children instead of the employment of clerks to do this.

'No sergeants' (Figure 139f)

The doctor who works without help from the paramedical or technical disciplines of nursing, radiology, etc. The rehydration centre in South America, which functions with only doctors and women skilled in methods of scalp vein infusion techniques, but with no full-time trained nurses. The pathologist who is expected to run a laboratory with assistants but no fully trained technician.

'No corporals' (Figure 139g)

The Under-Fives' Clinic with large attendances, in which only fully qualified nurses are allowed to care for children, instead of local less qualified auxiliary nurses who have undergone a special training to undertake this work.

'Too many generals' (Figure 139h)

The circumstance that exists in many Asian and South American hospitals, where there is pressure to employ the many doctors who have been trained to work in the cities and large towns, rather than in the rural areas where the people live. There is no one to teach and no one to delegate to. Much too much of the limited health budget is absorbed in paying the medical profession.

Divided loyalty (Figure 139i)

There may be other complications in the pyramid when the duties at the top become divided. An example of this is likely to occur when unskilled staff are under the direction of the hospital manager for hiring and discipline, but under the matron and sisters for their training and the supervision of their work. The difficulties that may arise in such a situation may be prevented if areas of responsibility and courses of action are discussed and defined before difficulties arise.

In many institutions there are likely to be more than one of these disorders of the pyramid. The idealized pyramid is something that can be striven for, but will hardly be reached, as the requirements of trained skill and their functions will continually alter. We must not forget the speed of change. The nurse with limited local training in an Under-Fives' Clinic can today save many more children's lives than could the best trained doctor thirty years ago. The speed of change is likely to be even more rapid over the next three decades.

THE PLACE OF MANAGEMENT IN THE FUTURE

A knowledge of management skills is likely to play a part in the future training of doctors in every medical school. However, the study of this discipline must take its place with others in the science and art of

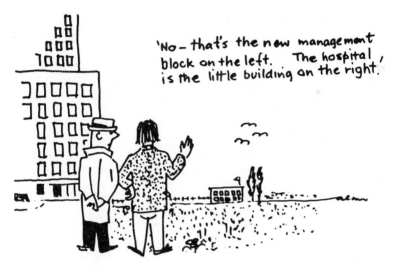

Figure 140. Management can be overemphasized

medicine. This, as every other discipline, can be overemphasized *(Figure 140),* but it will play a small but important role in the organization of child care.

CHAPTER 22

Communication and Learning

THOSE TO WHOM THE PAEDIATRICIAN COMMUNICATES

The value of good communication in making the doctor more effective in his job has been emphasized repeatedly in the preceding chapters. The original meaning of the word 'doctor' was 'teacher', which serves as a reminder of the doctor's responsibility and perhaps also of the inadequacy of his training in the field of communicating and learning. The doctor's ability to communicate effectively to parents is particularly important to the satisfactory care of children in the first five years of their life.

To his patients and to his staff the doctor is an exalted and busy man. Unless he is cautious he will repeatedly be accepting a 'yes' from people who do not really understand what he is saying. The doctor tends to follow the example of his own teachers. So often these teachers develop habits of mind which reduce their ability to communicate, and because of their senior position no one draws their attention to this. A simple and obvious example is handwriting. The medical profession, certainly in the UK, is notorious for its poor handwriting. Various excuses are put forward for this. The purpose of handwriting is to communicate accurately, and as accuracy in medicine is possibly more important than in any other profession, there can be little justification for continuing this impediment to good communication.

As mentioned in the last chapter, analysis of the work of managers showed that they spent around half their time communicating, and this will certainly be true of doctors. Teaching is a form of communication not only from teacher to student but also between students and from student to teacher. To make the most use of his time the doctor will attempt to use communication techniques as an essential part of learning, and this is why these have been grouped together. He will be communicating (and teaching) at a number of different levels, as shown in *Figure 141*. Each of these presents special problems. The majority of time may be spent in communicating with the mothers, who are likely to be illiterate in most developing countries. In achieving our objective of a change in behaviour, they will be more difficult to communicate with than any other group.

COMMUNICATING WITH ADMINISTRATORS AND POLITICIANS

Some visit to or inspection of health centres and hospitals is, or should be, carried out as a routine by those in charge of medical services, as one way in which they may keep in touch. The paediatrician expecting

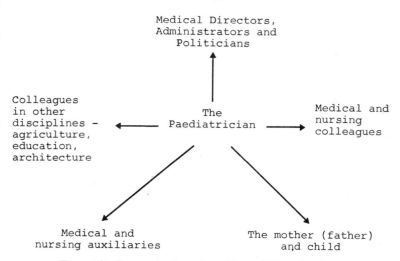

Figure 141. Communicating and teaching at different levels

an important visitor will plan well in advance to make the best use of such visits; he will know that it is unlikely that the busy visitor will carry away more than one idea, but that if this is well implanted, then he is likely to retain it. He may, for example, wish to show how serious whooping cough is in the area, and the need for adequate supplies of vaccine. The visitor's tour can be arranged so that time is left for him to sit down in front of a large chart showing the severity or mortality of whooping cough. If the necessary action that needs to be taken is clearly set out, he is more likely to understand the problem than if it is only discussed without a visual aid, or is the subject of a letter. After the visit, a follow-up letter covering the subject discussed and any plans made is essential.

Malnutrition is a problem in most countries of the developing world and in solving this problem the doctor has a special responsibility. As described in Chapter 8, overcoming malnutrition is a responsibility of many disciplines; however, it is the doctor's task to see that other disciplines realize the severity of the problem. Many lay senior people who have lived all their lives in a developing country have never seen children with severe malnutrition, such as those whom the doctor cares for every day. There can be few sights so disturbing as these children. The doctor must try to ensure that those in the many other professions whose activities may reduce the incidence of malnutrition are at least familiar with its appearance in local children, its catastrophic effects on a child's normal activities, and the possible long-term effect on physical and intellectual development (54, 328). The paediatrician who is anxious further the care of all the children in his community will muster the information about the major problems such as infectious disease and malnutrition in such a way that they may be readily understood by the visitors.

The paediatrician should spend some time in preparing good arguments to convince both committee and visitor. While he can, and should, delegate many aspects of child care to others, the preparation, planning and presentation of plans for improved child health services after adequate discussion with community leaders and other health workers can be done only by him and will remain one of his major responsibilities.

COMMUNICATING WITH COLLEAGUES IN OTHER DISCIPLINES

Such is the speed of the growth of knowledge that information outside the immediate field of medicine in which the doctor works is difficult for him to grasp, and almost non-existent from other disciplines such as agriculture and education. For many years, a department of agriculture in one state was completely absorbed in the task of persuading the local farmers to grow more cocoa. Some farmers were persuaded to turn their farms completely over to cocoa planting. As a result they were living off cassava bought in a nearby town – the cheapest food and one quite unsuited for the regular feeding of young children in their families. The medical profession had failed to make their voices heard and point out that this form of agriculture was likely to increase even further the considerable nutritional problems of the area. Efforts to increase economic growth must not be allowed to disrupt the feeding of children. However, this will repeatedly arise if there is not better team work and interdisciplinary liaison. The rapidly changing societies of developing countries are particularly vulnerable.

The need for locally prepared food-mixes such as the 'Hyderabad mix' has been described in Chapter 9. The design and preparation of such an infant food is important to the paediatrician, but its production and encouraging its use must be the joint effort of several disciplines. The doctor will remember the definition of management given in Chapter 21: 'Deciding what is to be done and getting others to do it'. He may find that the home economics, nutrition or other departments concerned with nutrition can be interested in undertaking the local preparation and distribution of an infant food such as this.

COMMUNICATING WITH TEACHERS

Contact with the teaching profession is equally important. The teacher may be unwilling to approach the doctor, but will frequently welcome an approach from him, and some ways in which this contact may develop are suggested here. An important aim of education should surely be to enable people to make better use of the environment in which they live. The teacher will therefore look for help from others, particularly those concerned with health.

If the child is to grow up to make the best use of the environment of a rural society, then an understanding of his own culture, child-rearing practices, the major diseases, their prevention, and parenthood, are all fields in which the teacher and doctor can work together. Such training, if well conceived, will help to retain the many beneficial child-rearing practices found in most developing countries. Ezekiel Mphahlele (196) wrote:

> These are the broad elements of the "African Personality" that we can be sure are common to most societies on this continent: the place of the extended family in the social stratum; the sense of communal responsibility; the tendency to gravitate towards other people rather than things and places; reverence for ancestral spirits; audience participation in entertainment activities.'

A better understanding of the values of these features of many Asian and South American as well as African societies in the developing world may prevent the young person forsaking them for the more tangible attributes of Western society, with its emphasis on material benefits.

To help a future parent in a rural (or urban) environment, teaching should provide some knowledge of the normal processes of growth and also the symptomatology and the stages in development of the common diseases that their children will contract. A simple description of the natural history of common illnesses, supported by the child's own experience, and how many of them can be prevented, should be part of the normal school programme. The picture of whooping cough in a child, how it is spread to other children, the story of the production of whooping cough vaccine and its use in preventing the illness, can be made a far more lively, interesting and useful subject for teaching in senior primary school classes than the rivers of another continent. Such teaching may be linked with practical activities involving the child in the overall health of the community in which he lives as described in Chapter 8. Any epidemic of disease should become a matter of concern to the whole community, including the school.

The doctor, unlike the teacher, sees the effects of ignorance of nutrition in his daily work, and it is his responsibility, through links with education, to ensure that the teaching of nutrition in schools receives adequate attention. This is a subject that can be brought into much of the teaching and also associated with school life. The following is a list of the ways in which it may be brought into all stages of schooling (233). These are the activities suggested for the senior class of a primary school.

(1) To weigh each other and for each to make his own pictorial growth record.

(2) To make visits to markets to price foods; make menus for good meals which can be bought at low cost; buy the selected foods; prepare meals and serve them to the class. If no kitchen is available, a stove or charcoal pot may be used inside, or a fire outside.

(3) To help prepare and serve school meals, or help provide a snack.

(4) To grow a school garden and keep small livestock (if suitable).

(5) To learn to preserve foods grown in the school garden.

(6) To prepare a good meal and invite parents to a party to share it.

(7) To prepare charts, posters, models on food and health and continue scrapbooks at a more advanced level.

(8) To carry out simple experiments on foods, such as separating milk into cream, curd and whey, or testing with blotting paper to find which foods contain fat, or with iodine for starch.

(9) To play team games for the selection of a good diet and hold competitions on food production and on other subjects concerned with nutrition.

(10) To study the food patterns of other lands.

(11) To prepare reports, plays and exhibitions on food and health and on the nutrition activities of the class.

Interest in good food habits and nutrition *(Figure 142)* may be increased in both school and community by activities which overlap to some extent; such as youth clubs, which may be attached to the school but accept children not attending; school producer and consumer co-operatives, which include the children's home garden products as well; the preparation in school of news-sheets, exhibitions and plays to inform the community about the programme, and parent—teacher associations and joint school—home projects.

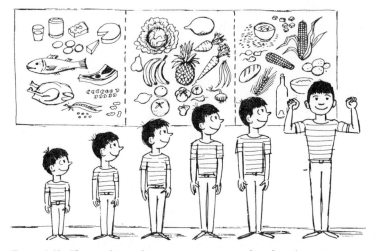

Figure 142. The teaching of nutrition must stress that there is a connection between good food and growing tall, strong and healthy (reproduced from Ritchie, 1967, by courtesy of the Food and Agriculture Organization of the United Nations)

A number of these activities are listed in an excellent nutrition textbook written for medical auxiliaries (141).

COMMUNICATING WITH ARCHITECTS

The failure of the doctor to communicate to architects the real needs of medical care is clearly seen on a visit to almost any hospital in the tropics. Specifically, the requirements for mothers and their small children are not met in the clinic or the ward (Chapters 19 and 20). This can only represent a failure to examine the requirements before and to analyse how successfully they have been met afterwards. This failure is seen not only in the small hospital but in the large hospital costing tens of millions of dollars. An example was provided when an architectural firm was designing their second vast hospital in Africa. In the first, the children's out-patient department had proved entirely inadequate and part of the old hospital had still to be used. In the second new hospital, the architect had not been told about the failure of his first design, nor had he received a specific 'paediatric brief', and he was in process of creating another department which would again prove quite unsatisfactory.

As in so many situations, no advantage can be gained by attempting to apportion blame between disciplines for this situation, which arises through their failure to achieve effective communication. Even where the doctor has been involved, other staff, particularly the nursing profession, may not have been considered. A theatre suite recently completed contained a satisfactory changing room for the surgical staff, but the nursing staff found they had to change in the room used for sorting dirty linen.

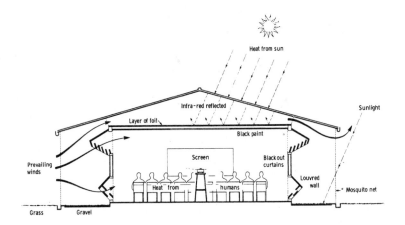

Figure 143. A design to allow lecture rooms to be darkened without a rise in temperature in a tropical country

In the field of visual communication the doctor has failed to inform the architect of the great need for a darkened room in which projected aids may be used. Due to influences from Europe, large glass windows and poor alternative ventilation make any attempt to black out many a tropical lecture room almost impossible. Light and heat go hand in hand, and a darkened but cool room should not be difficult to achieve. *Figure 143* shows one possible plan for a lecture room in a hot climate.

In this plan many louvres allow air to flow freely through the hall to remove the heat generated by the students. Gravel or grass and louvres will prevent light and heat being reflected in. The heat of the sun falls on the roof. The roof radiates infra-red rays which are reflected back by aluminium foil laid above the ceiling. As the air under the roof heats up, plenty of through ventilation is required. Lastly, as a darkened room is beloved by mosquitoes, the room may have to be screened. The gauze screening needs to be well away from the louvres if the flow of air is to be unrestricted. When light is required the curtains can be drawn from the fixed windows.

COMMUNICATION WITH NURSING COLLEAGUES

The failure of doctors to make effective communication with nursing staff has perhaps done much to inhibit medical care in many developing countries. This has already been referred to in Chapter 20.

COMMUNICATION WITH MEDICAL AND NURSING AUXILIARIES

The standard of work of the medical auxiliary will depend largely on the supervision he receives, and this can be more important than his original training. If the technique suggested for the Under-Fives' Clinic (see p. 328) is used, the auxiliary will continually learn on the job by in-service training. If the doctor can as a priority maintain this kind of communication, the teaching and supervision will be effective. Much of the supervision will be through working on sick children together. If the medical assistant is away from the doctor in a health centre in a village, it will be by visits, letters in reply to notes sent in with patients, possibly by wireless or telephone where these services exist. The regular refresher course will also offer opportunities for useful communication. The doctor will not only be offering further teaching to the assistant; he will also be learning about local attitudes, beliefs and customs, as described in Chapter 3.

In his communication with and supervision of nursing auxiliaries who are working away from the direct supervision of his senior nursing colleagues, the doctor must use tact and care, and he will need to be frequently in touch with these nursing colleagues to maintain their trust in his actions as they jointly supervise and improve the standard of care offered by peripheral workers (see *Figure 137*).

COMMUNICATING WITH THE MOTHER AND THE CHILD

The ancient Chinese proverb 'A picture is as good as a thousand words' is widely accepted, but only too often the greater difficulty that an illiterate person may have in comprehending a picture is overlooked.

This is an example of the problem, only now being appreciated, of our difficulty in communicating with mothers, many of whom will be totally or partially illiterate, and the majority of whom come from an entirely different cultural background. The present generation of young mothers in the developing countries is not only handicapped by physical ill-health, overwork and deprivation, but also lack the basic knowledge of how to rear a family. The training traditionally passed on by their grandmothers and mothers has for a number of reasons (including formal education) deteriorated and become less acceptable. The father as head of the family also needs health education. To provide this, the public health department in Nairobi issued Fathers' Newsletters, which proved popular, while in Zambia the medical assistants give health talks about children to the men waiting as out-patients.

In Chapter 5, difference in understanding of the cause of disease was emphasized. Even when the doctor takes this into consideration, he will have difficulty in speaking effectively to the mother about her sick child. To make the situation even worse, the doctor often gives the idea of communication scarcely any thought, as the following scene suggests.

It is set in the crowded out-patient department of a major hospital in Asia. Because of the large numbers that arrive daily, many interns have been drafted into the out-patient clinic each day to 'see' the children who attend. The interns sit round a table. There is no room for the mothers holding their children to sit down. They stand with their babies behind and to the side of the doctor, who writes on a 'bus ticket' and occasionally turns to feel a child, or perfunctorily to poke a stethoscope between the clothes of the dressed child.

In an effort to move away from the extreme situation such as this, the first consideration will be the position of the two people concerned. A familiar example of how furniture, full in-trays, the telephone, and many other things may inhibit communication is given in *Figure 144*.

The manager or doctor who wishes to communicate effectively can arrange an interview differently if he wishes to achieve a high level of communication *(Figure 145)*. There are possibly ten blocks to communication that have been removed in this figure. These are listed at the end of the chapter for those who wish to check their observations.

In the same way, a natural place for a small child is the lap of the mother seated opposite the doctor, without a table separating them. Many paediatricians prefer to sit down opposite the mother with the child on her lap during a ward round (see *Figure 121*).

Difficulties in communication lie just as much with the mother, as was found from investigation of a roadside clinic in India which has proved extremely popular. It was found that its popularity in part depended on the absence of any detailed questioning or examination of the child. The mothers' own traditional ayurvedic doctor did not need to ask many questions or examine the child, and they considered that a

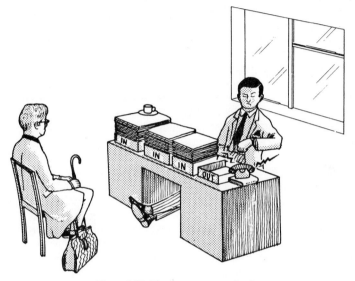

Figure 144. Blocks to communication

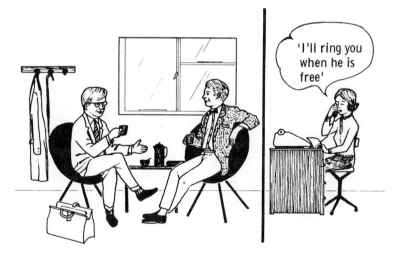

Figure 145. Facilitating communication

doctor who could treat their children without questioning and examination was preferable!

The traditional belief that associates cooling of the skin with the common cold, coryza or pneumonia is likely to last many decades. In areas such as Western Asia, where it is particularly strong, reluctance to undress the child will lead to difficulties. If the doctor insists, the mothers are less willing to come, while if he fails to see children undressed he is in danger of missing valuable information, and his physical examination, which is a complex process involving the senses of sight, touch, hearing and smell, will be inhibited.

The educational psychologists have drawn attention to the need for immediate feedback to improve the process of learning. The doctor sometimes needs to ask the mother to repeat to him in her own words the more important instructions that he gives on the management of her sick child, a process that is rarely possible, due to the large number of children to be seen. Once the doctor has delegated the care of the majority of children to auxiliaries, it is possible to spend more time talking with each mother. It is then even more important for the mother to repeat the instructions, as an example to the other members of the team to do the same when they are interviewing mothers.

In countries where the doctor divides his time between fee-paying private practice and government practice, he is in a particularly difficult situation. He has more time to spend with those culturally nearer to him, who can afford to pay his fees, and can usually talk effectively with them. The failure to communicate with his poorer patients he may put down to their 'stupidity', not realizing that the fault lies in the difference in culture and the difference in technique that may be required, rather than a difference in intelligence.

The meaning of words

In a recent study (181) a haphazard group of mothers attending an Under-Fives' Clinic with infants between the ages of 6 months and 1 year were asked if they had heard of a disease, and eight common diseases were given. They were then asked to describe the disease. The same was done with a group of health workers. The word for tuberculosis was understood by almost all the health staff as meaning tuberculosis, but two-thirds of the mothers considered that this was whooping cough. Similarly, the health workers all recognized the word for smallpox as this disease, but the mothers described a wide variety of conditions. Only two could describe smallpox; the majority described either a skin eruption or measles.

Clearly health workers should not assume that those listening understand what they are talking about, even when the vernacular terms are used. As in so many other fields, the medical people require help here from linguists, educationalists and other social workers. Staff involved in health education need to realize these difficulties, and local handbooks of vernacular terms need to be drawn up. The health educators must ascertain for themselves that their audiences are understanding them. Where interpreters have to be used, it will be very necessary to check that they understand these difficulties.

Communicating with the child

The fear that so many adults have of hospitals frequently originates from childhood experiences, many of which were unavoidable. However, the impact of many could have been reduced, both by the parents and through the actions of the doctor. The practice common at one time of saying to a child 'This will not hurt' before giving him a painful injection impressed the child that those who work in clinics were not to be trusted! The doctor will be in a dilemma in countries where private practice has fostered the idea that the best (often because for the doctor the most remunerative) method of giving medicine is by injection. Should he give the child an injection which is not necessary, or should he possibly lose the mother's confidence by relying on oral but equally effective therapy?

Much disease is crowded into the first five years of life in tropical countries and the paediatrician less frequently sees the older child with whom communication may be easier. Before the age of five years the young child and his mother may be considered as one, and if the confidence of the mother can be maintained, with some understanding of the disease process, she will pass this on to her child, rather than the 'spiritual' explanation that accounts for the cause of disease in traditional societies.

COMMUNICATING WITH THE 'ILLITERATE'

Many of the communication problems described here are quite unrelated to literacy, but are largely cultural in origin. In the absence of any other word, 'illiterate' will be used in inverted commas. The author hopes the use of the word in this way will not cause offence to readers whose revered and respected relatives cannot read or write.

Teachers all over the world are now more concerned and interested in how they can better communicate with undergraduates and graduates in the universities, but the problems that they meet are small compared with those that are met by the worker who wishes to communicate effectively with the 'illiterate' person. The problems coincidental with attempts to communicate with 'illiterates' have been little studied. The following section is largely derived from the work in Central Africa (87).

Communication must be a creative function, and it can be defined as the transportation of information from one individual to another, but to be effective there must be return messages. This is set out in *Figure 146.* In practice, the situation depicted in the tip half of *Figure 146* rarely exists in normal life, unless one is speaking on the telephone, and the other person is remaining mute, and then most conversations will not last long! Nearly always we are receiving some sort of reply and encouragement, particularly through the eye movements of the person with whom we are communicating, as in the audience in a lecture, or in the replies and comments that come in a normal conversation and encourage the speaker to continue.

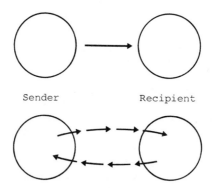

Sender   Recipient

Figure 146. Communication is two-way

Normal communication can usually be divided into that which involves thought and conception, and spontaneous exclamations. The patient may come along desiring an injection for his severe respiratory infection, and he has thought about this and evolved concepts which lead him to believe that he will be improved by receiving an injection. The second part may be the exclamation of pain as he receives the injection. These two are set out in *Figure 147.*

If we now consider the injection in rather greater detail, we can see the various steps that have taken place. In coming to ask for the injection, or for treatment, the patient has given thought to the action, and his concepts of medical care have led him to an intention which he expresses by coming and asking for treatment. When he has the experience of a previous injection, it may make him go tense, and the actual moment of injection may lead to an exclamation, and after he has received it he may show signs of pleasure at his desire having been fulfilled.

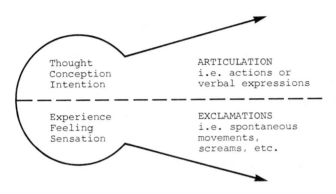

Figure 147. Two levels of communication

We already see here one great difficulty that may arise in any communication between cultures, namely that such expressions, exclamations and articulations may be different. An exclamation will always be accepted as a genuine expression, whereas articulation may not always be so considered. Is the expression given by articulation honest, or is it feigned? When we smile in the presence of a villager, he may take this in two ways. Are we smiling *at him* or *with him?* The 'illiterate' who has had no education in the academic sense is much *more* sensitive to the differences between exclamation and articulation. If we are to move some way towards the 'illiterate's' position, so that we can communicate better with him, this must then be the first step — a greater understanding of and sensitivity to expressions, exclamations and the tone of our voice, and our actions, to which he is highly sensitive. This may be but one of many advantages that the 'illiterate' has over those who read and write.

Communication must also involve touching

Those who have travelled in several countries will have noticed the considerable variations in the amount of touching involved between people and between the sexes. In some parts of the world, it is not uncommon to see adult men walking about hand in hand, and in others, two individuals during a conversation will touch each other many times. There are other areas of the world in which the amount of touching, particularly between the sexes, may be limited, or non-existent, except within the family. Willingness to touch and be touched is extremely important in child care. The author remembers a ward sister asking him, as he left a children's ward where he had been working, if he would touch the abdomen of a child in a certain cot, because he had felt the child's abdomen regularly up to that day, and the mother was anxious that her child should be touched by the doctor as on previous days.

Wishful thinking

The man who has had academic training usually has a clear distinction between thoughts and the actual occurrence. An immediate and important distinction for the doctor is between the facts of death or severe illness and their discussion with the mother. In an industrial society, a mother may expect a doctor to warn her that her child is dangerously ill and that a fatal outcome is not impossible, but in an 'illiterate' society the doctor may have to be more circumspect. The mere fact that he says a child may die may suggest to the 'illiterate' mind that he is wishing the child to die by mentioning the possibility. Let us look at this the other way round. In the many illnesses of childhood, the mother will indulge in wishful thinking that the child will get better, and her culture may suggest that, as part of this wishful thinking, she should offer sacrifices or go through various rituals. Statistically, children recover from the vast majority of illnesses, so that the mother will usually feel that her wishful thinking or ritual has been successful. This is an attempt by her to develop a model for causal relationships, and it must be considered a meaningful step in the development of man's mind.

In wishful thinking or 'magic thinking' there seems to be a relationship between cause and result. For example, mothers in some parts of the world who have lost children believe that they have gone to a sort of 'Peter Pan never-never land', and that they return with each succeeding birth. This belief is held very strongly even by many of the more educated people. It was expressed in the village by the symbolism of putting metal rings round the feet of children who were born after several deaths. Symbolically they were being chained down to stop them leaving the mother. There are excellent accounts of how symbolism and beliefs arise in cultures at all stages of development (126).

Decision-making

Coming to a decision between different lines of action may be much more difficult for a mother from an 'illiterate' society. She brings her sick child to the clinic with the firm idea that he will get an injection and will be made better. Before leaving home, she has gained the support of her family in this decision. However, when she arrives at the clinic, the doctor tells her that while an injection will improve the child's condition, it is important for him to be admitted to hospital so that he can be kept in a moist atmosphere and, should it be required, be given oxygen therapy. The mother has difficulty in understanding this situation and the different viewpoint expressed by the doctor. He must have great patience if he is to help her.

To the 'illiterate', the power of the environment is overwhelming, and success of failure does not seem to be related to their own free will, strength or abilities. Chronic illness is particularly difficult to bring for treatment, especially if progress is not rapid. They have come to expect Western medicine to work quickly. The 'illiterate' is much more interested in those pleasures of the moment, rather than in those which are greater and long-term (87). If the 'illiterate' is asked whether he would like to have one cigarette immediately or five cigarettes the day after tomorrow, even if he completely trusts the person making the offer he will almost certainly choose the one cigarette now. Perhaps this attitude offers some explanation for the problems of persuading patients to carry through prolonged treatment.

Concepts not easily accepted by the 'illiterate'

Many basic concepts that a literate person would not question are not necessarily accepted by the 'illiterate'. The following are examples of this.

Concept of quantity and mass

This can be demonstrated by small experiments, such as when two equally full bottles of Fanta orangeade are poured one into a tall thin and one into a short fatter cylinder. Although the 'illiterate' has seen the two equal bottles before they were emptied into the cylinders, he will still think there is more in the tall one. Similarly, if a large ball of plasticine is handled by him, and is then flattened on the table, he may consider that there is now more plasticine there.

He has the same problem over the concept of number. Twelve large stones are placed in a line in front of him, and he himself then places 12 small stones one in front of each of the larger ones. If now the small stones are drawn together in a line, he may state that there are fewer small stones than large ones, because they make a shorter line. His conception of number is different from our, but not 'wrong'.

Similar tests involving an understanding of the vertical and of the straight line have also shown the 'illiterate's' difficulty in understanding our concepts, which are taken for granted by people who have had only a few years' schooling.

Concept of perspective

Just as we have to learn to read, so we have to learn to understand pictures, and the 'illiterate' particularly has difficulty in understanding our 'rules' for perspective. The pictorial conventions depicting three dimensions in a two-dimensional picture came into European art during the Renaissance, and since then have been accepted as a matter of course. In our culture we learn at an early age to appreciate the third dimension through a series of clues.

However, these conventions are not obvious to someone unused to them (116). *Figure 148* is a picture of a man throwing a spear at an antelope. To an 'illiterate' person not used to pictures, the elephant in

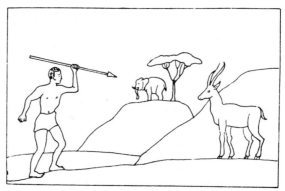

Figure 148. Concepts of perspective

the background is so small in relation to the man that it is usually considered to be an anteater, and the man is thought to be throwing the spear at the elephant rather than the antelope.

The ability to 'read' pictures may be quite unrelated to literacy, and difficulty in understanding pictures is being reduced by the influx of films and television.

Practical results of these investigations

From these and many other tests, it is clear that our ideas on the use of pictures in communicating with 'illiterates', and our whole methodology, need very careful study and continuous evaluation. Investigations were made to discover which of the following the 'illiterate' could understand most clearly.

(1) A simple line drawing.
(2) A silhouette.
(3) A 'block-out' of the subject, i.e. with the background on the photograph eliminated.
(4) A photograph.

The subject was told the following:
'These four pictures' (which were set out in the manner described above) 'show the same thing. Can you tell us what you see?'

When the subject had identified the picture satisfactorily, he was asked which picture showed him this first. The block-outs came out with a high majority, and this form of picture is now being widely used in health education in Zambia, with considerable success.* It is of course similar to pictures used in advertisements, in which the background is 'fogged' or out of focus.

There is clearly a need for stimulation if there is to be mental development. Even the stimulation of two years at a primary school was found to make a difference in these tests; the subject would score a high mark. Similarly, those who have lived near a town would score higher than those living in remote areas. Perhaps the advent of the low-price television set in the villages of rural areas will have a more decisive effect in producing stimulation than even the most optimistic of those concerned in spreading this form of education have hoped for.

Where do we and the 'illiterate' stand?

The mental processes of education can perhaps be represented as a straight line, starting off from situation A *(Figure 149)*. 'A' is the simplest form of stimulation producing some reaction, as in the famous conditioned reflex experiments of Pavlov, and this must be the starting point. We need not consider the various steps along this path until we come to the situation of the 'illiterate'. The 'illiterate' is in the situation of understanding that symbols can represent things which are not

---

*Examples of such material can be obtained from The National Food and Nutrition Commission of Zambia, P.O. Box 2669, Lusaka, Zambia

present. The symbol usually has a likeness to the thing that it represents. Dreams, imitation, gestures, ritual plays and dances are all of great significance, and perhaps we would say that this is the world of magic. The academic on the other hand, is in a stage further. He is concerned with handling and understanding a hypothetical world. The individual has liberated himself from the significance of the symbol,

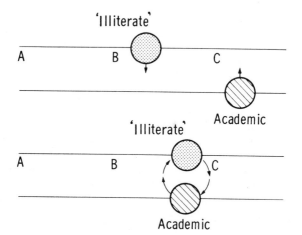

Figure 149. Communication between 'illiterate' and academic

and should have developed a philosophic scientific approach to problem-solving.

If the 'illiterate' and the academic remain in their relative positions, then there will be a low level of communication between them, and this leads to the well-known frustration which can so easily occur. For this reason, the 'illiterate' must be given educational stimulation sufficient for him to develop a series of concrete symbol processes and elementary abstract concepts, and the expert or academic must, for his part, recode his message in a form acceptable to the 'illiterate'.

The justification for writing so much on the theory of communication in a book on paediatrics lies in the belief that the doctor and the health team have in the past failed to communicate effectively, and that for them this is a high priority, particularly in child care. If in the future, communication is to be more effective the health workers must learn from the experts in this field. At the same time they need to discover and use methods by which they can obtain a feedback from the mothers on how their understanding, attitudes and behaviour have changed. This chapter cannot teach the necessary expertise, but attempts to suggest what is needed.

METHODS OF COMMUNICATION

Use of the spoken word

The spoken word will remain the most commonly used method of communication. A good example was found in the London teaching hospitals. At one time there was a tradition by which any senior person when undertaking a procedure would vocalize what he was doing, and why, so that those who were observing or helping could always be learning. This practice was not only excellent, but educational psychologists suggest that it should be extended to encourage any student to vocalize when he is practising the skill he is learning. Experimentally they have shown that skills are better learnt if there is vocalization of the steps by those undertaking them. This method may be of particular value in training auxiliaries who may not easily be able to visualize procedures which are written down.

The talk

Most societies in tropical countries have a tradition of communication through the spoken word, and for them, more than in industrial societies, more reliance can be placed on the spoken word. In the latter, due to the ever-increasing use of television, people are said to be becoming 'less literate and more picturate'. Talks need to be brief. Because the doctor has a captive audience in his clinic or the ward, he must not allow or encourage the nurse or health educator to speak for longer than they can keep the attention of their audience, which is unlikely to be more than ten minutes (see p. 335). The effective teacher in this and other situation will be the one who can achieve participation from the audience, particularly if this can take some traditional form as a song or lyric. The auxiliary needs to be reminded to keep his eyes looking around all his audience during a talk; if he does this, he is more likely to keep their attention, and will know if he has lost it. A worker in the Amazon area of South America made the interesting observation that mothers in her area would listen more happily and with more attention when occupied in sewing or some other activity.

A store of local proverbs can be most useful as a way of introducing a new idea and stimulating discussion. Their value has been described in these words (45).

> To 'illiterate' people the proverb is precious. Without the luxury of a library, wisdom has to be stored mentally and must be concise. Hence in proverbs the words are rich in meaning and the concepts expressed are a good starting point for conversation .

The recorded talk

A wider use of tape-recorded talks and songs in communicating at different levels is likely over the next decade. A paediatrician in Lagos wrote down (89) the major items of health information that he wished to pass on to the parents whom he saw in an overcrowded out-patient department. This was then translated into several languages used by the local populations, recorded on tape, and played regularly in the out-patients' waiting hall. This proved acceptable, and fathers would attend the children's out-patient department solely to hear the talk.

The small portable battery-operated tape-recorder may find a place in village work. If the education has to be undertaken largely by nurses, who as young women are less likely to be listened to, they can add to their authority by carrying a recording of some influential voice known to the community.

The lecture

The paediatrician in developing countries should be involved in the formal teaching of students, nurses or auxiliaries if he is to make the full contribution to the community that his own training warrants. Books and other sources of information are likely to be in short supply and, if available, difficult for the student to understand. For these reasons greater emphasis is laid on the lecture as a method of teaching. If there is a shortage of suitable books, the doctor may decide to prepare handouts, and a duplicator and an adequate supply of paper are essential teaching equipment. If the students make notes, these will be more valuable if the doctor can give the main headings on a blackboard.

Overhead projector

A valuable piece of equipment is the overhead projector *(Figure 150)*, which is becoming widely available and can be used in a well-lit room. The teacher can use the overhead projector facing the class. The transparency sheets can be prepared beforehand with a spirit-based felt pen, using either washed x-ray plates or polythene or acetate sheeting. (These pens can be differentiated from the water-based variety by their smell.) If the transparent sheets are placed over lined paper while being prepared, the results will be better. Diagrams may be easily copied from a book. The use of the overhead projector is one way by which the doctor can save time. If he has to give the same series of lectures on repeated occasions, the sheets of transparency, once prepared, can be used many times, saving the time taken by writing on a blackboard.

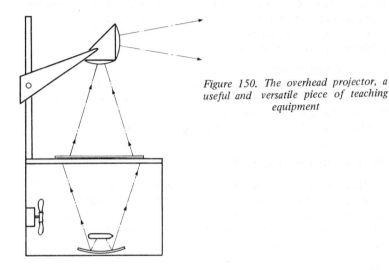

Figure 150. The overhead projector, a useful and versatile piece of teaching equipment

A useful monograph has recently appeared (22) which is helpful to lecturers. In this is assembled the evidence for and against different lecturing techniques. Activities which involve the audience are found to be both popular and efficient. The so-called 'split' lecture is an effective example of such an activity (324).

The split lecture

Observations during an hour's lecture period have shown that the level of attention reaches its highest level during the first ten minutes and remains high for the first 20–25 minutes, and then declines, to rise again towards the end of the lecture. For this reason a better use of the time may be possible. At present the lecture is frequently an inefficient method of learning; the student probably carries away no more than

*An excellent illustrated talk on the overhead projector is among the large collection of recorded material on a wide range of medical subjects available on loan or by purchase from The Medical Recording Service Foundation, Kitts Croft, Writtle, Chelmsford, Essex, CM1 3EI, UK

25–30 per cent of what has been said and is unlikely to retain more than half of this. Educational psychologists have also shown that the learning process may be more effective if there is both immediate feedback and discussion among the students, and that they are better at teaching each other than the teacher. The author has used the following 'split lecture' techniques successfully with nurses, medical students and postgraduates, on occasions in groups of over 100. Evaluation showed that they appreciated this as a variation from the normal lecture.

If the lecture period is for one hour, the time is divided into the following approximate periods.

(1)   A well-structured lecture – 25 minutes.
(2)   The students write answers to questions – 10 minutes.
(3)   They pass their answers to their neighbour for correction, and then discuss each other's corrections – 15 minutes.
(4)   The lecturer answers questions – 10 minutes.

The well-structured lecture (25 minutes)

Much of the art of lecturing is to be able to present the material in an ordered sequence and develop a well-reasoned argument. Bearing in mind that two-thirds of what is learnt is seen, and only a third through the ears, there is a good argument for the use of slides, or other visual aids, whenever possible.

The questions (10 minutes)

The student is reassured that he is not being 'examined'; if anyone is being 'examined' it is the lecturer. The questions should be designed so that approximately 80 per cent of the students will get 80 per cent of the answers right. They may be on a stencilled sheet with spaces to be filled in, or they may be written on the back of a blackboard which is turned over, or they can be written on a sheet of transparency and used with an overhead projector. The questions should cover the more important points in the lecture, those which the student should carry away with him. By getting him to answer these questions his brain is being asked to feed back information just fed into it; this process of feedback is the basis of methods of programmed learning.

Correcting answers, discussion (15 minutes)

This can be done in twos or threes; each student corrects the answers of a student sitting next to him, and they then discuss, if they have given different answers, which answers are likely to be correct. In this period of the lecture hour, discussions are being undertaken between the students in twos or threes. If there is a bright student sitting next to one not quite so bright, the more able student can explain any points and in so doing will himself learn the subject better.

Questions answered by the lecturer (10 minutes)

The standard of question is usually much higher than that raised after a normal lecture. Not infrequently the lecturer will find that he may not have included in his lecture one or two points required if the questions are to be answered satisfactorily. This missing-out of steps in developing an argument is not infrequent with a lecturer who may know his subject well, but tends to forget some of the steps necessary for the student to grasp if he is to understand it.

The split lecture is only one way in which the lecture 'hour' may be better used. Any means by which the participation of the student can be increased will lead to greater interest in the lecture. To be successful the lecturer will need to find a variety of methods suited to his personality and the group with whom he communicates. As long as he makes a point of always looking at his students when lecturing, he will soon discover how he can best maintain a high level of attention.

In the past the lecture was conceived as a method of 'pouring' information into the student *(Figure 151)*. Even with the use of visual aids, the lecture can be considered a relatively poor method of communication. Without the use of visual aids or when they are inappropriate its justification is even less.

> He never was heard
> And never was seen
> Who turned in the dark
> And read from the screen.
>
> His audience yawned
> It squirmed and it sighed
> He constantly put
> Too much on a slide. (320)

A lecturer speaks at around 100 words a minute; most students read in excess of 300 words a minute, particularly if they have studied fast reading techniques. Such students might well learn more by reading the subject three times rather than listening to it once.

The seminar

The seminar or small discussion group has greatly increased in popularity in the teaching of theoretical subjects. In bedside clinical teaching it has always had a major place. To be successful the number of participants must be limited — 12 is the maximum, and often this may be too many – and the students need to come prepared. The discussion should range between the students *(Figure 152)* and the good tutor's task will be to guide the discussion and to act as a 'resource person'. He will also try to draw in everyone; the less vocal

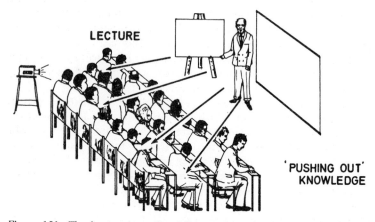

Figure 151. The lecture (reproduced by courtesy of Dr. S. Gauvain, formerly of the London School of Hygiene and Tropical Medicine)

can often contribute more of value than their more vocal colleagues. In *Figure 152* it is not possible to distinguish which of those sitting round the table is the lecturer; he should not play a central role. Such methods are well recognized in Islamic teaching, where the circle as a method of teaching is encouraged, and a relaxed posture for the participants is emphasized. Perhaps even the presence of a table is a deterrent to good communication.

Seminar teaching is expensive in terms of the time that the teacher has to devote to it. However, when well used the student will be asked regularly to present a subject logically, effectively and in a pre-determined time to his fellows. This experience is likely to be particularly useful to him in speaking and teaching when he works with a team in the future. The experience will also stand him in good stead when he becomes involved in committee work. This applies equally well to the auxiliary as to the doctor. If the care of children in a community is to reach a high level, auxiliaries who have had experience of child care must be encouraged to take their part in the local council or on any local committee in which the health care of the community's children may be influenced.

Individual study

Little attention has been spared in the past for the student's own method of study. Over several years the author has asked groups of international students how fast they read; only occasionally has a student known how fast he reads. The arguments in support of rapid reading are now well known (25). Here it must suffice to say that in the process of transferring information from the page of this book to the cells of the brain, the limiting factors are most certainly not the electrical reactions in the brain, but are more likely to be the speed of eye movement, the number of words recognized at one time, and perhaps unnecessary movement of the muscles of phonation. Clearly the doctor who can read and absorb what he reads quickly may be better able to care for children in the community than one who has not practised and improved this basic skill.

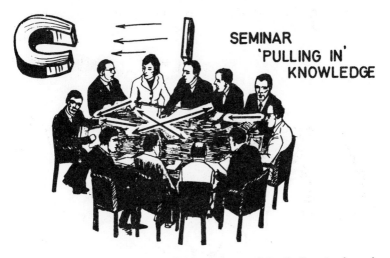

Figure 152. The seminar (reproduced by courtesy of Dr. S. Gauvain, formerly of the London School of Hygiene and Tropical Medicine)

The doctor who is attempting to help auxiliaries to learn more effectively may find that time devoted to their method of study early in the course may be well spent. As in the lecture, the individual may study more effectively if he participates in some way and uses visual aids.

Participation by the learner has been pioneered by the programmed

421

learning texts and teaching machines, but these have not been widely produced or used in medical training. Excellent examples are a book (214) on the ECG for medical students, and the programme on recognizing the *E. histolytica,* and a programmed text on statistics (201).

Bringing the student more information through the use of visual aids may be achieved by an increase in the number of illustrations in the texts he reads, as long as these are well chosen, relevant and well reproduced. Another way is through the use of transparencies and written or taped lectures. The use of slides and tapes in teaching is now well established (102). The author has attempted to evolve a machine for use in a library at relatively low cost *(Figure 153).* The slides and the cassette on which the lecture is pre-recorded are all stored in a plastic hanging folder *(Figure 154)* which the librarian can conveniently store in a filing cabinet. One side of the tape may have a talk and the other side a series of questions, so that the student can himself check whether he has learnt the main points of the lecture.

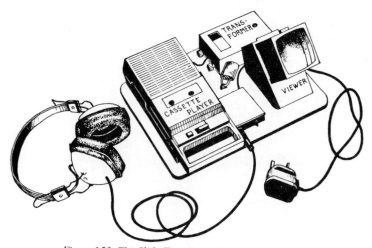

Figure 153. The Slide-Tape Tutor for individual study

INFORMATION, SKILLS AND ATTITUDE

Most attention has in the past been paid to the absorption of information by the student, and the lecture can rarely hope to achieve more than this. However, reading may be equally or more effective, in the view both of some teachers and, judging by their low attendance at non-compulsory lectures, of many university students.

Learning of skills usually requires individual study. However, the student may be helped by simulation. For example, the student is more likely to be able to appreciate the third heart sound if he listens to recordings in which this sound is first well separated from the other

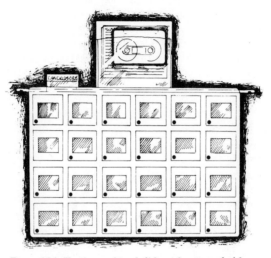

Figure 154. Plastic combined slide and cassette holders are supplied ready to hand in a hanging filing cabinet

heart sounds and then brought closer until he learns the time interval between the sounds necessary for his ear to pick up the third sound. As in all other steps in the learning process, the student needs to be able to check his skill against that of his fellow students and that of his teacher.

The paediatrician will attempt to teach the student not only the knowledge and the skills necessary to care for children, but also the attitude to his patients and his work among them. Of these, attitudes are not the least important, but in most forms of education little effort is made specifically to alter them, nor are they investigated by traditional methods of examination. The student is likely to absorb by example the attitudes of his teacher, but even more that of the group with whom he has studied. An attempt to develop a responsible and socially acceptable attitude in the group will be an objective of most teachers. This will develop most effectively in a group in which free discussion is expected and welcomed by the teacher. One way to stimulate discussion can be by having the student give his opinion on a number of questions. Examples of such questions for use in developing attitudes towards child health are shown in Table 55.

The students are asked to mark whether they agree, disagree or are uncertain, and the results are analysed by one of them. With a proportion of the questions there is likely to be considerable disagreement. In formulating the questions the objective will be to cause disagreement between the students, so that discussions between them can be encouraged. In the example cited the author disagrees with half the decisions shown by ticks. The students are grouped in some seating arrangement other than that of a lecture hall, and encouraged to debate the questions. As far as possible the teacher abstains from entering into

TABLE 55

Statement	Agree	Uncertain	Disagree
Well-baby clinics were set up to reduce the level of cross-infection.			✓
The solution to a given child health problem is the same in all communities.	✓		
Health education for mothers is concerned with the promotion of health and the prevention of disease and not with curative work.			✓
The common dish, where the meal is shared by a group or family, should be discouraged as an undesirable practice on grounds of hygiene.	✓		
If 70 per cent or more of the parents in a community see a nutrition education film, then this is a successful use of that film.	✓		
Non-medical healers and curers indigenous to the community should be prohibited from caring for children.			✓
The most successful person in teaching the mother is the doctor.	✓		
Once parents are shown how reasonable a suggestion is, they usually follow it.			✓

the discussion, even if asked for his opinion; he may however supply results of research that may be unknown to the students. No conclusion is likely to be reached on all the subjects, but the students may be found to continue their discussion after leaving the teaching session. In time a group attitude to these questions may develop. When the group breaks up and the individuals take up their work again, some of the attitudes developed by the group are likely to be maintained by the individuals.

VISUAL AIDS

The doctor has to communicate at many levels and in many ways, some of which have already been described. In achieving good communication use can be made of visual aids.

The film and television

These can be effective methods of communication, but unfortunately they have severe limitations, particularly in developing countries. A good film is expensive, and in most countries the world over only the good film will be acceptable, as the population has become used to commercially prepared films. Because of its expense, the producer attempts to make the film acceptable to as wide an audience as possible, and this will frequently result in the film being less suitable for teaching. When a film is shown, the teacher, so to speak, hands his audience over to the producer of the film. Clearly the film must be introduced and followed by discussion, but even with these the teacher has little influence on the impact which the film has on the audience. Again, experience in a number of developing countries has emphasized the difficulty of maintaining projection equipment in working order. As a result, a central film library of health films in one large developing country was distributing no more than 45 films a month for a population of several hundred million.

Those interested in communication in health have placed great hopes in the use of television and closed circuit television. The hopes for closed circuit television have still to be confirmed, even in the more developed areas of the world.

The slide

The 15 mm transparency (or 2 X 2 inch slide) is likely to remain the most widely used and versatile teaching aid. The basic cost of mass production in a cardboard mount is only 2 p ($0.05) and reproduction in colour costs no more than in black and white. This low cost encouraged the development of an organization (TALC)* that makes available 24 sets totalling over 600 transparencies. The majority of these sets are specifically intended for use in improving child health in developing

*Teaching Aids at Low Cost (TALC) is based on the Institute of Child Health, 30 Guilford Street, London WC1N 1EH, from which details may be obtained

countries. The mounted transparency in most instances is preferable to the film strip. The sprockets of the strip projector tend to damage the film strip with regular use, and the lecturer cannot vary the order of the slides he is using.

The slide is versatile, and it is already used extensively in most medical schools for lecturing. In the future it is likely that it will be used more for the seminar type of teaching and by the student studying alone, with either written or tape-recorded descriptions (see *Figure 148*).

A slide-tape automated lecture

Apparatus necessary for the use of a cassetted tape and slides to give a complete lecture is likely to become more widely used. The lecture and visual material can be more easily prepared than a film, cost less and can be updated. These presentations can also encourage participation with feedback from the student and discussion on individual slides.

The flannelgraph

The flannelgraph consists of a blanket or piece of winceyette pinned to a sloping board such as a blackboard on an easel. On this backing sheet of material, illustrated cut-outs may be placed. A variety of materials, including sandpaper or old pyjama cloth, may be stuck on the back of the cut-outs. An example of the use of a flannelgraph is the weight chart described in Chapter 7. On the background of the chart, enlarged and printed on winceyette, the progress of a child can be recorded by black dots. Other motifs may be laid on at the point where the child should receive inoculations, different foods, or at the time of developing new skills, such as that of holding a cube, or walking.

The flannelgraph is particularly valuable in that the student can participate in placing the motifs and building up a picture. For groups of more than 20 or 30 it is rarely satisfactory. It is particularly suited to training auxiliaries and it may be used in simple form for teaching mothers. Participation by the students in the use of the flannelgraph soon reveals their knowledge and understanding of the subject.

The poster

The poster was one of the earliest visual aids to be developed, but is still misused in many areas. Only too often the artist fails to evaluate and amend his picture to overcome misunderstandings. Good posters such as those produced by the National Food and Nutrition Commission of Zambia may be most effective as a starting point for a discussion.

Other visual aids

Many visual aids have been developed for different purposes, and those involved in teaching and education are well advised to familiarize themselves with some of the possibilities. One rule always persists, and that is that the actual article, e.g. vegetable or fruit, is the best visual aid. A number of countries are now setting up centres where teaching aids suitable to their own culture and with local languages can be produced. The best of these centres also train personnel in the production of their own teaching material. In London, the Centre for Educational Development Overseas (CEDO)*, formerly the Overseas Visual Aids Centre (OVAC), has a large display of the teaching aids mentioned here and many others, including flip charts and puppets. They also run short courses which are highly recommended for anyone in a teaching post in a developing country who is visiting London. They welcome enquiries by visitors or through the post.

BLOCKS TO COMMUNICATION AS ILLUSTRATED IN FIGURE 144

The following items in *Figure 144* may be considered as blocks to communication.

(1)   The doctor's facial expression.
(2)   The doctor is looking at his watch.
(3)   The way the doctor is sitting.
(4)   The telephone is interrupting them.
(5)   The doctor is obviously very busy.
(6)   Coffee for the doctor but not for his guest.
(7)   The desk acts as a barrier between them.
(8)   The visitor still has his coat on.
(9)   The visitor is sitting on an uncomfortable chair.
(10)   The light falls predominantly on the vistor's face.
(11)   The visitor's briefcase is closed; he has not produced any papers as a 'token' gift.

In *Figure 145* the doctor has attempted to overcome some of these barriers to communication.

*Centre of Educational Development Overseas, Tavistock House South, Tavistock Square, London WC14 9LG.

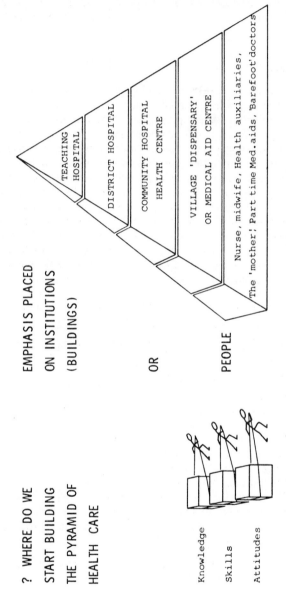

? WHERE DO WE START BUILDING THE PYRAMID OF HEALTH CARE

EMPHASIS PLACED ON INSTITUTIONS (BUILDINGS)

OR

PEOPLE

TEACHING HOSPITAL

DISTRICT HOSPITAL

COMMUNITY HOSPITAL HEALTH CENTRE

VILLAGE 'DISPENSARY' OR MEDICAL AID CENTRE

Nurse, midwife, Health auxiliaries, The 'mother', Part time Med.aids, Barefoot'doctors

Knowledge

Skills

Attitudes

Figure 155. Where do we start building the health pyramid?

WHERE DO WE START BUILDING THE HEALTH PYRAMID?

The last figure *(Figure 155)* is used to illustrate some final remarks on communication and to summarize much that is written in this book. The health services of a country have been likened to a pyramid with the teaching hospital at the top. If the Pharaoh's engineers had proposed building their pyramids starting at the top they would not have achieved much. Yet in health services in most developing countries it is the teaching hospitals that have received priority in development.

The health service will depend on the knowledge, skills and attitudes of its staff and not on the construction of large institutions. The introduction of the 'building blocks' of knowledge, skills and attitudes at the bottom of the pyramid must become a high priority. Most developing countries now have these large and phenomenally expensive teaching hospitals. In the future the successful of these institutions will not be those which do the most advanced surgery or develop emergency coronary units, but those which can provide 'packages' of training in health care for all levels of health workers and particularly those near to the base of the pyramid. For the highly specialized teaching hospital doctor to work out how health care can be provided at the base of pyramid will be difficult. Coming from a palace, only with difficulty will he understand the limitation of resources for the workers in the mud huts of rural society and at the same time be able to appreciate their advantages and opportunities. However, such a step is essential if the massive health care problems of the children and adults of any developing country are to be solved.

429

Appendix 1

ASSESSMENT QUESTIONNAIRE
(Please circle the appropriate figure or word)

Experience of commentator:

Initial training   Postgraduate   −5 years   5−20 years   20+ years

Medical   Paediatric   Nurse   Other (specify) . . . .

(Please circle your assessment)

Chapter

1 Guiding Principles	Useful	Fair	Not relevant to me	Not read
2 Economic Background	Useful	Fair	Not relevant to me	Not read
3 Beliefs and Attitudes to Child Rearing and Disease	Useful	Fair	Not relevant to me	Not read
4 Priorities: The Doctor's Dilemma	Useful	Fair	Not relevant to me	Not read
5 Care of the Newborn	Useful	Fair	Not relevant to me	Not read
6 Breast-feeding and Difficulties of Artificial Feeding	Useful	Fair	Not relevant to me	Not read
7 The Road-to-health Card	Useful	Fair	Not relevant to me	Not read
8 Home-based records and Levels of Care	Useful	Fair	Not relevant to me	Not read
9 The 'At-risk' Child	Useful	Fair	Not relevant to me	Not read
10 Diarrhoea	Useful	Fair	Not relevant to me	Not read
11 Acute Respiratory Infections	Useful	Fair	Not relevant to me	Not read
12 'Severe' measles	Useful	Fair	Not relevant to me	Not read
13 Whooping Cough	Useful	Fair	Not relevant to me	Not read
14 Malaria in Children	Useful	Fair	Not relevant to me	Not read
15 Tuberculosis	Useful	Fair	Not relevant to me	Not read
16 Common Skin Diseases	Useful	Fair	Not relevant to me	Not read
17 Common Anaemias	Useful	Fair	Not relevant to me	Not read
18 Birth Interval and Family Planning	Useful	Fair	Not relevant to me	Not read
19 The Under-Fives' Clinic − Comprehensive Child Care	Useful	Fair	Not relevant to me	Not read
20 Nursing	Useful	Fair	Not relevant to me	Not read
21 Management	Useful	Fair	Not relevant to me	Not read
22 Communication and Learning	Useful	Fair	Not relevant to me	Not read

431

APPENDIX

Please comment on material that you consider could be deleted, or with which you disagree. Also suggest additional material, giving references where possible.

Name and address if reply is desired

. . . .

. . . .

. . . .

. . . .

Appendix 2

433

APPENDIX

Other sets that are available are as follows:

BL   Burkitt's Lymphoma: its principal clinical features

CcO   Cancrum Oris: aetiology and management

ClG   Clinical Genetics: some of the ways in which a knowledge of genetics may help in clinical practice

CD   Contraceptive Devices: methods of family planning, prepared by the IPPF

Fwa   Foods of West Africa: (48 slides) foods commonly given to children, their preparation and nutritional value

GR   Growth: diagrams illustrating normal growth suitable for medical students

KwM   Management of Kwashiorkor: common causes of death and their prevention

Lp   Leprosy: a description of the disease with particular reference to childhood

Ml   Malnutrition: as seen in Indian children, but relevant to other areas

MR   Mental Retardation: (48 slides) common causes of mental retardation in the UK

PcD   Protein Calorie Deficiency: a description of the syndromes of kwashiorkor and marasmus

PEM   Pathology of Experimental Malnutrition: microscopic appearance of PCM in animals

SK   Skin Diseases in Temperate Areas: common skin conditions in children in Europe

SpC   Smallpox in Children: clinical description in African children and prevention

XrC   X-rays in Childhood: some diagnostic x-rays for students to study

Other material available from TALC includes weight charts, a flannelgraph, and transparent overlays to the chart which help to identify the state of nutrition of children.

The majority of these sets contain 24 slides. In 1973 they cost 50p a set for those working in developing countries. This price includes a script which describes each slide, and packing and postage by surface mail anywhere in the world.

An up-to-date list of material and an order form are available from Teaching Aids at Low Cost (TALC), Institute of Child Health, 30 Guilford Street, London WC1N 1EH.

References and Bibliography

1 Abbot, J. D. and Gillespie, E. H. (1972). 'Whooping cough. Cause and prevention.' *Trop. Doct.* **2,** 32
2 Abel-Smith, B., Ekholm, L., Klarman, H. E. and Rojo-Fernández, V. (1972). 'Can we reduce the cost of medical education?' *W.H.O. Chronicle* **26,** 441
3 Acheson, E. D. (1970). 'University, medical school and community.' *Br. med. J.* **II,** 683
4 Agadzi, V. K. (1972). Personal communication
5 Aguirre, A. and Wray, J. (1965). Unpublished data. Cited in Bryant, J. (1969). *Health and the Developing World.* Ithaca, N.Y.; Cornell University Press
6 Arole, R. S. and Arole, M. (1972). 'Comprehensive rural health project, Jamkhed.' *J. Christ. med. Ass. India Burma Ceylon* **47,** 177
7 Asahabi, P. V., Jacob, J. T. and Jayabal, P. (1969). 'The increase in severity of whooping cough in India.' *Vellore Alumni J.* **4,** 69
8 Asevkoff, B. and Bennet, J. V. (1969). 'Effect of antibiotic therapy in acute salmonellosis on the fecal excretion of Salmonellae.' *New Engl. J. Med.* **281,** 636
9 Axton, J. (1970). Personal communication
10 Babbott, F. L., Galbraith, N. S., McDonald, J. C., Shaw, A. and Zukerman, A. J. (1963). 'Deaths from measles in England and Wales in 1961. Section II. *Mon. Bull. Minist. Hlth* **22,** 167
11 Baird, D., Hytten, F. E. and Thomson, A. M. (1958). 'Age and human reproduction.' *J. Obstet. Gynaec. Br. Commonw.* **65,** 865
12 Balme, H. (1904). 'The signs and symptoms of measles in relation to diagnosis and prognosis.' *Practitioner* **2,** 504

REFERENCES AND BIBLIOGRAPHY

13 Barnett, C. R., Leiderman, H., Grobstein, Rose and Klaus, M. (1970). 'Neonatal separation. The maternal side of interactional deprivation.' *Pediatrics* **45**, 197
14 Barnes, T. E. C. (1972). 'Rural services for maternal and child health.' *Trop. Doct.* **2**, 79
15 Barnes, P. (1969). Personal communication
16 Barrie, H. (1963). 'Resuscitation of the newborn.' *Lancet* **I**, 650
17 Barrington, Kaye (1962). *Bringing up Children in Ghana.* London; Allen and Unwin
18 Biddulph, J. (1972). 'Standardised management of diarrhoea in young children.' *Trop.Doct.* **2**, 114
19 Biddulph, J. and Pangkatana, P. (1971). 'Weaning diarrhoea.' *Papua New Guin. med. J.* **14**, 7
20 Birmingham Survey (1951–55). *Maternity and Child Welfare Statistics.* Annual Report of the M.O.H.
21 Biviji, J. E., Shah, P. M. and Udani, P. M. (1972). 'Physical growth and complications following measles in an urban community.' *Indian Pediat.* **9**, 265
22 Bligh, D. (1971). *'What's the use of lectures?'* University Teaching Methods Unit, 55 Gordon Square, London WC1H ONT
23 Bolaji, L. (1970). *The Anatomy of Corruption in Nigeria.* Ibadan; Daystar Press
24 *Br. med. J.* (1970). 'Infection in the nursery.' (Editorial) **II**, 235
25 Brown, J. I. (1970). 'Diagnosing your reading problem.' *Mod. Med.* September, p. 843
26 Bruce-Chwatt, L. J. (1952). 'Malaria in African infants and children in Southern Nigeria.' *Ann. trop. Med. Parasit.* **46**, 173
27 Bruce-Chwatt, L. J. (1971). 'Some aspects of malaria and its control.' *Trop. Doct.* **1**, 147
28 Bruch, H. A., Ascoli, W., Scrimshaw, N. S. and Gordon, J. E. (1963). 'Studies of diarrheal disease in Central America.' *Am. J. trop. Med. Hyg.* **12**, 567
29 Brunser, O., Reid, A., Mönckeberg, F., Marconi, A., Contreras, I. and Trabucco, Edda (1966). 'Jejunal biopsies in infant malnutrition, with special reference to mitotic index.' *Pediatrics* **38**, 605
30 Bryant, J. H. (1969). 'The gap between biomedical technology and health needs in developing countries.' In *Science and Technology In Developing Countries.* Ed. A. B. Zahlan and Claire Nader. Cambridge; Cambridge University Press
31 Bryant, J. H. (1971). Reproduced in Hellberg, J. H. *Community Health and the Church.* Geneva; Christian Medical Commission, World Council of Churches
32 Bryant, J. H. (1969). *Health and the Developing World.* Ithaca, N.Y.; Cornell University Press
33 Buchan, W. (1797). *Buchan's Medicine*, p. 240. London; Strahan, Cadell and Davies

REFERENCES AND BIBLIOGRAPHY

34 Bullen, J. J., Rogers, H. J. and Leigh, L. (1972). 'Iron-binding proteins in milk.' *Br. med. J.* **I**, 69

35 Burgess, Anne (1957). 'Traditional systems of child care.' *J. trop. Pediat.* **3**, 118

36 Bwibo, N. O. (1971). 'Whooping cough in Uganda.' *Scand. J. inf. Dis.* **3**, 41

37 Bwibo, N. O. (1973). 'Management of respiratory infections in infancy and childhood.' *Trop. Doct.* **3**, 61

38 Cannon, D. S. H. (1958). 'Malaria and prematurity in the Western Region of Nigeria.' *Br. med. J.* **II**, 877

39 Cannon, D. S. and Hartfield, V. J. (1964). 'Obstetrics in a developing country.' *J. Obstet. Gynaec. Br. Commonw.* **71**, 940

40 Castle, Winifred M. (1972). *Statistics in Small Doses.* London; Longmans

41 Chalmers, A. K. (1930). *The Health of Glasgow, 1818–1925,* p. 340. Glasgow; Bell and Bain

42 Chen, P. C. Y. (1970). 'Indigenous concepts of causation and methods of prevention of childhood diseases in a rural Malay community.' *J. trop. Pediat.* **16**, 33

43 Chou En Lai (1972). Quoted in *The Sunday Times* (London), 30 April 1972

44 Church, M. A. (1972). 'Fluids for the sick child. A method of teaching mothers.' *Trop. Doct.* **2**, 119

45 Church, M. (1972). Personal communication

46 Coghill, N. P. (1969). 'Change and growth in hospitals.' *Lancet* **II**, 1058

47 Cole-King, S. M. (1972). Personal communication

48 Conco, W. Z. (1970). *An analysis of the Traditional Beliefs of the South African Bantu and their Relation to Health and Disease.* Dissertation for D.T.P.H. London School of Hygiene and Tropical Medicine

49 Cook, R. J. (1971). 'Is hospital the place for the treatment of malnourished children?' *J. trop. Pediat. envir. Child Hlth* **17**, 1 15

50 Cooper, Christine (1965). Personal communication

51 Court, S. D. M., Jackson, H. and Knox, G. (1953). 'The recognition of whooping cough.' *Lancet* **II**, 1057

52 Court, S. D. M. (1963). *The Medical Care of Children.* London; Oxford University Press

53 Court, S. D. M. (1971). 'Child health in a changing community. Charles West Lecture, Royal College of Physicians.' *Br. med. J.* **II**, 125

54 Cravioto, J., Delicardi, Elsa R., Pinero, Carmen, Lindoro, Martha, Arroyo, Margarita and Alcarde, Emma (1971). 'Mental development and malnutrition, neuro-integrative development and intelligence in school children recovered from malnutrition in infancy.' *Proc. Nutr. Soc., India* **10**, 192

55 Cruickshank, R. (1963). 'Diarrhoeal diseases in the United Kingdom.' In *Epidemiology*, p. 62. Ed. J. Pemberton. London; Oxford University Press

56 Cunningham, N. (1969). 'An evaluation of an auxiliary-based child health service in rural Nigeria.' *J. Soc. Nigerian Hlth* **3**, 21

57 Cunningham, N. (1971). *Report to the U.S. A.I.D. Conference on the Use of Weight Charts.* (Duplicated report). Washington

58 Cutting, W. A. M. (1972). 'The Under-Fives' Clinic.' *J. Christ. med. Ass. India Burma Ceylon* **47**, 160

59 Cutting, W. A. M. (1972). Presentation at Washington Conference on Under-Fives' Clinics

60 Daniell, W. F. (1852). 'On the epidemic rubella of Accra, West Coast of Africa.' *Dubl. J. med. Sci.* **14**, 25

61 Davie, R., Butler, N. and Goldstein, H. (1972). *From Birth to Seven*, Chapter 16. London; Longmans

62 Davies, D. F. (1971). 'Milk protein and other food antigens in atheroma and coronary heart disease.' *Am. Heart J.* **81**, 289

63 *Demographic Year Book of the United Nations* **(1967)**. 'Infant mortality.'

64 Dingle, J. H., Badger, G. F. and Jordan, W. S. (1964). *Illness in the Home: Study of 25,000 Illnesses in a Group of Cleveland Families.* Cleveland, Ohio; Press of Western Reserve University

65 Dissevelt, A. G. and Vogel, L. C. (1971). 'An analysis of the operations of the medical assistant in an out-patient department, with emphasis on administrative procedures.' In *Health and Disease in Africa. Proceedings of 1970 East African Medical Research Council Scientific Conference.* Ed. G. C. Gould. Nairobi; East African Lire:ature Bureau

66 Dixon, J. M. S. (1965). 'Effect of antibiotic treatment on duration of excretion of *Salmonella typhimurium* by children.' *Br. med. J.* **II**, 1343

67 Dobbing, J. (1971). 'Effect of nutrition on the nervous system.' *Proc. Nutr. Soc. India* **10**, 177

68 Donald, A. B. (1938). 'The diagnosis of whooping cough.' *Br. med. J.* **II** 613

69 Douglas, J. W. B. (1950). 'Some factors associated with prematurity.' *J. Obstet. Gynaec. Br. Commonw.* **57**, 143

70 Douglas, J. W. B. and Simpson, H. R. (1964). 'Height in relation to puberty, family size and social class in a longitudinal study.' *Milbank meml Fund q. Bull.* **42**, 20

71 Drinkwater, H. (1885). *Remarks upon the Epidemic of Measles Prevalent in Sunderland*, p. 45. Edinburgh; James Thin

72 Eaves, W. (1970). 'Technical and economic feasibility study for the setting up of a local manufacturing complex to supply hospital equipment.' *Intermediate Technology Development Group Publication* No. 70/35

73 Edington, G. M. (1967). 'Pathology of malaria in West Africa.' *Br. med. J.* **I**, 715

74 Eppink, H. (1968). *An experiment to determine a basis for nursing decisions in regard to time of initiation of breast feeding.* E.D.D. dissertation. Detroit; Wayne State University. Univ. Microfilms Inc. No. 69–14 668

75 Elias-Jones, T. F. (1970). 'Antibiotics in diarrhoeal illnesses.' *Lancet* **II**, 1308

76 Elwood, P. C., Waters, W. E., Greene, W. J. and Woods, M. M. (1967). 'Evaluation of a screening survey for anaemia in adult non-pregnant women.' *Br. med. J.* **IV**, 714

77 Elwood, P. C. (1970). 'Some epidemiological aspects of iron deficiency relevant to its evaluation.' *Proc. R. Soc. Med.* **63**, 1230

78 Erlich, P. (1972). 'Britain and the population crisis. Presidential Address to the Conservation Society.' Reported in *Lancet* **I**, 189

79 Evans, R. L. (1971). Personal communication

80 Foll, C. V. (1959). 'An account of some of the beliefs and superstitions about pregnancy, parturition, and infant health in Burma.' *J. trop. Pediat.* **5**, 51

81 Fawcitt, J. and Parry, H. E. (1957). 'Lung changes in pertussis and measles in childhood.' *Br. J. Radiol.* **30**, 76

82 Fomon, S. J. (1967). *Infant Nutrition.* Philadelphia, Pa. and London; W. B. Saunders

83 *Food and Agriculture Organization of the United Nations.* (1962). Sixth Report of the Joint FAO/WHO Expert Committee on Nutrition. *Tech. Rep. Ser. Wld Hlth Org.* No. 245, 25, 27

84 Forbes, C. E. and Scheifele, D. W. (1972). 'The management of measles in Nairobi and current concepts.' *E. Afr. med. J.* **50**, 159

85 Fox, W. (1964). 'Realistic chemotherapeutic policies for tuberculosis in the developing countries.' *Br. med. J.* **I**, 135

86 Freedman, R. (1963). *The Sociology of Human Fertility. A Report and Bibliography.* Oxford; Blackwell

87 Fuglesang, A. (1970). *Communicating with the Illiterate.* Mimeographed study from the National Food and Nutrition Commission, P. O. Box 2669, Lusaka, Zambia

88 Galbraith, N. S. and Cockburn, W. C. (1963). 'Deaths from whooping cough in England and Wales in 1960 and 1961.' *Mon. Bull. Minist. Hlth* **22**, 54

89 Gans, B. (1963). 'Some socio-economic and cultural factors in West African paediatrics.' *Archs Dis. Childh.* **38**, 197

90 Garby, L., Irnell, L. and Werner, I. (1969). 'Iron deficiency in women of fertile age in a Swedish community.' *Acta med. scand.* **185**, 113

91 Gelfand, M. (1964). *Medicine and Custom in Africa.* Edinburgh and London; E. and S. Livingstone

92 Ghai, O. P. (1971). Personal communication

93 Ghosh, Shanti, Bhargava, S. K. and Bhargava, Vyaga (1971). 'Growth pattern of babies in the Delhi area in the first year of life.' *Proc. Nutr. Soc. India* **10**, 82

94 Gibbs, F. A. and Rosenthal, I. M. (1962). 'Electroencephalography in natural and attenuated measles.' *Am. J. Dis. Childh.* **103**, 395

95 Gish, O. (1970). 'Health planning in developing countries.' *J. dev. Stud.* **6**, 67

96 Goldschmidt, B. (1966). 'Practical infant feeding, with special reference to the instruction of mothers of low socio-economic status.' *S. Afr. med. J.* **40**, 71

97 Goodhart, J. F. and Still, G. F. (1921). *The Diseases of Children*, p. 223. Eleventh ed. London; J. and A. Churchill

98 Gopalan, C., and Visweswara Rao, K. (1969). 'Nutrition and family size.' *J. Nutr. Diet.* **6**, 258

99 Gorbach, S. L. (1970). 'Acute diarrhoea. A 'toxin' disease?' *New Engl. J. Med.* **283**, 44

100 Gordon, J. E., Guzman, M. A., Ascoli, W. and Scrimshaw, N. S. (1964). 'Acute diarrhoeal disease in less developed countries.' *Bull. Wld Hlth Org.* **31**, 9

101 Gothi, G. D., Savic, D., Baily, G. V. J. and Samuel, R. (1970). 'Cases of pulmonary tuberculosis among the out-patients attending general health institutions in an Indian city.' *Bull. Wld Hlth Org.* **43**, 35

102 Graves, J. (1970). Reports on the First, Second and Third Conferences on the Use of Audio Tape in Medical Education, available from the Medical Recording Service Foundation, Royal College of General Practitioners, Kitts Croft, Writtle, Chelmsford, Essex, CM1 3EI, UK

103 Griffith, L. S. C., Fresh, J. W., Watten, R. H. and Villaroman, M.P. (1967). 'Electrolyte replacement in paediatric cholera.' *Lancet* I, 1197

104 Hamilton, P. J. H., Gebbie, D. A. M., Wilks, N. E. and Lothe, F. (1972). 'The role of malaria, folic acid deficiency and haemoglobin AS in pregnancy at Mulago Hospital.' *Trans. R. Soc. trop. Med. Hyg.* **66**, 594

105 Hamilton, P.J.H.(1964). An Analysis of Basic Data on Admissions in 1963 and 1964 to Mulago Hospital, Kampala. Report for Ministry of Health, Uganda, 1965

106 Hanks, J. R. (1963). 'Maternity and its rituals in Bang Chan.' *Interim Rep. Ser.* No. 6, Data Paper No. 51. Ithaca, N.Y.; Cornell University Press

107 Hardy, A. V. (1959). 'Diarrheal diseases in infants and children.' *Bull. Wld Hlth Org.* **21**, 309

108 Harfouche, J. K. (1970). 'The importance of breast feeding.' *J. trop. Pediat.* **16**, 135

109 Hellberg, J. H. (1972). *Christian Medical Commission Document* CMC/72/8, W.C.C., 1211 Geneva 20, Switzerland

110 Hendrickse, R. G. and King, M. A. R. (1958). 'Anaemia of uncertain origin in infancy.' *Br. med. J.* **II**, 662

111 Hendrickse, R. G. and Sherman, P. M. (1965). 'Morbidity and mortality from measles in children seen at University College Hospital, Ibadan.' *Arch. ges. Virusforsch.* **16**, 27

112 Hendrickse, R. G., Hasan, A. H., Olumide, L. O. and Akinkunmi, A. (1971). 'Malaria in early childhood.' *Ann. trop. Med. Parasit.* **65**, 1

113 Herzberg, H., Mausner, B. and Snyderman, B. B. (1959). *The Motivation to Work.* New York; John Wiley

114 Hirsch, A. (1883). *Handbook of Graphical and Historical Pathology.* Translated by C. Creighton. London; The New Sydenham Society

115 Holdaway, D., Romer, A. C. and Gardner, P. S. (1967). 'The diagnosis and management of bronchiolitis.' *Pediatrics* **39**, 924

116 Holmes, A. (1964). *Health Education in Developing Countries.* London; Thomas Nelson

118 Hytten, F. E. and Leitch, Isabella L. (1971). *The Physiology of Human Pregnancy.* Oxford; Blackwell Scientific

119 Illich, I. (1971). *Deschooling Society.* Harmondsworth, Middx; Penguin Books

120 Illingworth, R. S. (1972). *The Normal Child.* Fifth ed. London; J. and A. Churchill

121 Imperato, P. J. (1968). Personal communication

122 Imperato, P. J. (1970). 'Indigenous medical beliefs and practices in Bamako, a Moslem African city.' *Trop. geogr. Med.* **22**, 211

123 Jacob John, T., Montgomery, E. and Jayabal, P. (1971). 'The prevalence of intestinal parasitism and its relation to diarrhoea in children.' *Indian Pediat.* **8**, 137

124 Jacob John, T. (1972). 'Problems with oral polio vaccine in India.' *Indian Pediat.* **9**, 252

125 Jacob John, T. (1968). Duplicated report

126 Jahoda, G. (1969). *The Psychology of Superstition.* Harmondsworth, Middx; Penguin Books

127 James, W. P. T., Draser, B. S., Miller, C. (1972). 'Studies in the physiological mechanism and pathogenesis of weanling diarrhoea.' *Am. J. Clin. Nutr.* **25**, No. 6, 564

128 Jelliffe, D. B. and Jelliffe, E. F. (Eds) (1971). 'The uniqueness of human milk.' *Am. J. clin. Nutr.* **24**, 968, 1013

129 Jelliffe, D. B. (1966). 'The assessment of the nutritional status of the community.' *Wld Hlth Org. Monograph Series* No. 53 Geneva; World Health Organization

130 Jelliffe, D. B. (1967). 'Approaches to village level infant feeding.' *J. trop. Pediat.* **13**, 119

131 Jolly, H. (1971). *Diseases of Children.* Second ed. Oxford; Blackwell Scientific Publications (also in ELBS low-cost edition)

132 Kakar, D. N., Srinivas Murthy, S. K. and Parker, R. L. (1972). *People's Perception of Illness and their Use of Medical Care Services in Punjab.* Mimeographed report of a paper presented in the Seminar on Behavioral Research in Health and Medical Care sponsored by the Indian Council of Medical Research, New Delhi, March 1972

133 Kamath, K. R., Feldman, R. A., Sundar, Rao P. S. S. and Webb, J. K. G. (1969). 'Infection and disease in a group of South Indian families. General morbidity patterns in families and family members.' *Am. J. Epidemiol.* **89**, 375

134 Kark, S. L. and Steuart, C. W. (1962). *A Practice of Social Medicine.* London; E. and S. Livingstone

135 Kellmer Pringle, M. L. (1971). 'Policy implications of child development studies.' *Assign. Child.* **15**, 113

136 Kempe, C. H. (1968). *The Biologic Basis of Pediatric Practice*, p. 586. Ed. R. E. Cooke. New York; McGraw Hill

137 Kenny, Jean F., Boesman, Mary I. and Michaels, R. H. (1967). 'Bacterial and viral coproant bodies in breast-fed infants.' *Pediatrics* **39**, 202

138 Kerr, D. N. S. (1970). Reported in *The Guardian,* 9 September 1970

139 King, M. (Ed.) (1966). *Medical Care in Developing Countries.* Nairobi; Oxford University Press

140 King, M. (1970). 'The auxiliary. His rôle and training.' *J. trop. Med. Hyg.* **73**, 336

141 King, M., *et al.* (1973). *Nutrition in Developing Countries.* London; Oxford University Press

142 King, M. (1972). 'Medicine in Red and Blue.' *Lancet* **1**, 679

143 Kinnear-Brown, J. A., Stone, Mary M. and Sutherland, I. (1968). 'BCG vaccination of children against leprosy in Uganda. Results at end of second follow-up.' *Br. med. J.* **I**, 24

144 Klaus, M. H., Kennell, J. H. and Plumb, Nancy Zuehlkes (1970). 'Human maternal behavior at the first contact with her young.' *Pediatrics* **46**, 187

145 Kline, P. (1972). *The Scientific Study of the Freudian Theory.* Speech to the British Association. Exeter

146 Knox, G. and Morley, D. C. (1960). 'Twinning in Yoruba women.' *J. Obstet. Gynaec. Br. Emp.* **LXVII**, 6, 981

147 Krugman, S., Giles, J. P., Friedman, H. and Stone, S. (1965). 'Studies on immunity to measles.' *J. Pediat.* **66**, 471

148 Lagrisse, M. (1970). 'Absorption of dietary iron.' (Editorial) *J. trop. Pediat.* **16**, 29

149 Laing, J. S. (1900). *The Prevalence and Mortality of Whooping Cough in Aberdeen from 1882–1900.* Thesis. Aberdeen

150 *Lancet* (1875) **I**, 865. 'Measles in the Southern Hemisphere.' (Leading article)

REFERENCES AND BIBLIOGRAPHY

151 *Lancet* (1965) **I**, 791. Leading article quoting Stewart, J. B. (1962). Am. J. Obstet. Gynec. **83**, 430

152 Lathem, W. and Newberg, A. (1970). *Community Medicine, Teaching Research and Health Care.* New York; Appleton Century

153 Laugesen, B. M. (1972). Presentation at Workshop on Under-Fives' Clinics, Hyderabad, October 1972

154 Lees, R. E. M. (1966). 'Malnutrition: the infant at risk.' *W. Indian med. J.* **15**, 211

155 Leitch, I. (1945). 'Diet and tuberculosis.' *Proc. Nutr. Soc.* **3**, 156

156 Lloyd, A. V. C. (1968). 'Bacteriological diagnosis of tuberculosis in children.' *E. Afr. med. J.* **45**, 140

157 Lucas, A. O., Hendrickse, R. G., Okubadejo, O. A., Richard, W. H. G., Neal, R. A. and Kofie, B. A. K. (1969). 'The suppression of malarial parasitaemia by pyrimethamine in combination with dapsone or sulphormethoxine.' *Trans. R. Soc. trop. Med. Hyg.* **63**, No. 2, 216

158 Mabogunje, A. L. (1971). *Development of Small Scale Industries. A Challenge to 'Aid Donors'.* Report from Swedish International Development Authority, Stockholm

159 MacFayden, D. M. (1964). 'Childhood mortality in Swaziland.' *Cent. Afr. J. Med.* **10**, 8

160 Mahler, M. (1966). *Proc. 18th Int. Tub. Conf.*, p. 77. Amsterdam; Excerpta Medica

161 Marsden, P. D. (1964). 'The Sukuta Project.' *Trans. R. Soc. trop. Med. Hyg.* **54**, 455

162 Marsden, P. D. and Marsden, S. A. (1965). 'A pattern of weight gain in Gambian babies during the first 18 months of life.' *J. trop. Pediat.* **10**, 89

163 Martin, W. J., Morley, D. C. and Woodland, Margaret (1964). 'Interval between births in a Nigerian village.' *J. trop. Pediat.* **10**, 82

164 Maslow, A. H. (1954). *Motivation and Personality.* New York; Harper

165 Mather, R. J. and Jacob John, T. (1973). 'Popular beliefs about smallpox and other common infectious diseases in South India.' *Trop. geogr. Med.* **25**, 190

166 Matthews, T. S. (1966). 'Difficult transfusions.' *E. Afr. med. J.* **43**, 464

167 Maxwell, C. J. M. (1970). Personal communication

168 McCullough, B. L. (1972). 'A contribution from Congo.' *Trop. Doct.* **2**, 93

169 Mcgregor, D. (1960). *The Human Side of Enterprise.* New York; McGraw Hill

170 MacGregor, I. A., Gilles, H. M., Walters, J. H., Davies, A. H. and Pearson, F. A. (1956). 'Effects of heavy and repeated malarial infections on Gambian infants and children.' *Br. med. J.* **II**, 686

171 MacGregor, I. A. (1964). 'Measles and child mortality in the Gambia.' *W. Afr. med. J.* **13**, 251

172 MacGregor, I. A., Rahman, A. K., Thompson, Barbara, Billewicz, W. Z. and Thomson, A. M. (1968). 'The growth of young children in a Gambian village.' *Trans. R. Soc. trop. Med. Hyg.* **62**, 341

173 McKigney, J. (1971). 'Economic aspects.' *Am. J. clin. Nutr.* **24**, 1005

174 Mead, Margaret (1954). *Growing up in New Guinea,* Harmondsworth, Middx; Penguin Books

175 Medical Research Council (1964). *Br. med. J.* **I**, 413

176 Millar, J. D. (1968). *Measles. An Epidemic Model for Planning Vaccination Programs in West Africa.* Presented at E.I.S. Conference, National Communicable Disease Center, USA

177 Miller, F. J. W., Seal, R. M. E. and Taylor, Mary D. (1963). *Tuberculosis in Children.* London; J. and A. Churchill

178 Miller, F. J. W. (1973). 'Regional differences in tuberculosis in children.' *Trop. Doct.* **3**, 66

179 *Milton Keynes: A Health Service for.* (1968). Department of Health and Welfare, Aylesbury, Bucks.

180 Moffat, M. (1969). *Mobile Young Child's Clinics in Rural Uganda.* Mimeographed report available from the Ankole Preschool Protection Programme, P. O. Box 221, Mbarara, Uganda, East Africa

181 Moffat, W. M. U. and Nganwa-Bagumah (1971). 'Do we mean what they say?' *J. trop. Pediat. envir. Child Hlth* **17**, 47

182 Moraes, N. L. de A. (1962). 'Medical importance of measles in Brazil.' *Am. J. Dis. Childh.* **103**, 233

183 Morley, D. C., Woodland, Margaret and Martin, W. J. (1963). 'Measles in Nigerian children.' *J. Hyg., Camb.* **61**, 115

184 Morley, D. C. (1963). 'A medical service for children under five years of age in West Africa.' *Trans. R. Soc. trop. Med. Hyg.* **57**, 2, 79

185 Morley, D. C., Woodland, Margaret and Cuthbertson, W. F. J. (1964). 'Controlled trial of pyrimethamine in pregnant women in an African village.' *Br. med. J.* **I**, 667

186 Morley, D. C. (1964). 'The severe measles of West Africa.' *Proc. R. Soc. Med.* **57**, 846

187 Morley, D. C., Martin, W. J. and Woodland, Margaret (1966). 'Whooping cough in Nigerian children.' *Trop. geogr. Med.* **18**, 169

188 Morley, D. C., Martin, W. J. and Allen, Irene (1966). 'Measles in West Africa.' *W. Afr. med. J.* **16**, 24

189 Morley, D. C., Woodland, Margaret, Martin, W, J. and Allen, Irene (1968). 'Heights and weights of West African village children from birth to the age of five.' *W. Afr. med. J.* **17**, 1, 8

190 Morley, D. C., Martin, W. J. and Allen, Irene (1967). 'Measles in East and Central Africa.' *E. Afr. Med. J.* **44**, 12

191   Morley, D. C. (1968). 'A health and weight chart for use in developing countries.' *Trop. geogr. Med.* **20**, 101

192   Morley, D. C., Bicknell, Joan and Woodland, Margaret (1968). 'Factors influencing the growth and nutritional status of infants and young children in a Nigerian village.' *Trans. R. Soc. trop. Med. Hyg.* **62**, 2, 164

193   Morley, D. C. (1968). 'Prevention of protein—calorie deficiency syndromes.' *Trans. R. Soc. trop. Med. Hyg.* **62**, 2, 200

194   Morley, D. C. (1971). 'Shopping around for measles vaccine.' (Editorial) *J. envir. Child Hlth* **17**, 45

195   Morris, J. N. and Heady, J. A. (1955). 'Social and biological factors in infant mortality. Objects and methods.' *Lancet* **I**, 343

196   Mphahlele, E. (1964). 'The future of African Cultures.' *Foreign Aff.* **42**, 614

197   Mulligan, T. O. (1971). 'Typhoid fever in young children.' *Br. med. J.* **IV**, 665

198   Myrdal, G. (1970). *The Challenge of World Poverty.* Harmondsworth, Middx; Penguin Books

199   Nagpaul, D. R. (1967). 'District tuberculosis control programme in concept and outline.' *Indian J. Tuberc.* **14**, 186

200   Naish, F. C. (1956). *Breast Feeding – A Guide to the Natural Feeding of Infants.* London; Lloyd-Luke (Medical Books)

201   National Communicable Diseases Center (1964). *Identification of Intestinal Amebae. Amebiasis Laboratory Diagnosis.* Public Health Service Publication No. 1187, U.S. Department of Health, Education and Welfare, Washington D.C., USA

202   National Communicable Diseases Center (1967). 'Measles eradication 1967.' *Morbid Mortal.* **16**, No. 15 (Suppl.)

203   Nelson, W. E. (Ed.) (1966). *Textbook of Pediatrics*, p. 48. Eighth ed. Philadelphia, Pa.; W. B. Saunders

204   National Communicable Diseases Center (1968). Reports of E.I.S. Conference

205   Nestart, A. and Harrison, Irene (1964). 'Treatment of progressive primary tuberculosis with isoniazid alone.' *Lancet* **I**, 1068

206   Newsom, J. and Newsom, E. (1965). *Patterns of Infant Care in an Urban Community.* Harmondsworth, Middx; Penguin Books

207   Norman-Taylor, W. (1961). 'Witchcraft, sorcery and mental health.' *Hlth Educ. J.*

208   Nyboe, J. (1960). 'The efficacy of the tuberculin test.' *Bull. Wld Hlth Org.* **22**, 5

209   Nyerere, M. J. K. (1969). Speech to T.A.N.U. Conference

210   Odhiambo, T. R. (1967). 'East Africa. Science for development.' *Science, N.Y.* **158**, 876

211   Office of Health Economics, London (1971). *Cost of Medical Care,* No. 15, Dec. 1971

212 Oomen, H. A. P. C. and Malcolm, S. H. (1958). 'Nutrition of the Papuan child.' *S. P. C. techn. P.* No. 118
213 Ortiz, J. S., Firiklea, J. F., Potter, Elizabeth, Poon-King, T. and Earle, D. P. (1970). 'Epidemic nephritis and streptococcal infection in Trinidad.' *Archs intern. Med.* **126**, 140
214 Owen, S. G. (1966). *Electrocardiography.* London; English University Press
215 Panum, P. L. (1846). *Observations made during the Epidemic of Measles on the Faroe Islands in the Year 1846.* Translated by Delta Omega Society, Cleveland, Ohio 1940
216 Parker, R. L., Srinivas Murthy, A. K. and Bhatia Jagdish, C. (1972). 'Relating health services to community health needs.' *Indian J. med. Res.* **60**, 1835
217 Parkin, J. M. (1973). *E. Afr. med. J.* (in press)
218 Davies, T. P. and Parkin, J. M. (1972). 'Catch up growth following early childhood malnutrition.' *E. Afr. med. J.* **49**, 672
219 Pasachoff, J. M., Cohen, R. J. and Pasachoff, N. W. (1970). 'Belief in the supernatural among Harvard and West African university students.' *Nature, Lond.* **227**, 971
220 Paul, D. B. (1955). *Health, Culture and Community.* New York; Sage Foundation
221 Wong, H. B. (1964). 'Hyperbilirubinaemia and kernicterus in Singapore.' *J. Singapore paediat. Soc.* **6**, 1
222 Pierce, N. F., Banwell, J. G., Mitra, R. C., Caranasos, G. J., Keimowitz, R. I., Manji, P. M. and Mondal, A. (1968). 'Effect of intragastric glucose—electrolyte infusion upon water and electrolyte balance in Asiatic children.' *Gastroenterology* **55**, 333
223 Powell, M. (1970). 'The eternal triangle.' *Br. med. J.* **II**, 416
224 Preston, N. W. (1970). 'Technical problems in the laboratory diagnosis in prevention of whooping cough.' *Lab. Pract.* **19**, 482
225 Pringle, G., Busvine, J. R., Charmot, G., Rocossé J. H. *et al.* (1969). 'Experimental malaria control and demography in a rural East African community. A retrospect.' *Trans. R. Soc. trop. Med. Hyg.* **63**, No. 4, Suppl. 2–18
226 Puffer, Ruth, R., Serrano, C. V. and Dillon, Ann (1971). 'The Inter-American investigation of mortality in childhood.' Interim report of Pan-American Health Organization reproduced from *Assignm. Child.* Paris; UNICEF
227 Raju, V. B., Narmada, R., Shanmugasundram, R. and Sambandham, C. T. (1971). 'Crude mortality and tuberculosis morbidity among infected and uninfected children.' *Indian Pediat.* **8**, 11
228 Rea, J. N. (1965). *Morbidity in Relation to Social Class and Nutritional State in Nigerian Children.* Dissertation for the D.P.H., London School of Hygiene and Tropical Medicine
229 *Reports of the Local Government Board, Public Health and Medical Subjects* (1918). New Series No. 115, p. 7. London; H.M.S.O.

230 Rhazes, (A.D. 850). *A Treatise on the Smallpox and Measles.* Divisio Morborum, Cap. 149. London; New Sydenham Society (1848)

231 Rifkin, Susan and Kaplinsky, R. (1972). *Health Strategy and Development Planning.* Mimeographed report available from the Tropical Child Health Unit, Institute of Child Health, London

232 Ristori, C., Boccardo, H., Borgono, J. M. and Armijo, R. (1962). 'Medical importance of measles in Chile.' *Am. J. Dis. Childh.* **103**, 236

233 Ritchie, Jean (1967). *Learning Better Nutrition.* FAO Nutritional Studies No. 20. Rome; Food and Agriculture Organization of the United Nations

234 Rogers, K. B. and Koegler, S. J. (1951). 'Inter-hospital cross-infection of epidemic gastro-enteritis associated with type strains of *B. coli.*' *J. Hyg. Camb.* **49**, 152

235 Rosenheim, M. (1970). 'The role of the United Kingdom in medicine.' *Proc. R. Soc. Med.* **63**, (Suppl.), 1208

236 Salber, E. J. (1956). 'The effect of different feeding schedules on the growth of Bantu babies in the first week of life.' *J. trop. Pediat.* **2**, 97

237 Salk, L. (1962). 'Mother's heart beat as an inspiratory stimulus.' *Trans. N.Y. Acad. Sci.* **24**, 753

238 Schoemaker, E. (1971). Personal communication

239 Schofield, F. D., Tucker, W. M. and Westbrook, G. R. (1961). 'Neonatal tetanus in New Guinea.' *Br. med. J.* **II**, 785

240 Scott, Reginald (1584). *The Discoverie of Witchcraft.* London. Quoted in Parrinder, E. G. (1958). *Witchcraft.* Harmondsworth, Middx; Penguin Books

241 Scott, R. B., Jenkins, M. E. and Kessler, Althea D. (1951). 'Erythroblastosis fetalis in the Negro infant.' *J. Pediat.* **39**, 680

242 Scrimshaw, N. S., Gordon, J. E. and Taylor, C. (1968). *The Interaction of Nutrition and Infection.* WHO Monograph Series No. 57. Geneva; World Health Organization

243 Segall, M. (1972). 'The Politics of Health in Tanzania.' In *Towards Socialist Planning.* Dar-es-Salaam; Tanzania Publishing House

244 Senanayake, P. (1973). *Evaluation of Under-Fives' Clinics.* Ph.D. Thesis (in preparation)

245 Senecal, J. (1959). 'Alimentation de l'enfant dans les pays tropicaux et subtropicaux.' *Courr. Cent. int. Enf.* **9**, 1

246 Shattock, F. M. (1971). 'Disease prevention and health promotion.' *J. Coll. gen. Practnrs* **21**, 393

247 Sheifelle, D. W. and Forbes, C. E. (1972). 'Prolonged giant cell excretion in severe measles.' *Pediatrics* **50**, 867

248 Shennan, T. (1914). 'The morbid anatomy of tuberculosis in man.' *Lancet* **I**, 595, 673

249 Sheridan, M. D. (1962). 'Infants at risk of handicapping conditions.' *Mon. Bull. Minist. Hlth* No. 21, 238

250 Shrank, A. B. (1965). 'A field survey in Nigeria.' *Trans. a. Rep. St John's Hosp. derm. Soc., Lond.* **51**, 85

251 Skorov, G. and Knoppers, A. (1970). *International Aspects of Technical Innovation.* UNESCO Symposium, Paris

252 Solon, F. S. (1970). 'Rural internship in community medicine.' *Santo Tomás J. Med.* **23**, 171

253 Spence, J. (1960). *The Purpose and Practice of Medicine,* p. 274. London; Oxford University Press

254 Staff, T. H. E. (1968). 'Treatment of severe kwashiorkor and marasmus in hospital.' *E. Afr. med. J.* **45**, 399

255 Stanfield, J. P. (1971). 'The Luteete family health centre. Nutrition rehabilitation in a rural development strategy.' *J. trop. Pediat. envir. Child Hlth* **13**, 67

256 Stanfield, J. P. (1970). 'Levels of care.' *J. trop. Pediat. envir. Child Hlth* **18**, 75

257 Stanfield, J. P. (1969). 'Fever in children in the tropics.' *Br. med. J.* **I**, 761

258 Stanfield, J. P. (1968). 'The "At Risk" Concept.' *J. trop. Pediat.* **14**, 201

259 Stewart, Rosemary (1967). *Managers and Their Jobs.* London; Macmillan

260 Swift, P. N. (1972). 'The effects of organisation, Mbale, Uganda.' *J. environ. Child Hlth* **18**, 87

261 Swift, P. N. (1972). Personal communication

262 Takulia, H. S., Taylor, C. E., Sangal, S. P. and Alter, J. D. (1967). *The Health Center Doctor in India.* Baltimore, Md; The Johns Hopkins Press

263 Tanner, J. M., Whitehouse, R. H. and Takaishi, M. (1966). 'Standards from birth to maturity for height, weight, height velocity and weight velocity. British children 1965.' *Archs Dis. Childh.* **41**, 454

264 Tanner, J. M. (1968). 'Earlier maturation in man.' *Science, N.Y.* **218**, 21

265 Taylor, Joan (1970). 'President's Address. Infectious infantile enteritis, yesterday and today.' *Proc. R. Soc. Med.* **63**, 1297

266 Tempest, M. N. (1966). 'Cancrum Oris.' *Br. J. Surg.* **53**, 11

267 Thompson, Barbara and Baird, D. (1967). 'Some impressions of childbearing in tropical areas, II.' *J. Obstet. Gynaec. Br. Commonw.* **74**, 4

268 Thompson, B. (1966). 'The first fourteen days of some West African babies.' *Lancet* **II**, 40

269 Thomson, A. (1970). 'The evaluation of human growth patterns.' *Am. J. Dis. Childh.* **120**, 398

REFERENCES AND BIBLIOGRAPHY

270 La Torre, T. A. (1956). *Boln méd. Hosp. infant., Méx.* **13**, 785
271 Trousseau, A. (1869). *Lectures on Clinical Medicine,* p. 228. Volume 2. London; New Sydenham Society
272 *Tuberculosis in India: a Sample Survey.* (1959). Indian Council for Medical Research, Special Report No. 34
273 Uttley, K. H. (1960). 'The epidemiology and mortality of whooping cough in the Negro over the last 100 years in Antigua, British West Indies.' *W. Indian med. J.* **9**, 77
274 Van Roy, E. (1970). 'On the theory of corruption.' *Econ. Dev. cult. Change* **19**, 86
275 Viswanathan, D. M. (1936). *Rec. Malar. Surv. India* **6**, 239
276 Wald, N. (1972). 'Morbidity and mortality in relation to social class.' *Lancet* **I**, 259
277 Watson, G. I. (1956). 'The complications of measles.' *J. Coll. gen. Practnrs Res. Newsl.* Suppl. No. 11
278 Webb, J. (1970). *Diseases of Children in the Tropics.* Second ed. Ed. D. B. Jelliffe, London; Edward Arnold
279 Weinstein, L. (1955). 'Failure of chemotherapy to prevent the bacterial complications of measles.' *New Engl. J. Med.* **253**, 679
280 Welbourn, H. F. (1959). 'Backgrounds and follow-up of children with kwashiorkor.' *J. trop. Pediat.* **5**, 84
281 Wilkins, J., Williams, F. F., Wehrle, P. F. and Portnoy, B. (1971). 'Agglutinin response to pertussis vaccine.' *J. Pediat.* **79**, 197
282 Williams, Cicely D. (1955). 'The organisation of child health services in developing countries.' *J. trop. Pediat.* **1**, 3
283 Williams, Cicely D. (1963). 'The story of kwashiorkor.' *Courr. Cent. int. Enf.* **13**, 361
284 Williams, Cicely D. and Jelliffe, D. B. (1972). *Mother and Child. Delivering the Services.* London; Oxford University Press
285 Wilson, M. (1971). *The Hospital – A Place of Truth.* Birmingham; University of Birmingham
286 Wilson, J. (1973). 'The management of febrile convulsions.' *Trop. Doct.* **3**, 58
287 Wittmann, W. and Hanson, J. D. L. (1965). 'Gastroenteritis and malnutrition.' *S. Afr. med. J.* **39**, 223
288 Woodruff, A. W. and Dickinson, C. J. (1968). 'Use of dexamethasone in cerebral malaria.' *Br. med. J.* **III**, 31
289 W.H.O. Expert Committee (1965). 'Nutrition in pregnancy and lactation.' *Tech. Rep. Ser. Wld Hlth Org.* No. 302
290 World Health Organization (1967). *Serological Study of Respiratory Diseases.* Geneva
291 W.H.O. Expert Committee on Health Statistics (1966). Tenth Report. 'Sampling methods in morbidity surveys and public health investigations.' *Tech. Rep. Ser. Wld Hlth Org.* No. 336
292 World Health Organization (1972). 'Nutritional anaemias.' *Tech. Rep. Ser. Wld Hlth Org.* No. 503
293 *World Medicine.* Editorial, 15 December 1971

294 Worsley, P. (1972). Reported in *The Guardian*, 19 August 1972

295 Wraith, R. and Simpkins, E. (1963). *Corruption in Developing Countries.* London; Allen and Unwin

296 Wray, J. D. and Aguirre, A. (1969). 'Protein—calorie malnutrition in Candelaria, Colombia.' *J. trop. Pediat.* **15**, 76

297 Wray, J. D. (1971). 'Population pressure on families. Family size and child spacing.' In *Rapid Population Growth: Consequences and Policy Implications.* Volume 2. Baltimore, Md; The Johns Hopkins Press

298 Wray, J. D. Reported in Bryant, J. (1969). *Health and the Developing World,* p. 240. Ithaca, N.Y.; Cornell University Press

299 Wyon, J. B. and Gordon, J. F. (1971). *The Khanna Study.* Cambridge, Mass.; Harvard University Press

300a Yerushalmy, J., Bierman, M. D., Kemp, D. H., Connor, A. and French, F. E. (1956). 'Longitudinal studies of pregnancy on the island of Kauai, territory of Hawaii.' *Am. J. Obstet. Gynec.* **71**, 80

300b Yerushalmy, J. (1945). 'On the interval between successive births and its effect on the survival of infant. An indirect method of study.' *Hum. Biol.* **17**, 65

301 Zaki-Amin, Zaman, Taj-Eldin, Allos and Al-Rahim, Q. (1971). 'Infantile diarrhoea in Iraq.' *Pakist. pediat. J.* **1**, No. 3—4

302 Cravioto, J. (1970). 'Mental performance in school age children.' *Am. J. Dis. Childh.* **120**, 404

303 Kleevens, J. W. L. (1971). 'Housing, urbanisation and health in developing (tropical) countries.' *Trans. R. Soc. trop. Med. Hyg.* **65**, Suppl. 30

304 Leary, P. M. (1966). 'A pattern of measles among some Africans in a Bantu Reserve.' *S. Afr. med. J.* **40**, 293

305 *The Work of Health Visitors in London* (1971). Research Report No. 12. Greater London Council Department of Planning, County Hall, London

306 Spence, J., Walton, W. S., Miller, F. J. W. and Court, S. D. M. (1954). *A Thousand Families in Newcastle-upon-Tyne.* London; Oxford University Press

307 Perry, Caroline and Frey, Susanne (1971—72). Personal communications

308 Dick, G. (1966). 'Combined vaccines.' *Can. J. publ. Hlth* **57**, 435

309 Stanfield, J. P., Bracken, P. M., Waddell, K. M. and Gall, D. (1972). 'An intradermal diphtheria-tetanus-pertussis immunisation schedule.' *Br. med. J.* **II**, 197

310 Schulman, I. (1961). 'Iron requirements in infancy.' *J. Am. med. Ass.* **175**, 118

311 Cantwell, R. J. (1972). 'Iron deficiency anaemia of infancy.' *Clin. Pediat.* **11**, No. 8, 443

312 King, M. (1973). *The Laboratory in Developing Countries.* London; Oxford University Press

REFERENCES AND BIBLIOGRAPHY

313 Berghost, C. (1972). *Thoughts on Community Services in Low Production, Physically Deprived Nations.* Duplicated report available from World Neighbours, Chimaltenango Development Programme, Guatemala

314 Nugorohi, Gunawan (1972). *An Insurance Based Health Service in Central Java.* Mimeographed report available from Jl. Brigjen Soediarto 484, Solo, Indonesia

315 Hammam, M., Allah, A. F. A., Hammouda, A. M. and Shaurawz, A. E. A. (1973). 'Field training in family health care for medical students in Assuit University.' Presented at a *Conference on the Teaching and Practice of Family Health, Benghazi*

316 Fendall, N. R. E. (1972). *Auxiliaries in Health Care.* Baltimore, Md; Johns Hopkins Press

317 King, F. (1973). Private communication

318 Cockrane, A. L. (1972). *Effectiveness and Efficiency.* Nuffield Provincial Trust

319 Morley, D. C., Abayomi, I. and Woodland, Margaret (1973). *J. trop. Pediat.* (in press)

320 Hewitt, R. M. (1951). 'Legible lantern slides.' *Pediatrics* 7, 145

321 Arnhold, R. (1972). 'What do you do all day?' *J. trop. Pediat.* 18, 225

322 Gish, O. (1973). 'Resource allocation. Equality of access and health.' *Int. J. Hlth Services* (in press)

323 'Hexachlorophene. Its usage in the nursery.' (1973). *Pediatrics* (Suppl.) 51, 329

324 Beard, R. (1970). *Teaching and Learning in Higher Education.* Harmondsworth, Middx; Penguin Books

325 Nalin, D. R., Richardson, S. H. and Bhattacharjee, A. K. (1973). 'Diarrhoea resembling cholera introduced by Escherichia coli culture filtrate.' *Lancet,* 1, 885

326 Cash, R. A., Toha, K. M. M., Nalin, D. R., Huq, Z. and Phillips, R. A. (1969). 'Acetate in the correction of acidoses secondary to diarrhoea.' *Lancet* II, 302

327 Whittle, H. C., Abdullahi, M. T., Fakunle, F., Parry, E. H. O. and Rajkovic, A. D. (1973). 'Scabies, pyoderma and nephritis in Zaria, Nigeria. A clinical and epidemiological study.' *Trans. R. Soc. trop. Med. Hyg.* 67, 349

328 *Nutrition, the Nervous System and Behavior* (1972). PAHO Scientific Publication No. 251, Washington D.C.

Index

Croup, 196, 205
Cuba, doctor's salaries, 32, 75
Cultural aspects of child health, 43
Culture
  child-rearing and, 51
  epidemiological approach to beliefs, 53
  good and bad customs, 52
  measles and, 212
  relation to health, 45
  understanding of, 44, 46

Decision-making, 365
  'illiterate', by, 411
Dehydration, 142, 152, 188, 344, 357, 374, (see also Rehydration)
  diarrhoea, in, 172, 174, 186
  measles, in, 223
  pneumonia, in, 202
  treatment, 186, 188 (see also Rehydration)
Delegation
  communication and, 388, 389
  results of, 388
Denmark, training of medical students, 73
Dental problems, 62
Diarrhoea, 142, 170–194, 357
  aetiology of, 174
  anaemia caused by, 290
  antibiotics in, 192
  'at-risk' child and, 165, 167
  cessation of breast-feeding and, 181
  clinical picture, 171
  definition, 170
  dehydration in, 172, 174, 186
  diagnosis, 191
  diet in, 192
  disaccharidase deficiency in, 192

epidemic, 170
epidemiology, 179, 180
E. coli causing, 174, 182
family size and, 300
frequency of different infections, 175
general considerations, 170
growth failure and, 182
infants and young children, in, 171
isolation of pathogens, 176
kwashiorkor following, 129, 134
malaria and, 252
malnutrition and, 180
measles and, 176, 214, 216, 221, 224, 252
mortality rate, 171, 318
mother's attitude to, 172
neonatal, 170
nutrition and, 181, 194
prevention, 68, 184
priorities, 194
Proteus morganii, 179
recurrent form, 165, 172
respiratory tract infection and, 172, 191
Salmonellae infection in, 175, 179
Shigella infection in, 175, 185
teething and, 173
treatment, 185
  drugs in, 191
  intravenous rehydration, 189
  oral fluids, 191
  rehydration centres, 193
weanling, 171, 180
weight loss in, 127
whooping cough and, 252
Diet in diarrhoea, 192
Diphtheritic corynebacteria, 281
Disaccharidase deficiency in diarrhoea, 192

Faith healing, 53
Family, diarrhoea in, 180
Family planning, 70
  Asia, in, 298
  birth interval and, 296
  clinics, 317
  involvement of father, 313
  national attitude towards,
    314
  Under-Fives' Clinic, role of,
    313
Family size
  agricultural areas, in, 8
  Asia, in, 63
  morbidity and, 300
  physical growth and, 302
Farmers, 25
Fees, 35, 41
Femoral head, infections of,
  76
Fever
  malaria, in, 250
  tuberculosis, in, 266
Fiji, measles epidemics in,
  208
Films in teaching, 425
Flannelgraph in teaching,
  426
Folic acid deficiency, 288
Foreign body, inhalation of,
  200
Fungal infections, 282

Gambia, measles in, 209, 210
Giardiasis, 179
Glucose-6-phosphate dehydrogenase deficiency, 252,
  286
Griseofulvin, 282
Ground nuts (peanuts), 134, 200
Growth
  breast milk and, 110
  diarrhoea and, 182
  family size and, 302
  kwashiorkor and, 182

  maintaining adequate rate of,
    134
  measurement of, 124
  recording, 324
Growth charts, 137
  kept in homes, 151
  reference lines in, 138
  rehydration requirements and,
    190

Haemoglobin
  anaemia, in, 292, 293
  birth, at, 284
Haemoglobinopathies
  'at-risk' child and, 166
  malaria, in, 252
Haemophilus influenzae, 205
Haemopoiesis, 284
Haemoptysis in whooping cough,
  241
Haemorrhage, ante- and postnatal,
  66, 67
Harvard mean, 138
Heaf test, 267
Health clinics, 3 (see also Under-
  Fives' Clinics)
  contact with mothers in, 28
  financial aspects of, 19, 27
  health education in, 15
  India, in, 20
  management of anaemia in, 295
  need for, 13
  objectives, 11, 366
  Tanzania, in, 18
Health education
  health clinics, in, 15
  nurse–midwife's role in, 71
  respiratory infection and, 199
  role of, 14
  Under-Fives' Clinic, in, 334
Health pyramid, 428, 429
Health service
  development of, financial
    aspects, 16
  users of, 57

Mother-child relationship (*cont.*)
  premature infants, in, 92
  rural areas, in, 77
Mother–nurse relationship, 329
Mouth, changes in, in measles, 214

Neomycin, 282
Neonatal mortality (see also
      Infant mortality and Child
      mortality)
  Nigeria, in, 93
  reduction of, 77, 78
Neonatal period, 76–99
  care of eyes, 82
  care of orphans during, 96
  congenital abnormalities (see
      Congenital abnormalities)
  delayed clamping of cord, 84
  diarrhoea in, 170
  environment of child during, 91
  general observations on care,
      76
  hyperpyrexia during, 88
  hypothermia during, 88, 91
  immunization during, 98
  jaundice in, 98
  need for warmth and moisture,
      91
  nursing position of infant, 94
  paediatrician–obstetrician
      co-operation during, 81
  physical contact between
      mother and child, 92, 95
  prevention of umbilical stump
      infection, 89
  resuscitation methods, 85
  skin infections in, 282
  special care units, 94
  sucking baby out, 83
  tying of cord, 84
  washing facilities for
      attendants, 90
Nephritis, scabies and, 281
Newborn (see Neonatal period)

Nigeria
  economics of Under-Fives'
      Clinics, 339
  hospital costs in, 28
  measles in, 209, 214, 218
  medical care in, 50
  relation between birth weight
      and survival, 93
  respiratory infections in, 198
  stillbirth statistics in, 93
  training of doctors in, 21
  tuberculin reaction in, 270
  twinning in, 97
  weight records in, 125
Noma, 215
Nurse(s), 341–363
  clinic, in, 342, 361
  communication, 403
  consultations, role in, 328
  control of admission and
      discharges by, 350
  home-visiting by, 342, 362
  hospital, in, 342, 345
    assignment of duties, 351
    control of admissions and
        discharges, 350
    imbalance between doctors,
        administrators and,
        346
  observations made by,
      356
  personal relationships of,
      345
  problems, 361
  ratio to doctors, 346
  relationship with doctors,
      347, 362, 403
  relationship with mothers,
      329
  responsibilities, 350
  role of, 14, 341, 362
    caring, 343
    child feeding, in, 354
    children's nursing, in, 349
    humanizing agent, 345
    medicine giving out, 338

Schools, home-based medical
    records and, 151, 152
Scurvy, 288
Shigella infection in diarrhoea,
    175, 176, 185
Sickle cell anaemia, 290
Skill pyramid, 389
Skin diseases, 279—283
    doctor's responsibility,
        283
    fungal, 282
    incidence, 280
    infections, 279
    parasitic, 283
Small bowel infection in
        malnourished child, 182
Smallpox, 69, 318
Smoking during pregnancy, 80
Social workers, 155
South America
    birth interval in, 306, 309
    measles mortality in, 211
    population growth in, 298
    rehydration centres in, 193
Sputum examination in tubercu-
        losis, 271, 272
Spleen
    malaria, in, 251
    tuberculosis, in, 263
Split fees, 35
Staphylococcal infection of skin,
        281
Steroid therapy in malaria, 255
Stilbirths, Nigeria, in, 93
St. Lucia, 'at-risk' child in,
        165
Streptococcal infection of skin,
        281
Streptomycin in tuberculosis, 266
Sulphonamides in pneumonia, 201
Superstition, illness and, 47
Swaddling, 52

Tanzania
    cost of health service in,
        18, 31

malaria in, 249
president's statement on family
    planning, 314
village medical helpers in,
    15
Tape recorders, use of, 416
Teachers, communication with, 399
Teaching
    by nurses, 349
    children's ward, in, 357
    communication and, 409
    different levels, 397
    doctor's role, 359
    methods, 415—429
        films and TV, 425
        flannelgraphs, 426
        individual study, 421
        lectures, 416
        posters, 426
        programmed learning,
            421
        recorded talks, 416
        seminars, 419
        slides, 425
        talks, 415
        visual aids, 416, 425
    skills and attitudes, 422
    Under-Fives' Clinics, in,
        335
Teething, diarrhoea and, 173
Television in teaching, 425
Tetanus, 80, 384
Tetmosol, 283
Tetracyclines in whooping cough,
    241
Thailand
    brain drain from, 33
    corruption in, 42
Thiacetazone in tuberculosis,
    276
Thiamine in breast milk, 112
Throat infections, 205
Thumb sucking, 107
Tinea capitis, 282
Tinea corporis, 279
Tine test, 267
Tonsillitis, 195, 196